DATE DUE

WORLD MEDICINE

To our fathers

Who never met, but might have liked to

WORLD MEDICINE

Plants, Patients and People

DAVID BELLAMY

AND

ANDREA PFISTER

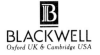

BLACKWELL
Oxford UK & Cambridge USA

First published 1992

Blackwell Publishers
108 Cowley Road,
Oxford, OX4 1JF,
UK

Three Cambridge Center
Cambridge, Massachusetts 02142,
USA

British Library Cataloguing in Publication Data

A CIP catalogue record for this book is available
from the British Library.

Library of Congress Cataloging-in-Publication Data
Bellamy, David J.
World medicine: plants, patients, and people / David Bellamy and Andrea Pfister.
p. cm.
Includes bibliographical references and index.
ISBN 0–631–16933–4 (alk. paper)
1. Materia medica, Vegetable – History. 2. Medicine – History. 3. Alternative medicine
– History. I. Pfister, Andrea. II. Title.
RS164.B412 1992
610–dc20

Typeset in 11 on 13pt Sabon
by Hope Services (Abingdon) Ltd
Printed in Great Britain by Biddles Ltd., Guildford

This book is printed on acid-free paper

CONTENTS

CONTENTS

List of Illustrations

Prefaces: Why This Book?

Well, I am a botanist and my dad was a pharmacist, manager of Boots Cash Chemists in Cheam in Surrey, England. His shop was a model of polished mahogany drawers and ground-glass-topped jars and the prescription book was copperplate and leather-bound, and when he came home at night he smelt, well, of chemists' shops. His mum was very proud of him, and so were we. Granny always smelt of lavender or linseed or liquorice and chlorodyne or pennyroyal and she used to tell us of the herbalists' shops of her youth in London, like the one described by Sir E. A. Wallis Budge in his fascinating little book, *The Divine Origin of the Craft of the Herbalist*, published at Culpeper House in 1928.

> Many of my contemporaries will remember a herbalist's shop which was situated in a popular street near King's Cross in the year 1865, and its dirty and unkempt appearance. The shop proper was about 8 feet wide and 20 feet long. Its window front was glazed with small panes of bottle-green glass, which were seldom washed or cleaned, and on the brightest day very little light entered the shop through them; during the winter months, and especially in foggy weather, the shopkeeper was obliged to carry on his business by the light of two or three guttering 'dips', i.e. tallow candles. A long narrow counter took up much of the floor space. On one end of this stood a rickety glass case containing small bowls of seeds and berries, which were well coated with dust, and on the other stood a pair of rusty iron scales and a huge glass bowl of a mixture called 'sarsaparilla wine'.

Men and women, as well as the children, who came in and spent their halfpennies and pennies freely drank this wine out of teacups of various sizes and shapes and makes, which were rarely rinsed in water, and were usually turned bottom upwards on the counter to dry. A large cardboard label was tied round the bowl, and on this were written in large capitals the names of all the ailments and sicknesses which this particular brand of sarsaparilla wine was said to cure.[1]

On the end wall was a shelf whereon stood a couple of ostrich egg-shells, and several bottles containing 'preparations' of various kinds, of a most uninviting appearance, and two human skulls. Below the shelf, nailed to the wall, was a small dried crocodile or lizard, and below this a miscellaneous collection of dried 'specimens', all richly coated with dust. On another shelf was a series of small bottles and flasks which contained extracts, or decoctions, of herbs, medicated unguents and perfumes and vegetable oils. Another shelf was filled with bottles of medicated sweets, such as paregoric drops, squills, lozenges, sticks of horehound candy, 'stick liquorice', etc., and these sweets were in great demand by juvenile customers. From the ceiling and on the wall in front of the counter hung bundles of dried herbs, lavender, rosemary, mint, camomile, dandelion, sorrel and many others, all well covered with dust. Under the counter were wooden boxes containing poppy-heads, senna leaves, marsh-mallow, linseed meal, etc., and a stock of paper bags and phials of various sizes.

The proprietor sold his wares rather by 'rule of thumb' than by measures or scales, and he eschewed the writing of directions for the use of his patients. He was old and very shabby, but kindly, and many of his customers were evidently friends and acquaintances, judging by the way in which he advised them as to their ailments. His shop was well patronized by children, who came there to see him exhibit 'Pharaoh's serpents'. He would set on a plate a lump of some brown substance rather like chocolate, and when he applied a lighted match to a certain part of it, the lump changed its shape and heaved, and from its sides several spirals emerged and went wriggling across the plate like worms, to the great delight of the onlookers. When asked why these wriggling things were called 'Pharaoh's serpents', he said that he did not know, but that his father and his grandfather had always called them by this name. When he was unable to advise a customer, he used to knock the counter with a weight, and then his wife, a little old wizened woman, would appear from behind the shop and take charge of the case. It was generally thought that she was the real herbalist to the establishment, and certainly her reputation in the neighbourhood was great.

My dad still demonstrated Pharaoh's Serpents and sold horehound candy, stick liquorice, rolled his own pills and made his own tinctures, elixirs, tisanes and a very potent personal hair grease, for managers of Boots in those days were not allowed to sport the frivolity of curly hair. In fact I only found out his hair did curl after he had retired.

I will always remember his excitement when he came home with the news that penicillin was being prescribed. I used to watch with awe as he prepared it under a glass canopy held together with Elastoplast, with a bunsen burner under one corner to keep the air rising and the whole thing sterile. I can also remember his slow disillusionment as sales reps rolled up with an ever-increasing plethora of patent medicines which eventually relegated his knowledge and skills of pharmacy to the boredom of management.

Yet I can never forget his knowledge of materia medica and his special smell, of chemists' shops. That is why I had to write this book, to say thank you to my father for a life-long interest and to all those plants which for so many millennia helped to keep the human world healthy in mind and body.

DAVID BELLAMY
Bedburn, 1990

P.S. I can also remember that when I was taken to the doctor, suffering from boils or carbuncles or worse, before the days of penicillin, I was always dressed in my best clothes and I believed in the fact that he would make me well. What is more, he did, saving my life on at least two occasions.

Notes

1 Sir E. A. Wallis Budge, *The Divine Origin of the Craft of the Herbalist* (London: Culpeper House – The Society of Herbalists, 1928).

2

Brickbats are fully expected. When a botanist and an ecologist – and the former a media personality to boot – dare step into the hallowed fields of medicine, they should hardly be surprised at the noise of lancets being sharpened. And yet, what we have come to intend by the word medicine may well be ripe for a bit of judiciously aided introspection.

I owe my life to modern, 'Western', medicine: in general terms, due to the higher standards of health, and directly in person more than once. On the other hand, it is a chiropractor who occasionally keeps my damaged back in running order after 'regular' medicine (*and* acupuncture) gave it up as a bad job, and I have at times made use of Traditional Chinese Medicine in preference to its Western counterpart. As we are trying to say, there is room for both. More than that; there is need for both.

When David Bellamy and I originally set out to write this book, we thought at first about all those splendid medicinal plants found in Earth's forests and fields. What we soon discovered was that the plants were there all right, but that their medicinal properties depended in a sizeable measure on the beholder. The plant itself might or might not contain chemicals capable of interacting visibly with the body and the mind controlling it, but whether this turned the plant into 'medicine', whether the interaction constituted 'healing', or indeed what constituted the 'disease' requiring such 'healing', was to a considerable extent decided upon by the potential patient's beliefs and attitude, and those of his community and culture. It was the difference between 'illness' – you or me feeling ill – and 'disease' – you or me being considered ill by our friends and neighbours and society at large, with all its customary consequences, positive or negative as they may be.

How these concepts, at times widely differing from culture to culture, developed and evolved makes a fascinating study and in its finer details – tribal ethnomedicine – needs the pen of an anthropologist to best describe it. What attracted our interest was a more specific aspect of the process, namely, how did the whole panoply of beliefs present in the precursors of Western civilization, continuously enriched first by empirical knowledge, later by scientific thought, and periodically subjected to massive transfusions of 'foreign' facts and ideas, gel into what is now referred to as 'regular' Western Medicine? Also, could this end result really be said to satisfy growing humanity's health requirements? These are not just a botanist's questions, for they involve all of us, but what better thread is there with which to follow this process than the knowledge of medicinal plants, the common link joining our pre-hominid ancestors with today's (and presumably tomorrow's) physician, let alone the alternative healer to the laboratory-bound medical researcher?

There is currently in the West a malaise, a growing dissatisfaction with 'regular' medicine, which puts pressure on the observer to take sides in a clash between mainstream and alternative practices. In this book we maintain that such a divide is not particularly useful, largely artificial and only relatively short-lived at that. Western Medicine, both in its curative aspects – scientific medicine and pharmacology – and in its socially preventive ones – hygiene and sanitation – has given humanity immensely powerful tools and techniques over the relatively short timespan of some three centuries. Its very success has played no little part in the present spectacular population growth which threatens to swamp both mankind and the environment on which it depends, and indeed has increased our expectations to the point that we are ready to find fault in side effects where not too long ago any cure or improvement at all would have been considered little short of a miracle. Still, it may be that it is high time for 'regular' medicine to merge again with the other streams of healing from which it separated a few short centuries ago.

Both the traditional 'health maintenance' crafts of the herbalist and the wise woman and the still traditional but otherwise highly structured and long-established non-Western medical systems such as Traditional Chinese Medicine and Ayurveda are part of a continuum of healing skills, essentially based on accumulated knowledge concerning medicinally active plants and plant products. Out of this background 'regular' medicine arose, adding scientific rigour and much else new, but remaining to a great extent ultimately dependent on the selfsame patrimony of medico-botanical knowledge.

What for centuries have been the scourges of humanity – transmissible diseases and acute infections – have by and large been reduced to controllable entities, and the tools with which at least to understand novel outbreaks are at hand. What mankind now faces is a new class of problems: widespread degenerative and environmentally caused diseases, and generalized health maintenance in a vastly inflated population. It is my belief that only by reintegrating Western-style 'regular' medicine with its traditional counterparts will we be able to utilize to its full extent the potential of our accumulated healing skills, and thereby provide for mankind's growing needs at an acceptable cost. This book traces my and David's route to this conclusion. I hope that it will also show the interest and the fascination which carried us along it.

ANDREA U. PFISTER
London, 1991

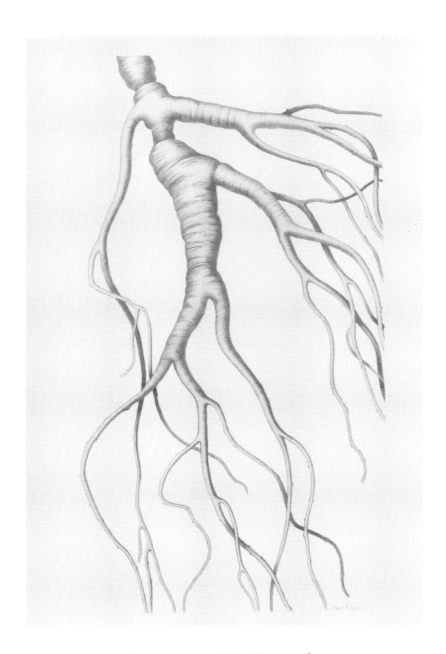

The root system of the Ginseng plant.

Acknowledgements

Over and beyond those contributions which we gratefully acknowledge in the text, we would like to express our thanks to the following for their help throughout the parturition of this book.

In Australia: The Australian Institute of Aboriginal Studies, Canberra.

In Hong Kong: Dr Paul But, CMMRC, The Chinese University, Sha Tin; Dr Ming Hung Wong, Baptist College; Dr H. W. Yeung, CMMRC, The Chinese University, Sha Tin.

In Sri Lanka: Dr Vinya S. Ariyaratene, Sarvodaya, Moratuwa; Mrs Sharmini Luther Block, Colombo; Mr I. K. G. Chandrasena, Sarvodaya, Moratuwa; Professor Arthur C. Clarke, Colombo; Dr N. P. Games, Wedagama, Meetiringale; Dr A. Liyanagamage, Colombo; Dr D. G. A. Perera, IFS, Kandy; Dr P. D. A. Perera, MARGA Institute, Colombo; Dr O. S. Peries, IFS, Kandy; Dr Upali Pilapitiya, BMARI, Maharagama; Professor Cyril Ponnamperuna, IFS, Kandy; Mr M. Rajasingham, Environmental Laboratories Ltd, Maharagama; Dr E. I. L. Silva, IFS, Kandy; Dr Anuradha Sirisena, Wedagama, Meetiringale; Mr L. Sugunadasa, Department of Ayurveda, Colombo; Mrs Kamini Vitrana, Ruk Rekagano, Colombo; Mr W. K. Wickramasekera, Department of Ayurveda, Colombo.

In Switzerland: Dr Barbara Fischer, Zürich; Professor Ian Fischer, Zürich.

In the United Kingdom: the staff of the British Library, Lending Division, Boston Spa; Mr and Mrs D. Bullock, Selby; the staff of Durham University Library, Durham; Miss Juliet Stoy, Woodland; and last but by far not least, Rosemary and Henrietta Bellamy, for their patience.

Dawn

From Self-heal to Family Doctors – or, How Did Medicine Come About?

Our household has, or rather had, seven cats. One was ours, an indoor cat of high breeding and well inoculated against the problems of disease. The others we had inherited with the rambling garden and they all lived outside. The continual struggle of five of them centred around attaining the status of an indoor cat, so they were petted and wormed each in due season. The seventh, called Panda, was a wild individualist, unapproachable by all except one of my children and then only at arm's length. It was great to watch arthritic, ageing Panda, always first to, and king of, the warmest sunsoaked spot. When suffering fron a flu-like malaise he would only take cold water and part of his routine was to chew grass and vomit. Only in his last days did he come into the house, where he was consoled not only by the Bellamy clan but by all the cats too, until he passed away purring – a toothless veteran of self-survival in a society overflowing with hygienic cat-lit, worm powders and all the other paraphernalia of twentieth-century peticare.

People, whether they like cats or not, are also social animals. Since their eruption here on Earth some five million (the figure is changing all the time, so let us stick with five million) years ago, the family and gradually the larger social groups have been their units of survival – units in which healing, or at least attempts at healing, accidents or illness must have taken place long before Alexander Fleming changed my dad's opinion of things. When a

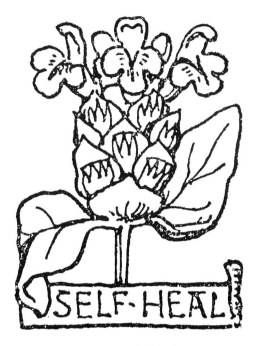

FIGURE 1.1 Self-heal.

patient bled, they would have done their best to stop the bleeding, when burned to cool the pain; when cold the patient would be kept warm, when hot with fever kept cool. Illness would often climax in vomiting or diarrhoea; some would recover. So as new foods were tried and tested, the knowledge of which made you sick or explosively defecate would have been stored away for future use: a quick cure, or kill.

Those mums, wives, widows, aunties and their male kin who absorbed more of the local plant lore than others would have been in great demand in the clan or tribe. Success would have engendered both praise and jealousy, and protectionism of knowledge; failure would have brought claims of witchcraft. The most sought-after of these self-taught physicians may well have been individuals who had themselves recovered from symptoms from which all others had died. He or she may have been desperately ill, even comatose for some time, all hope gone, then suddenly, miraculously they

6

were on the mend. Themselves seeking an explanation, they may have quoted dream experiences from that comatose state, and so the whole concept of the healing shaman could have arisen. Recovery from epileptic attacks could have played a similar role. The linking of healing and some form of mystic, religious thought must have been there since Animism proposed that there existed a soul or spirit in man, animals and all important artefacts. In eastern Asia and the Orient, Shamanism and Animism predate the more familiar mainstream religions like Buddhism and Confucianism. In China, shamanic vestiges remain in the Taoist tradition which is still served by monastries and temples throughout the country, even though ecstatics, shamans and diviners were banished when Confucianism was established as the state religion in the first century BC.[1]

Similarly, in Borneo, the Dayaks refer in their legends to a somewhat shamanic journey to the sky. The god Tupa-Jing noticed that the Dayaks were on the verge of destroying themselves because they had no cures for sickness and were cremating ill people out of necessity. He therefore saved a woman from the funeral pyre as she ascended in clouds of smoke, took her to heaven, and instructed her in the skills of medicine. With these, she was able to return to earth and pass on the precious knowledge she had obtained.[2]

It could well be that the shaman/healer was the first focal point for the bonding of families into clans, and the first dichotomy in medicine, a dichotomy between the family herbalist who used the plants to hand, upon which they had come to rely, and the shaman with his or her 'sacred plants': plants which open the door to a greater reality of the supernatural. For example, it has been told how the Chumash medicine woman Chequeesh told researcher Will Noffke in 1985 that she had learned of her native heritage by utilizing the 'dream herb', Mugwort, *Artemisia vulgaris*. For the Jivaro of Ecuador the familiar world is 'a lie' and there is only one reality, that of the supernatural – a reality onto which a window could be opened by using certain plants which have come to be known as hallucinogenic and which, at least in the modern world, have given a whole new and sinister meaning to the word 'drug'. To the Western mind, there is little distinction between curative

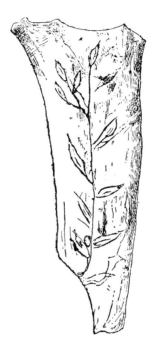

FIGURE 1.2 Paleolithic representation of a plant on bone. It was the reindeer that provided the bone, but the plant was important enough to be carved on it – the first prescription?

and hallucinogenic or recreational 'drugs'; to a shaman, Aspirin might be a drug, but Peyote (or whatever other hallucinogenic plant is being referred to) is sacred.[3]

Hallucinogenic plants and, in the single case of the toad *Bufo marinus*, an animal, contain complex chemicals, mainly alkaloids, which are also the active ingredients of most toxic and medicinal plants. It is of great interest to note that dosage is often the only factor between a return and a dead-end trip.

Administered by embalming the skin, by enema, by wound infusion, smoked, snuffed, eaten and drunk, such ingredients soon go to work. Once inside, they produce a variety of effects, often revolving around a dreamlike state with dramatic alteration in the sphere of experience, in the perception of reality, with changes even of space and time and in consciousness of self. They invariably induce a series of visual hallucinations, often in kaleidoscopic movement, and usually in indescribably brilliant and rich colours, frequently accompanied by auditory and other effects.

To date about 120 hallucinogenic plants have been identified worldwide, most of them in the New World and many in tropical forests and their derivative vegetation. The reason that none have been identified in the similarly diverse vegetations of the Old World tropics is a mystery. All evidence would indicate that the locals have never bothered to look, for by the laws of plant dispersion, evolution and average, they must be there. Evidently the Amerindian peoples, moving rapidly through the New World over the past ?30,000 years, found a way to commune with God through their knowledge of the flora. The tribes of Africa have their shamans, and through spirit possession and other ritual dances and practices effectively alter their consciousness, during which time they become God. It is of great interest to see in the more liberated Christian churches of today communicants 'taking a trip' into the ecstasy of belief without resorting to drugs or dance, but to the ritual experience of worship alone. It is also of interest to watch the reactions of the less liberated, who go to church expecting only to talk and sing about God.

There is no getting away from the fact that the vast majority of the alkaloids and hence the hallucinogens researched to date are found in the upper crust of the plant kingdom, the Angiosperms or flower-bearing plants, and a few in the lower-crust group, the Fungi, mushrooms and toadstools. There is also good evidence indicating them to be luxury plant products, or at least products of plants which enjoy high nitrogen input, such as those living in tropical rainforests, and of course plants with built-in nitrogen production like the Fabaceae, the Pea and Bean family.

Although Europe lacks tropical rainforests, it has plenty of nitrogen-fixer-rich flora and nitrogen-rich habitats, and yet few hallucinogenic plants have been researched. The most famous of all is the toadstool *Amanita muscaria* or Fly Agaric, used from Siberia southwards by shamans and others, toasted at the fire – its very bitter taste perhaps a built-in warning of the danger within – or made into a decoction with reindeer milk and Blueberries.

Knowledge of its efficacy spread far and wide, for it was the origin of the sacred Soma plant of the Vedic Indian tradition. *Amanita* has one unique property, in that it acts as a catalyst, the drug itself passing unharmed through the shaman's or patient's body ready to be recycled for ritual or medical use via the urine.[4]

Europe's main plant family with hallucinogenic connections is the Solanaceae, the Potato Flower family. Four plants, all of which today grow in disturbed field/woodland edge, nitrogen-rich habitats, complete the coven: Deadly Nightshade (*Atropa belladonna*), Henbane (*Hyoscyamus niger*), Mandrake (*Mandragora officinarum*) and *Datura*; all were used by witches, probably since they were first discovered. The danger of all these highly poisonous plants is that their poisonous principles can enter the human body through the skin, and so they must be handled with great care. It is said that the flight of witches was probably a flight through the mind of the initiate and that the broomstick provided inflight assistance by being covered with creams containing the hallucinogenic plants. One can only guess at the number of luckless test cases before the witch got her dose rate right.

The same must be true of the New World, for some of the plants here are dangerous in the extreme. For example, the Peyote of Mexico (*Lophophora williamsii* and other cactuses) contains at least thirty different nasties with a really foul taste. Yet someone at some time discovered that the sun-dried plant can be eaten whole with psychedelic effects. Likewise the seeds of Morning Glory (*Ipomoea violacea* amongst others), used as a sacred preparation by the Aztecs, are now known to contain alkaloids very similar to the synthetic LSD. Did South America have sacrificial as well as real guinea pigs? The San Pedro curative cults of Peru were based on the mescaline-rich Cactul (*Trichocereus pachanoi*), prepared as a tea and administered at all-night sittings during which the patients' problems were diagnosed. At dawn they were sent off on long pilgrimages to bathe in a number of sacred lakes high in the Andes: real kill or cure stuff, especially for the weak of heart.[5]

The list of methods of preparation, administration and mixing to fine-tune and prolong the desired results make fascinating reading, and shows that the early Amerindians were not only skilled plant taxonomists but pharmacologists too. Was it just that the vast resources of the New World, opened up late to the explosive migration of human kind, provided such easy pickings for the hunting-gathering clans that they had time on their hands, time to be laid back and to experiment?

Perhaps the most fascinating thing in all this is that none of the psychoactives used by the shamans appeared to be addictive in the hard drugs sense of today. Coca (*Erythroxylum coca*) leaves are served as tea to ageing tourists in the High Andes, while cocaine refined from the same plant is at present smacking the world in its addicted teeth.[6]

One rule, however, seems to apply to all these hallucinogens – including *Datura*, which, if administered over a long time, produces effective amnesia – is that ceremony or at least environment appears to be a critical fact in the psychoactive procedure: the hype appears to be part and parcel of the result.[7] In early eastern North American cultures, adolescent males were confined to a long-house for two weeks, during which time they imbibed a beverage containing *Datura*. During the extended period of amnesia they forgot what it was like to be a child and learned what it meant to be a man – perhaps the nearest equivalent in man to metamorphosis in the insect world. And over on the Pacific coast in Oregon, mycophages who consume the wrong mushrooms by accident end up having their stomachs pumped, while those who go out to feast on the same mushrooms for hallucinogenic purposes appear to enjoy their trip with no immediate nasty side effects.[8]

The rights and wrongs of ritualistic medicine and of the use and abuse of psychoactive drugs will continue, I am sure, as long as there are people and plants left on this Earth. However, in the meantime, over the millennia and down the centuries the local herbal practitioner must have continued to do a good job, making use of everything that was to hand and so doing sterling work for human society. Medicine was here to stay.

There are of course no written accounts of these origins of the herbalist or the shaman, but there is some archaeological evidence. This comes to us in the form of burials in which the internee had been laid to rest prepared for afterlife, with food and medicine: grave-goods which link both the practice, the profession and the conflict of eternity. The most ancient evidence unearthed to date

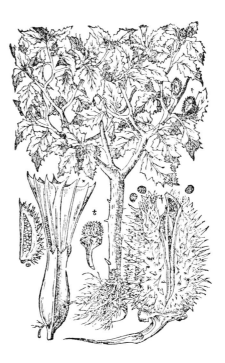

FIGURE 1.3 Thorn-apple or *Datura stramonium*: *Datura* played a significant role in both the Old and the New World, from witches' brews to initiatory rites.

comes from Iraq, from a district with the haunting name of Shanidar. There, some 60,000 years ago, a man of Neanderthal lineage was put to rest in a shallow grave, which already contained the remains of two adult females and a baby. The soil which had so long enclosed his bones bore fingerprints, not his but equally telltale, fingerprints of pollen in such abundance that the flowers which produced them must have been laid to adorn the body of the dear departed. The shape and form of the pollen grains allow no less than eight genera of plants to be identified, all of which still grow in abundance in the woods and fields around the grave site. Seven species belonging to those genera are all used to this day in local herbal medicine, and all appeared in the *British Pharmacopoeia* of the twentieth century. They include members of the full diversity of the healing flower families from the Ephedraceae, a non-missing link between the cone-bearers and the flower-bearers, the Compositae or Daisy Flower family and the Liliaceae or Lily Flower family, both somewhere near the top of evolutionary advancement of the two main lines of flower-bearing plants.

It may well be that the grave flowers were no more than decoration and had no medical significance. However, it is unlikely that all would have been flowering in the same locality at the same time; for example, the Grape Hyacinth (*Muscari* spp.) is an early flowerer, while the Mallows (*Althaea* spp.) would flower in early summer. Some may well have been taken from stocks specially dried for some purpose, and what better purpose than their healing powers?[9]

Notes

1 Nevill Drury, *The Elements of Shamanism* (Longmead, Shaftesbury, UK: Element Books, 1989).
2 Ibid.
3 Ibid.
4 Wade Davis, 'Hallucinogenic plants and their use in traditional societies – an overview', *Cultural Survival Quarterly*, 9.4 (1985), pp. 2–5.
5 Ibid.
6 Ibid.; W. Golden Mortimer, *History of Coca – The 'Divine Plant' of the Incas* (1901; San Francisco: Fritz Hugh Ludlaw Memorial Library Edition, 1974).
7 Davis, 'Hallucinogenic plants', pp. 2–5.
8 Ibid.
9 Ralph S. Solecki, 'Shanidar IV, a Neanderthal flower burial in northern Iraq', *Science*, 190 (28 Nov. 1975), p. 880; and Arlette Leroi-Gourhan, 'The flowers found with Shanidar IV, a Neanderthal burial in Iraq', *Science*, 190 (7 Nov. 1975), p. 562.

General information

Barbara Griggs, *Green Pharmacy – A History of Herbal Medicine* (London: Robert Hale, 1981, 1987).

The Pharmaceutical Society, *The Pharmaceutical Codex* (London: The Pharmaceutical Society, 1987).

The British Pharmacopoeia Commission, *The British Pharmacopoeia* (London: HMSO, 1988).

2

Onions, Pyramids and Clay Tablets – The Egyptian Heritage

'Praise to thee O Nile, that cometh forth from the Earth to nourish
the dwellers of Egypt'

Song of the Nile – Anon[1]

Put in a somewhat less reverent way by one Will Cuppy:

'Egypt has been called the gift of the Nile. Once every year the river
overflows its banks depositing a layer of rich alluvial soil on the
parched ground. Then it recedes and soon the whole countryside as
far as the eye can see is covered with Egyptologists'

– and, it goes without saying, with green plants.[2]

Thanks to the awesome presence of the Aswan Dam, the annual
miracle of cost-free fertilizers and irrigation is no more, but thanks
to that annual crop of Egyptologists the miracles of the civilization
which prospered between 3000 and 1000 BC live on. Amongst all
the facts and artefacts uncovered over more than a hundred
seasons of excavation are eight papyri which provide us with the
world's first written accounts of medicine and medicines, many of
which are still in use today.

Papyrus is a type of paper made from the fibres of *Cyperus
papyrus*, a member of the Sedge family. It is found growing in its
natural state alongside fresh water throughout North Africa and
also graces homes and open-plan offices as a so-called house plant,
one of a group which go under the collective name of the Umbrella
Grass Reeds. To confuse the terminology even further, there is little

doubt that it was the biblical Bulrush amongst which the infant Moses was hidden. Sedge, Grass, Rush, three different common names all applied to one plant, are in fact names applied to three different families of plants. The Grass family, or Gramineae, provides much of the human population with its staple food such as Rice, Wheat and Corn. The Rush family, or Juncaceae, are waterside plants which apart from their role in the productivity of wetlands serve few direct human purposes. The Sedge family, or Cyperaceae, is a very diverse family with at least 3,000 species found worldwide, which though important components of much grazing provide the human race with little of direct importance other than papyrus. It is thanks to this one plant and to the dry climate of Egypt that we have a permanent record of medicine as practised as far back as perhaps 3300 years BC.

The most important of the eight medical papyri was discovered by an Arab, purportedly in Thebes in 1862, and was sold to one of that annual rash of Egyptologists by the name of Professor Ebers. The papyrus, which must be regarded as the first edition of a Pharmacopoeia, starts with these lines: 'Here begins the book of the preparation of medicines for all parts of the human body.' On the back it is dated 1555 BC, although it refers to prescriptions from more remote times. In all it identifies some 160 vegetable drugs, and from it we can be certain that the ancient Egyptians were fully conversant with the use of *Acacia* gum, castor oil, Colocynth, Henbane, Indian Hemp, linseed, Mandrake, Mint, Pomegranate bark, Poppy, Senna, Squill, Thyme, turpentine and yeast. According to the *British Pharmaceutical Codex*, written at the turn of this century, most were still in use, so it is of little wonder that Homer sang thus of opium in the *Iliad*:

> The drug, of such sovereign power and virtue, had been given to Helen by Polydamna wife of Thon, a woman of Egypt, where there grew all sorts of herbs, some good to put in the mixing bowl and other poisonous. Moreover, every one in the whole country is a skilled physician, for they are of the race of Paeon.[3]

Of the race of Paeon they may have been, but as documented by paintings in the Valley of the Queens at Luxor, they showed enough initiative of their own without divine help. A short time before the writing of the Ebers Papyrus, Queen Hatshepsut in 1493 BC sent an expedition to Africa. The expedition included doctors, and returned with various drugs. These included Broomcorn (*Sorghum vulgare*), myrrh gum and *Ammi majus*, the root of which was eaten by caravaneers to protect themselves from the burning sun and which has been shown to contain 8-methoxysporalen, which promotes pigmentation of the skin, a built-in sunshade called a tan.

Of the other seven medical papyri, perhaps the most interesting is the so called Hearst Papyrus, eighteen coarse brown sheets of papyrus covered with heavy black and red hieratic script and comprising a series of medical prescriptions. This papyrus was named in honour of Mrs Phoebe Apperson Hearst, who financed an Egyptian expedition from the University of California from 1899 to 1905. The leader of the expedition, Dr George A. Reisner, states that:

> In the spring of 1901, a roll of papyrus was brought to the camp of the Hearst Egyptian Expedition near Der-el-Ballas, by a peasant of the village as a mark of his thanks at being allowed to take *sebah* from our dump-heaps near the northern *kom*'. When questioned, the peasant stated that 'he had found the roll while digging for *sebah* two years before, that he had put it away in a cupboard in his house and forgotten it'. When pressed further, he said that the roll was discovered in a pot among the house walls between the southern *kom* and the southern cemetery. Reisner goes on to say that the roll was brought to the camp 'tied up in the end of a native head-cloth (*suga*) and had, of course, been carried in a similar manner from the place where it was found to the village. The damage done to pages XVI to XVIII which were on the outside of the roll was due to this treatment.' On examining the papyrus, Reisner noted that 'the roll had not been opened since antiquity as was manifest in the set of the turns, the fine dust, and the casts of insects. The beginning of the roll was inside. In the middle of the first page preserved, the papyrus has been torn in two in antiquity and rolled up with the torn page inside.'[4]

Over a third of the 260 prescriptions detailed in the Hearst document are mentioned in the much larger and more authoritative Ebers Papyrus, which is thought to be contemporaneous with it.

The really fascinating thing about these eighteen papyrus sheets is that they appear to be the working manual of a local practising physician. It would seem that he went along to a medical centre and with the help of a scribe copied down all the useful prescriptions from a number of different sources. Although they are set out in no particular order, analysis of the contents of this key record of the past allowed the recognition of at least five distinct categories of illness or complaint:

1 Internal diseases, including fevers, urinary disorders and ailments of the stomach and heart: here, apart from many prescriptions for dispelling evil which are probably remedies for the relief of general malaise, there are four for constipation, two for heart diseases and no less than eight for curing fluid accumulation or dropsy. Of the 65 prescriptions to be taken orally, 81 per cent are quantified, so here we already see the very laws of pharmaceutical science.

2 Cutaneous ailments are dealt with in many prescriptions, from wounds and abrasions to insect and animal bites and burns, and so are irritations of the anal region and boils, abscesses and carbuncles. Detailed study of this and other material led to the conclusion that the physicians of those far-off days understood quite a lot about blood poisoning. They may not have linked symptom with cause, but they knew that if full healing was to be achieved then every trace of 'pus in the blood' had to be eliminated. There is no doubt that this semi-systematized knowledge could have in part been gained from and certainly must have helped in the preservation of bodies during mummification. Frankincense was a popular ingredient in most of these recipes, which not only must have helped prolong active life but also the attainment of bodily immortality. Its sweet smell must also have made the tasks of both physician and mortician a little more pleasant.

3 Orthopaedic conditions are covered under the heading 'pains and sickness in the limbs'. This included sprains and fractures, and where 'throbbing of muscles and conduits' was mentioned it probably referred to arthritic and rheumatic conditions. Inunctions for bruises and casts for broken limbs indicate a well-developed first-aid practice.

4 Cosmetics and beauty products for the young and would-be young abound, from skin creams to remedies for balding, dandruff and greying hair. Some dental prescriptions which also can be included in this category indicate that the problems of scurvy were not unknown.

5 Recitals, whose modern equivalent might be advertising hype, comprise eight prescriptions with 'magical implications'. Whether they were used by the physician with a basis of belief on his part or simply to ensure public placebo we will never know.[5]

Turning to the materia medica in order of popularity, we find some firm favourites. Gourd, be it the edible or the bitter variety which is also known as Colocynth, is mentioned no less than 33 times. Its use ranges from that of a bland pasty material for external application to purgative action when used in controlled quantified amounts. *Acacia* is listed 20 times, in all but three as a paste for poultices and dressings. Its limited use internally was probably as a bland bulk purgative or carrier for other more active ingredients. From other sources we know that *Acacia* spikes finely ground with dates and honey were used as a contraceptive and abortifacient. It is now known that *Acacia* gum dissolved in water produces lactic acid, a component of many modern contraceptive gels. Figs also figure in a number of purgative remedies and in quantitative prescriptions for 'removing noxious matter from the body'. Barley, Beans, Peas and Wheat, all of which were important components of a 'healthful diet', are cited as ingredients for soothing mucilaginous poultices. Cinnamon, one of the spoils of the expedition to Ethiopia, was also used in this way.

Carminatives include Anise, Coriander and Cumin, and were used both externally and internally, while dermal astringents, especially for insect bites, included Garlic and Leek. From other sources we know that during the building of the pyramids the slaves were given enormous amounts of Radishes, Garlic and Onions. Whether this was purely due to overproduction of these annual crops on those freely irrigated soils or to their antibiotic properties due to the bacteriostatics raphanin, allicin and allistatin which they are now proven to contain, is not known. Juniper is included in twenty prescriptions used in urinary disorders and the expelling of fluid accumulation. A diuretic property of dates is also

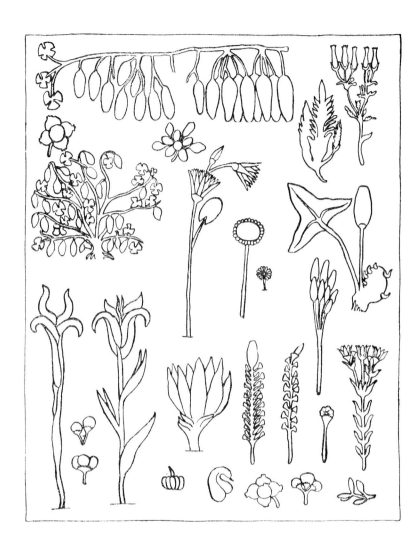

Figure 2.1 The first gardener's catalogue and/or pharmacopoeia: the plants gathered by Thothmes III in his Syrian campaign (see p. 102 for a translation of the inscription)

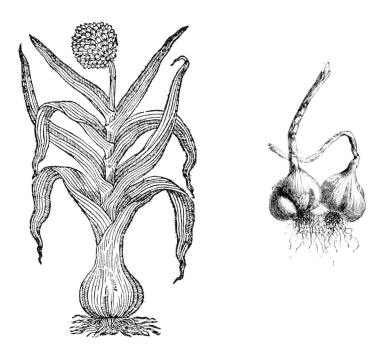

Figure 2.2   Garlic, hated by some but loved by many through the ages.

indicated, along with that of the petals and leaves of the Castor Oil Plant; castor oil, however, was not used as it was in my young days as the most noxious-tasting but highly effective purgative, along with syrup of figs (ugh). Perhaps they had not learned the art of cold expression of the oil from the seed, which leaves the toxic ricinoleic acid behind in the skin. Or again, perhaps they had more feeling for their patients, a supposition borne out by the use of the sweet taste of honey in 77 of the formulations, including no less than five for treating afflictions of the toenails. Other carriers include oil – presumably olive oil – in 40, beer in 27, water in 24, wine in 12 and milk in 11.

In conclusion, C. D. Leake in his book *The Old Egyptian Medical Papyri* states that, taken as a whole, certain generalizations may be made:

1 The relatively large number of drugs recommended by the old Egyptian physicians for the treatment of various diseases seem to have a rational basis. They are the sensible applications to diseased conditions of the readily observable action of crude animal, plant and mineral materials occurring in the environment, materials which must have been noted in the continuous search for food, or as a result of accidental contact;

2 no significant poisonous or toxic agents are recommended in the old Egyptian medical texts, in spite of the considerable number of such materials which occur naturally in the Egyptian environment; and

3 the various drugs recommended for therapeutic use in the old Egyptian papyri would seem to tend toward beneficial results, as judged on the basis of modern knowledge.

There is little doubt that medical science in ancient Egypt reached its most developed stage during the Eighteenth Dynasty, the so-called 'New Kingdom' (1590–1320 BC). During this time commerce flourished, giving a firm economic basis which saw the flowering of the arts and the standardization of hieroglyphic inscription; expeditions were sent out and monotheistic worship was attempted. Perhaps most significant of all, the land was at peace. During this time up to 72 per cent of all prescriptions in the papyri were quantified. Towards the end of it, in medical documents like the London Papyrus, dated 1350 BC, no quantification is found amongst the spells and recitals. However, all was not lost, for in the London Demotic Papyrus of the third century AD, amongst divinations, spells and erotica 20 per cent of the recipes are quantified.

At about the same time as the compilation of the Ebers Papyrus, some thousand kilometres to the east in Mesopotamia, modern-day Iraq, Iran and part of Syria, another branch of the medical tree was making use of many of the same plants. From Campbell Thomson's mammoth study of 660 cuneiform tablets we have a list of some 250 drugs used by the Assyrians. Those in common use include Carob, Colocynth, Indian Hemp, Juniper, Mandrake, Myrrh, Saffron and Thyme. Back in those days there was no need for animal rights groups to complain about the malpractices of medical rsearch. The tablets provide ample evidence of the use of slaves to test the efficacy and the non-lethal dose of poisonous plants before they were used on the king. It was in this way that very poisonous plants like Deadly Nightshade could be used to counteract bladder spasms, persistent coughing, asthma and excessive salivation. There is also ample evidence that in both countries pharmaceutical practice was developed to a high level of technical competence by a priesthood. They practised what they preached in the temples, religiously healing both the body and the soul with recitals, recipes and well-tested prescriptions.[6]

And if you weren't a king? Well, amateur medicine seems to have been developed to an equally high degree. In an interesting passage of his *History*, Herodotus mentions that in Babylon

> they have no physicians, but when a man is ill, they lay him in the public square, and the passers-by come to him, and if they have ever had his disease themselves or have known any one who has suffered from it, they give him advice, recommending him to do whatever they found good in their own case, or in the case known to them; and no one is allowed to pass the sick man in silence without asking him what his ailment is.[7]

Notes

1 Chauncey D. Leake, *The Old Egyptian Medical Papyri*, Logan Clendening Lectures on the History and Philosophy of Medicine, Second Series (Lawrence, KAN: University of Kansas Press, 1952), p. 3.
2 Will Cuppy, *The Decline and Fall of Practically Everybody* (New York: Holt, 1950), in *The Old Egyptian Medical Papyri*, p. 3.
3 Homer, *The Iliad*, trans. S. Butler (Chicago: Encyclopedia Britannica Inc., 1952), IV: 228.
4 Leake, *The Old Egyptian Medical Papyri*, pp. 47–8.
5 Ibid.
6 Campbell Thompson, *Assyrian Medical Texts* (Oxford, 1923) and *Assyrian Herbal* (London, 1924), in Sir E. A. Wallis Budge, *The Divine Origin of the Craft of the Herbalist* (London: Culpeper House – The Society of Herbalists, 1928).
7 Herodotus, *The History of Herodotus*, trans. George Rawlinson (Chicago: Encyclopedia Britannica Inc., 1952), I: 197.

3

THE GOOD LIFE – OR,
THE JEWISH HERITAGE

In between Egypt and Mesopotamia, another system of medicine arose, which in one way or another closely influenced the concept of healing in the Western world up to our day. The Jews collected and applied skills and knowledge from the civilizations surrounding them, but only in so far as they fitted into their own overwhelming cultural identity and strict monotheistic scheme of things. This could at times create problems, as 'healing' true and proper was seen primarily as God's prerogative, and the physician's role purely that of helping the patient and easing his trials and tribulations. Other factors, however, such as their strict concept of religious purity and the unparalleled rules of practical hygiene developed over a long period of nomadic existence, distinctly favoured the development of the art of maintaining health; and their strong concept of the sanctity of life probably made the physician's help as efficient as it could be at the time. Nevertheless, it is interesting to see that in early times physicians who called themselves 'rofe' – healer – were more often than not foreigners, and the term often had derogatory overtones, regardless of the high consideration given to the preservation of life and the care of the sick. It would appear that although most of the prophets knew the techniques of healing, they merely attended/ treated the patient and were never styled 'rofe'.[1]

The literary documents which first recorded the history of and later incorporated the culture of the People of Israel, the Bible and the Talmud, abound with passages referring to health and hygiene. The Bible mentions a sizeable number of plants, and amongst those used for food and shelter, those with religious significance and those useful as paragons and examples good or bad, there are a number of them specifically mentioned as having medicinal properties which are still being recognized today. Their exact identification is not always easy, and the vagaries of translators, intentional or not, are sometimes unhelpful, as the cautionary tale of Charles Foster Kent, Professor of Biblical Literature at Yale University, shows: the good professor managed to produce an *Alcohol-free Bible*, in which the word 'wine' was replaced by 'raisin-cakes', 'grapejuice' or 'juice', and from which the entire New Testament passages concerning the wedding at Cana were conveniently omitted.

Using the Moldenkes' work, *The Plants of The Bible*,[2] as a guide, we see for instance that the plant referred to as Aloes in the Old Testament was most probably not *Aloe sucotrina*, but Eaglewood, *Aquilaria agallocha*; Sandalwood, *Santalum album*, has also been suggested. *Balanites aegyptica* is probably the source of the 'balm' mentioned as a medicinal agent in Jeremiah, though the mention of 'balm' in Genesis 37:25 has no medicinal connotations, and could equally well be referring to *Pistacia lentiscus*, as the spice trade to Palestine would have hardly been flourishing yet in Jacob's days. This is a native of the area, and its resin, mastic, is used as an astringent, aromatic and masticatory as well as a fragrance. The various species of *Boswellia* are the main source of frankincense, mentioned abundantly throughout the Scriptures. *Balsamodendron kataph* and *Balsamodendron myrrha* are the true sources of myrrh and were used, apart from embalming and perfumery, as an astringent tonic and as a cleansing agent. Several of the references to 'myrrh' in Genesis, on the other hand, seem to be mistranslations of the Hebrew word for ladanum, which would refer to one of the species of *Cistus*, possibly *Cistus ladaniferus*. *Ferula galbanifera* is the source of galbanum, another of the frequently mentioned aromatic resins, used both ritually and for purification, and as an antispasmodic. Throughout the Bible, there are references to 'gall', 'bitter galls', 'grapes of gall' and other such vegetable unpleasantness. A probable candidate is *Citrullus colocynthis*, the Bitter Gourd, the creepers of which abound throughout Palestine and whose attractive fruit is indescribably bitter, and used medicinally as a violent cathartic. The Mandrake's aphrodisiac properties are mentioned in Genesis 30:14–16, and it is probable that the narcotic and purgative properties of *Mandragora officinarum* were known from fairly early times as well. A final plant, important throughout the Mediterranean area, is the Olive, *Olea europaea*. Olive oil, apart from constituting a major component of the diet and being used for ritual anointment and as a lamp fuel, was also used medicinally as a vehicle and during surgery as a cicatrizant.

The material contained in some parts of the Pentateuch is perfectly factual and accurate, and rules such as those concerning the prohibition against the consumption of blood and quarantines for infectious diseases are unique and do not seem to appear in any

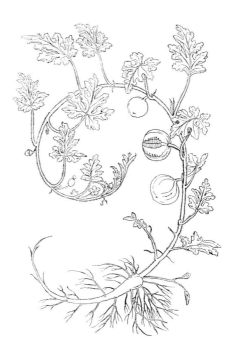

FIGURE 3.1 Colocynth (*Citrullus colocynthis*), improbable gift of the desert, referred to in the Bible as the 'grapes of gall'.

of Israel's neighbours.[3] Some of the most indicative passages are those of Leviticus 13 concerning the identification of leprosy (though there was considerable confusion over the use of the terms 'plague' and 'leprosy', the latter covering a variety of skin diseases as well as yaws and leprosy – indeed, the Midrash states that there were actually twenty-two different sorts of 'leprosy' mentioned in the Scriptures).[4]

45 And the leper in whom the plague is, his clothes shall be rent, and his head bare, and he shall put a covering upon his upper lip, and shall cry, unclean, unclean.

46 All the days wherein the plague shall be in him he shall be defiled; he is unclean: he shall dwell alone; without the camp shall his habitation be.

47 The garment also that the plague of leprosy is in, whether it be a woollen garment, or a linen garment;

49 And if the plague be greenish or reddish in the garment, or in the skin, either in the warp, or in the woof, or in any thing of skin, it is a plague of leprosy, and shall be shewed unto the priest:

50 And the priest shall look upon the plague, and shut up it that hath the plague seven days:

51 And he shall look on the plague on the seventh day: if the plague be spread in the garment, either in the warp, or in the woof, or in a skin, or in any work that is made of skin; the plague is a fretting leprosy; it is unclean.

52 He shall therefore burn that garment, whether warp or woof, in woollen or in linen, or any thing of skin, wherein the plague is: for it is a fretting leprosy; it shall be burnt in the fire.

53 And if the priest shall look, and, behold, the plague be not spread in the garment, either in the warp, or in the woof, or in any thing of skin;

54 Then the priest shall command that they wash the thing wherein the plague is, and he shall shut it up seven days more:

55 And the priest shall look on the plague, after that it is washed: and, behold, if the plague have not changed his colour, and the plague be not spread; it is unclean; thou shalt burn it in the fire; it is fret inward, whether it be bare within or without.

56 And if the priest look, and, behold, the plague be somewhat dark after the washing of it; then he shall rend it out of the garment, or out of the skin, or out of the warp, or out of the woof:

57 And if it appear still in the garment, either in the warp, or in the woof, or in any thing of skin; it is a spreading plague: thou shalt burn that wherein the plague is with fire.

58 And the garment, either warp, or woof, or whatsoever thing of skin it be, which thou shalt wash, if the plague be departed from them, then it shall be washed the second time, and shall be clean.

59 This is the law of the plague of leprosy in a garment of woollen or linen, either in the warp, or woof, or any thing of skins, to pronounce it clean, or to pronounce it unclean.

Leviticus 13[5]

Altogether these seem a useful set of rules for the control and prevention of mycoses and cloth moulds, apart from the more serious pathogens. Indeed, the Pentateuch contains many such directives for the disinfection of all contaminated clothes and furnishings by burning or fumigation. In Deuteronomy 23:13−14 we find that as part of his sanitary gear, every soldier had to carry in his belt a small shovel or paddle, 'and it shall be, when thou sittest down abroad, thou shall dig therewith, and shall turn back and cover that which comes from thee.'[6]

It is not easy to identify Jewish Medicine according to the classical 'schools', though if passages such as Genesis 7:22 – 'all in whose nostrils was the breath of life . . . died' – had any formative effect, it probably came close to the 'pneumatic' school, which maintained Air to be the vehicle of life. More probably, any principle or school of thought which did not have a Biblical or Talmudic origin had to stand on its own merits, with no uniform rule or regulation. In fact, the Jewish Law's respect for life was such that magical and occult practices might be given the benefit of the doubt, and frequently tolerated even against religious injunction. Nevertheless, one can imagine that practical considerations and empirical knowledge would have played the most important part, and that this knowledge was far from trivial is shown by the records concerning Mar Samuel (c. AD 165−257, practising in Persia), who stressed the need for strict cleanliness in all persons and objects coming in contact with the 'os uteri' during childbirth.[7] The historian Josephus mentions that the Essenes, a mystic splinter of the Pharisees, devoted part of their activities to helping the sick, for which they would use herbs and roots; nevertheless, these were seen only as aids in bringing the soul nearer to perfection, healing being in the hands of God.[8]

The classic Talmudic Era can be roughly dated between 200 BC and AD 700, a period which covers the tribulations of the second Jewish Commonwealth and of the second Diaspora following the second fall of Jerusalem in AD 70. Throughout this period, the Written Law and the Oral Tradition became the spiritual home of the Jews.[9] The Talmud includes a complex set of laws relating to everyday life from getting up in the morning to retiring at night. Detailed laws relate to hygiene and a healthful diet and lifestyle, all of which if followed religiously must have greatly reduced the need for medicine. For example, cleanliness in general and the washing of hands before meals in particular was elevated to the dignity of a religious ceremony, for which only clean and unpolluted water (or, in case of emergency, deep snow) was suitable. Equally, there is an absolute prohibition on the consumption of food, drink or water which has been contaminated by worms or mites, a measure of primary importance considering the abundance of parasitic diseases in hot countries – and the limitations of filters seem to have been recognized at an early stage. The same sort of prohibition applies to

> The black spots, sometimes found in fruit and in such vegetables as beans, peas, and lentils, [which] are the breeding places of worms and may not be eaten. When such spots are found in fruit, they may be cut out and the rest of the fruit may be eaten; but when found in a bean, pea, or lentil, the whole must be discarded.[10]

It is evident that if mycotoxins were unknown, their effects were known all too well. Equally, salting and even freezing of foods were touched upon, in a manner equally applicable to today's fast food society:

> Frozen meat must be allowed to thaw out before being soaked, but it must not be placed near a hot stove nor put in hot water, lest the

blood become hardened. In cases of emergency, the frozen meat may be soaked in tepid water.[11]

The Talmud is as much (or as little) a medical text as is the Bible, but medical matters are discussed in it on occasions. There are also accounts of medical texts and even of a pharmacopoeia which, however, have not survived in any recognizable form. Julius Preuss has pointed out, though, that even though the dietary laws may serve a hygienic purpose, they are not meant as 'hygienic laws', but as divine commands.[12] There is little reference in the Talmud to therapeutic diet, probably because it was something on which the rabbi's opinion was seldom required. Also, it should be kept in mind that most dietary laws involved meat products, which were a relatively small part of the usual diet. Generally speaking, the same rules apply as for the healthy, except of course if life is endangered; rabbinically banned substances may be used for the cure of the sick without restriction, as long as they are not actually consumed. Herbs and other edible substances grown for exclusively medicinal purposes are not generally regarded as human food in a technical sense, and do not incur the usual dietary and purity laws: the original Talmudic ban on taking medicines on a Sabbath was introduced to guard against the possibility of pounding spices on the Sabbath, and not in connection with their use.[13]

Constipation was treated with herbs ('Abodah Zarah 11a) and if necessary with purging, unless the patient was pregnant (Pesahim 42b). The rabbis of the Talmud knew of the analgesic and hypnotic properties of opium and cautioned against overdoses.[14] Two remedies for 'heaviness of the heart', interpreted alternatively either as asthma or as melancholy, are described in the Talmud. In one, 'hiltit', probably Asafoetida, is dissolved in water and three gold dinar weights thereof taken on three consecutive days; for some reason, omitting the last dose was considered detrimental to the patient's health. Here, too, the interpretation of medical terms can at times be a problem: the term 'heart' (Hebrew *lev*, Aramaic *libba*) was frequently used in a generic way meaning chest or breast. Similarly, a therapy for heart pain (perhaps heartburn?) consists of the ingestion – but not the inhalation – of Black

Cumin: 'one who regularly takes Black Cumin will not suffer from heart pain . . . The mother of Rabbi Jeremiah used to take bread for him and stick Black Cumin on it [so that it should absorb the taste] and then scrape it off [to remove the smell]' (Berakhot 40a).[15] As a final fling, reminiscent of the narcotic use to which Mandrake wine has been put, the Talmud states: 'the condemned are given wine containing frankincense to drink so that they should not feel aggrieved' (Semahot 2:9).[16]

Regardless of the nature of the treatment offered, there was a strong practical bent in attitudes towards the medical profession. The Talmud advises the reader not to live in a town without a physician (Sanhedrin 17b), nor in a town where the leader of the community is a physician (Pesahim 113a) – he is too busy with his medical practice to devote himself to community affairs. In the same vein, patients are advised in the Baba Kamma 85a not to consult a transient physician, as he would not have an adequate knowledge of local conditions. Was this a safeguard against quackery or was it professional protectionism?[17]

The foremost authority on the history of Jewish Medicine is Julius Preuss (1861–1913), and in his *Biblisch-Talmudische Medizin* we have a compendium of his published works and ideas. Amongst them one finds interesting hints of advanced practical knowledge, such as that the second-century Talmud recognized the inheritability and sex-linkage of haemophilia: if two sisters each lost a son through bleeding, the third sister did not have to circumcise her son. Plant lore is also present, though to a more limited extent: in a chapter on obstetrics Preuss mentions contraception by a 'potion of herbs' (or 'cup of roots') prepared with Alexandrian gum, liquid alum and Garden Crocus, mixed with beer or wine (Shabbat 110a). Preuss also points out that one of the consequences of the importance of hygienic laws to the Jewish community was that Jewish doctors made far less use of the *Dreckapotheke* – the collection of remedies containing dung, faeces, menstrual blood, human parts and other such components having more magical than medicinal properties, which one finds in such abundance in medieval medicine. In the final chapter on dietetics, he deals with rules of lifestyle and preventive medicine, going far beyond the question of food intake.

The general rules of health and nutrition, amongst others, are: eat moderately, eat simply, eat slowly, and eat regularly . . . Do not sit too much, for sitting provokes haemorrhoids; do not stand too much, for standing is harmful to the heart; do not walk too much, for excessive walking is harmful to the eyes.[18]

The latter point possibly relates to the high light levels in lands which were slowly but surely being denuded of their natural vegetation and inexorably moved towards desertification, an interesting point considering the number of laws pertaining to conservation, especially of trees. But more important is the basic concept mentioned, that of moderation. An attitude which left healing to God and the maintenance of health to Man was highly likely to bring about an effective code of 'Good Life', suitable for the entire variety of lifestyles with which the Jewish people were faced throughout the Diaspora; and this is exactly what we find. In Hyman E. Goldin's *The Jew and his Duties*, an English abridgement of the *Kitzur Shulhan Arukh*, the compilation of codes and obligations originally codified by Joseph Karo in the sixteenth century, which is still being used today in its modernized form, we find this code expressed clearly and succinctly, in a manner that is well worth quoting at length:

1 It is the command of the Almighty that one must keep one's body healthy and strong. One should therefore shun anything which tends to injure the body, and strive to acquire habits that help develop the body to its full vigour.

2 One should therefore adopt the happy mean, eating neither too little nor too much. Excessive eating can be as harmful as malnutrition.

3 When a person is young his digestive system is strong; therefore he is in greater need of regular meals than the middle-aged person. The aged man, because of his weakness, requires light food, little in quantity and rich in quality to sustain his strength.

4 On hot days the digestive system is weak, therefore less food should be consumed than on cool days. And the medical scientists have suggested that in the summer a person should eat only two-thirds of the amount he eats in the winter.

5   It is a known rule in medical science that before eating, a person should take some exercise, by walking or by working, until the body becomes warm. While eating, he should be seated or recline on his left side; and after the meal, he should not move about too much, so that the food may not reach the stomach before it is well digested and cause him harm, but he should walk a little and then rest.

6   A person should eat only when he has a natural desire for food and not an unnatural one. A natural desire for food is called 'hunger', and occurs when the stomach is empty; an unnatural desire is a longing for a particular kind of food, and is called 'appetite'. In general a healthy, strong person should eat twice a day, and the feeble and the aged should eat little at a time several times during the day, because excessive eating weakens the stomach. It is best to omit one meal during the week, in order that the stomach may have a rest from its work and its digestive power may thus be strengthened.

7   It is advisable that every person should become accustomed to have breakfast in the morning.

8   Since the digestive process begins with the grinding of the food with the teeth and by mixing it with the juice of the saliva, therefore one should not swallow any food without masticating it well, so as not to overtax the stomach.

9   Water is the natural drink for a person and is healthful for his body. If it is clean and pure, it is helpful in that it preserves the moisture of the body and hastens the expulsion of worthless matter. One should select cool water for drinking, because it satisfies the thirst and helps the digestion more than water which is not cold. But the water should not be too cold, because it quenches the natural warmth of the body; especially when a man is tired and weary, he should be very careful not to drink very cold water.

10   A person should eat only when he is hungry, and drink when he is thirsty, and should not neglect the call of nature even for one moment.

11   Weariness in a moderate degree is good for the physical health, but weariness to an excess, as well as inactivity, are injurious to the body. In the hot season, a little exercise will suffice, but in the

cold season, more is required. A fat person needs more exercise than a lean one.

12 He who desires to preserve his health, must learn about his psychological responses and control them; joy, worry, anger, and fright are psychological actions. A wise man must always be satisfied with his portion during the time of his vain existence and should not grieve over a world that does not belong to him. He should not look for superfluities, and he should be in good spirits and joyous to a moderate extent at all times.

13 A person should endeavour to dwell where the air is pure and clear, on elevated ground, and in a house of ample proportions.

14 The air best for the physical well-being is that of even temperature, neither too hot nor too cold. Therefore precautions should be taken not to heat the house too much in the winter time as many senseless people do, because excessive heat occasions many illnesses. A house should be heated just enough so that the cold may not be felt.[19]

The rules and laws went far beyond those of personal health, covering Man's duties towards animals: 'The Law of God forbids the infliction of needless pain upon any living creature. On the contrary, it is our duty to relieve any living creature of pain, whether it is ownerless or not'[20] – which shows that the fundamental tenet 'What is hateful to thee, don't do to another; this is the basis of the entire Jewish Law, while the rest is a mere commentary thereon. Go and complete its study' (Babli, Shabbat 31a)[21] does not apply to Man alone, but to all creatures of God. Likewise respect for the fruits of the Earth as expressions of the Divine is shown in the following passage and the Blessing which it contains:

We are not permitted to enjoy a beautiful sight in nature, without thanking the Almighty for it. On seeing fruit trees in blossom we must say the benediction: 'Blessed art Thou, O Lord our God, King of the universe, who hath made the world wanting in nought, but hath produced therein goodly creatures and goodly trees wherewith to give delight to the children of men.' This benediction should be said only once a year. If we have delayed saying the benediction past blossom time, we should not say it at all.[22]

Notes

1 Fred Rosner, *Medicine in the Bible and the Talmud* (New York: Ktav Publishing House, Yeshiva University Press, 1977).
2 Harold N. Moldenke and Alma L. Moldenke, *Plants of the Bible* (Waltham, MA: Chronica Botanica Co., 1952).
3 Rosner, *Medicine in the Bible and the Talmud*.
4 Moldenke and Moldenke, *Plants of the Bible*.
5 *The Holy Bible*, King James' Authorized Version (London: Oxford University Press).
6 Ibid.
7 *The Holy Bible*; and Immanuel Jacobovits, *Jewish Medical Ethics* (New York: Bloch Publishing Co., 1975).
8 Rosner, *Medicine in the Bible and the Talmud*.
9 Ibid.
10 Hyman E. Goldin, *The Jew and his Duties – The Essence of the Kitzur Shulhan Arukh* (1953; New York: Hebrew Publishing Co., 1984), p. 69:16.
11 Ibid., p. 70:5.
12 Rosner, *Medicine in the Bible and the Talmud*.
13 Jacobovits, *Jewish Medical Ethics*.
14 Rosner, *Medicine in the Bible and the Talmud*.
15 Ibid., p. 83.
16 Ibid., pp. 217–18.
17 Ibid.
18 Ibid., p. 35.
19 Goldin, *The Jew and his Duties*, pp. 210–12.
20 Ibid., p. 212.
21 Ibid., p. 179.
22 Ibid., p. 64:1.

4

CLASSICAL MEDICINE

Latin may be the language of botany but many of the terms it uses have their roots in the language of that Greek culture which laid the foundations of Western civilization between the seventh and third centuries BC, and whose roots are themselves found in the settling of the eastern Mediterranean by Indo-European peoples over the preceding millennium or so. The background of their healing crafts was the same North Asian Shamanic corpus of knowledge and myth which gave rise to Central and South Asian medicine, and indeed the similarities are apparent over a long period of time; further east, in China and beyond, the relationships may well be there but have become too remote to be readily recognized.

Every schoolboy used to know and quote from Homer's *Iliad*, and it is there that we find some of the first references to European materia medica. In Book IV: 188, 'and Agamemnon answered "I trust dear Menelaos, that it may be even so, but the surgeon should examine your wounds and lay herbs upon it to relieve your pain." '[1] And in Book XVI: 842, 'he then crushed a bitter herb, rubbing it between his hands and spread it upon the wound. This was a virtuous herb which killed all pain, so the wound presently dried and the blood left off flowing.'[2]

Homer was not a man known to have existed, but a hypothesis constructed to account for the existence and quality of the *Iliad* and *Odyssey*, the Homeric Poems – indeed Samuel Butler contended that the *Odyssey* was written by a woman, though the most likely source would be someone's compilation of a series of pre-existent orally transmitted poems. As to dates, earlier than the sixth century BC must suffice. Their importance, apart from their literary quality, lies in the glowing picture they draw of this period and of the beliefs which ruled the Greeks' lives at the time. At this stage, healing was almost entirely concerned with the repair of traumatic injuries; diseases were considered to be punishments sent by the Gods, and were by definition unhealable. What healing crafts existed were given divine origin as well, and invariably seen as a special favour granted by the Gods to the healer.

Typical of the passage from mythical to empirical medicine was the development of the figure of Asklepios. Initially a demigod son of Apollo and a nymph, who was taught medicine by the centaur Chiron, he is referred to in the *Iliad* simply as a healer; later he inspired a divine cult centred around temples of healing such as the sanctuary at Epidauros, where the patients/suppliants could rest, be cleansed and restored by a medically trained priesthood, and undergo the healing rite of Incubation. In this process, the patient would, after suitable ritual preparation, spend one or more nights inside the temple, at times in underground chambers. Afterwards, he would discuss his dreams with the priest/healer, who would interpret them, providing both diagnosis and, if possible, a cure. What knowledge of herbal medicine lay behind such a rite is unknown, but whatever it was it certainly drew considerable assistance from the setting, which must have acted both as a psychoanalysis and as a spur towards psychosomatic healing. The cult has parallels throughout Asia Minor, had already been transferred to Rome in Republican times (293 BC), and was probably the ground out of which subsequent medical schools arose – and in many Mediterranean countries, the belief that spending a night in a church will cure a persistent disease is still far from gone.[3]

It was through the evolution of philosophical concepts that medicine lost its supernatural overtones. Certainly, the help of the Gods was both necessary and welcome, and the healer was impotent against fate, but disease itself gradually came to be seen as a purely natural phenomenon, and hence amenable to natural treatment. In particular, it was recognized as a deviation from the natural state of health, and hence the role of the healer became

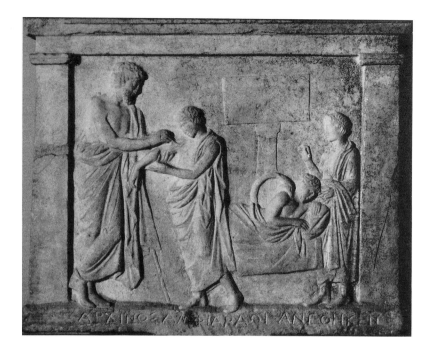

FIGURE 4.1   A fourth-century BC Greek vase painting showing Asklepios, the
personification of Western medicine, treating Archinos.

more and more that of one who restores (or at least tries to
restore) the natural balance of things.

Thales of Miletus (*c.*630 BC), generally considered to be the first
Greek philosopher of note, introduced the concept of Physis – the
physical essence out of which and into which all things transform
and evolve, with no supernatural involvement. For him, this
primordial element was Water, from which Air, Earth and Fire
were derived. All other matter was but a manifestation of a
combination of these elements. Anaximenes (*c.*545 BC) defended a
similar system, but substituted Air for Thales' Water and
introduced the crucial point that this primitive element persisted
throughout its transformations, remaining the fundamental principle of matter – the first rudiments of the principle of conservation
of matter and energy.[4]

At about the same time, Pythagoras was trying to find a definition of the universe in mathematical and geometrical terms, laying the foundations of plane geometry in the process. He also laid the roots of the Humoral Theory by postulating the *Enantioses*, the ten paired and opposite principles which compose every entity:

Finite	*vs.* Infinite
Even	*vs.* Odd
Unity	*vs.* Plurality
Right	*vs.* Left
Male	*vs.* Female
Fixed	*vs.* Mobile
Straight	*vs.* Curved
Light	*vs.* Darkness
Good	*vs.* Evil
Regular	*vs.* Irregular

At about the same time, Empedocles of Acragas reduced these opposite pairs to two, Hot and Dry *vs.* Cold and Moist, defining these as properties of the four root Elements – Fire, Air, Earth and Water – themselves qualified in the human body by the four Humours: Phlegm, Yellow Bile, Blood and Black Bile.[5]

These concepts were elaborated further and applied to human health in the Hippocratic corpus of writings, and rigidly systematized by Galen. By this time the idea of Temperaments – bodily states created by the balance or imbalance of the Humours – had also appeared, and eventually Empedocles' idea of 'Likes attract, opposites repel' transformed itself in Galen's dictum that diseases are best treated by their opposites; in other words, that medicinal substances can be classified according to Element, Humour and Temperament, and that they are best suited for the treatment of dysfunctions of opposite nature.[6] These two figures, Hippocrates and Galen, were to become the dominant influence on medicine and the healing arts in general until well into the modern age.

Hippocrates may or may not have been a single individual. It is generally believed that he was born around 460 BC on the island of Cos, and that he practised medicine there and elsewhere; on the other hand, the myth of the Father of Medicine has long overwritten the history of the man. The works generally ascribed to him may be the work of an individual, or may be the compilation of the products of the medical school of Cos. Whichever the case may be, their influence was enormous. He developed the concepts of Humours and Temperaments, setting out a true theory of medicine, but he never lost sight of the fundamental goal, the patient's wellbeing. He recognized that illness was an interaction between the patient as a whole person, the disease, the healer and the environment surrounding them, and that the process of healing must involve all of these; he also had considerable faith in the healing powers of nature, which the healer had to aid rather than replace, concentrating on the prognosis rather than on the disease,

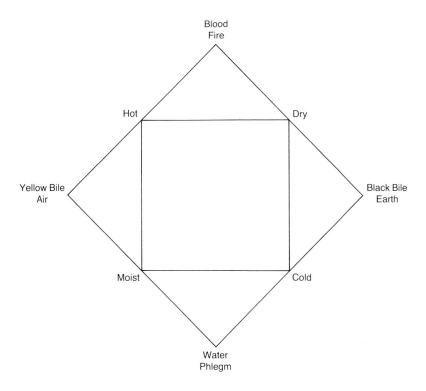

FIGURE 4.2 The Empedoclean view of the elemental structure, which in the form of Hippocrates' writings permeated European thought and health care from around the fifth century BC until modern times.

and using the diagnosis as a tool to this end. His writings range from the philosophy of medicine to human ecology, but the best known, and probably most influential, were the *Aphorisms* and the Hippocratic Oath. The *Aphorisms* were a collection of short comments and observations which were part of the Western medical curriculum right up to the nineteenth century. The one most frequently quoted is probably the famous opening one, 'Ars longa, vita brevis': 'Life is short, and Art long; the crisis fleeting; experience perilous, and decision difficult. The physician must not only be prepared to do what is right himself, but also to make the patient, the attendants, and externals cooperate.'[7]

The Oath, on the other hand, was and is a statement of the healer's mission, expressed in terms of the welfare of the patient, which in one form or another is still recognized as the conceptual basis of the medical profession.

The Hippocratic Oath

I swear by Apollo the physician, and Aesculapius, and Health and All-heal, and all the gods and goddesses, that, according to my ability and judgment, I will keep this Oath and this stipulation – to reckon him who taught me this Art equally dear to me as my parents, to share my substance with him, and relieve his necessities if required; to look upon his offspring in the same footing as my own brothers, and to teach them this art, if they shall wish to learn it, without fee or stipulation; and that by precept, lecture, and every other mode of instruction, I will impart a knowledge of the Art to my own sons, and those of my teachers, and to disciples bound by a stipulation and oath according to the law of medicine, but to none others. I will follow that system of regimen which, according to my ability and judgment, I consider for the benefit of my patients, and abstain from whatever is deleterious and mischievous. I will give no deadly medicine to any one if asked, nor suggest any such counsel; and in like manner I will not give to a woman a pessary to produce abortion. With purity and with holiness I will pass my life and practice my Art. I will not cut persons labouring under the stone, but will leave this to be done by men who are practitioners of this work. Into whatever houses I enter, I will go into them for the benefit of the sick, and will abstain from every voluntary act of mischief and corruption; and, further from the seduction of females or males, of freemen and slaves. Whatever, in connection with my professional practice or not, in connection with it, I see or hear, in the life of men, which ought not to be spoken of abroad, I will not divulge, as reckoning that all such should be kept secret. While I continue to keep this Oath unviolated, may it be granted to me to enjoy life and the practice of the art, respected by all men, in all times! But should I trespass and violate this Oath, may the reverse be my lot![8]

Galen (Claudios Galenos, latinized into Claudius Galenus, AD *c.*130–*c.*200) was a teacher of medicine more than a physician. Born in the ancient centre of culture of Pergamum in Asia Minor, he grew up in a scholarly household and studied medicine, probably also under the influence of Pergamum's temple of Asklepios. After lengthy travels, which included a period of study at the medical school of Alexandria, then still a major centre of learning, he practised first in Pergamum as physician to the gladiators, and then in Rome. Here his reputation soared, both as teacher and as personal physician to the emperors Marcus Aurelius and Commodus. Galen was a teacher, and a pugnacious one. He followed the Humoral Theory, and owed most of his learned knowledge to the Hippocratic school; his 500 or so treatises aren't just medical texts, but the classification and systematization of Hippocrates' work, and its passionate (and vituperative) defence against any competing medical theories which had grown since. As a structured corpus of medical knowledge it had no precedent in the West, and it was to remain the fundamental medical text until the seventeenth century. Regrettably, though, the teacher overtook the healer. Hippocrates' concept of treating the whole person, his recognition of the interactions between the patient and his surroundings, his faith in nature and his preference for an observational and pragmatic approach did not survive intact Galen's intellectual regimentation. His *magnum opus* eventually smothered initiative and inventiveness as well as the opposition, and the cultural withdrawal of the late Roman Empire failed to produce any alternative views. As a result, over a millennium would have to pass before the words *ipse dixit*, 'He [Galen, in this case] says so', would cease to be treated as undisputable proof in medical arguments.[9]

Not that nothing happened in between. The Greek civilization peaked and was followed first by Alexander's supremacy and by that mix of Greek and Asian culture referred to as Hellenism, then by Rome. Athens long remained the cultural centre before being overtaken by Alexandria, and it is around the Athenian schools – nominally of philosophy, but in fact involved in all existing branches of knowledge – that the basis of natural science was laid. The figures who left the greatest mark on our subject were the three generations of teachers at Athens' centre of learning, the Academy.

Plato (*c*.427–347 BC), the founder of the Academy, through whose writings we are aware of most of what we know of the preceding generations of philosophers – Socrates foremost amongst them – was mainly involved in philosophy and in political theory, but did devote considerable thought to science. His *Timaeus* was an exposition of cosmology and natural history, which he collated from both Greek and Egyptian sources; it was also to some extent an attempt at finding a structure in nature, by attempting to fit Empedocles' biology into the rigid mathematical view of the Pythagorean school. It was, however, Plato's pupil Aristotle (384–322 BC) whose treatises on nearly every aspect of the knowable were to become as much an authority on the natural sciences as Hippocrates' and Galen's were on medicine. He spent twenty years at the Academy, leaving after Plato's death. After a few years of wandering, he became tutor to the young Alexander of Macedonia. In 336 BC he returned to Athens and set up the Peripatetic school of philosophy, a name derived from the path in the garden of the Lyceum where he walked and talked with his pupils – a foretaste of Carolus Linnaeus, who formalized the Greek-rooted Latin nomenclature of plants and animals two millennia later, teaching his students while walking around botanic gardens. The Lyceum was a permanent institution of learning, complete with library and lecture timetables, and it is believed that the majority of Aristotle's extant works have been derived from lectures given there.[10]

A sizeable proportion of these works verges on biological subjects, ranging from medicine through to marine biology. Amongst his descriptions of animals and their habits he mixes tales – such as the claim that the bite of a shrewmouse is dangerous to a horse, and that of a pregnant shrewmouse more dangerous still – with precise descriptions and practical advice. In his *Parts of Animals*, II:1, he carries Hippocrates' classification into the realms of anatomy by establishing Degrees of Composition: the First Degree is the composition of primary substances out of the four Hippocratic Elements, Air, Water, Fire and Earth; the Second Degree is that in which homogeneous tissues are formed out of the primary substances; and the Third Degree is the formation of organs out of homogeneous tissues. His forays into veterinary science also mix some clearly unsupported tales with practical knowledge. For example, in the *History of Animals*, IX:6, he tells of the ways animals have of curing themselves, with some fantasy: that tortoises have to eat Marjoram when they have partaken of snake, that weasels will eat Rue before attacking a snake so as to gain a poisonous breath, and that storks and other birds will apply Marjoram to injuries. More realistically, in the *History of Animals*, VII: 21–6, he maintains that pigs can catch measles and foot-rot, and that the latter can be treated with excision of the affected part, warm baths, and by feeding of mashed mulberries. In an interesting passage on flatulence, diarrhoea and insomnia in elephants, he suggests dipping the beast's fodder in honey as a costive, and salt, olive oil and water rubs against insomnia; to top it off, he advises the application of slices of roast pork against the elephant's pains in the shoulders.[11]

Finally, it was Theophrastus (*c.*372–287 BC) who succeeded Aristotle at the Lyceum, and who himself was a great Peripatetic teacher. Under his direction enrolment of pupils at the Lyceum rose to its highest point. He was without doubt the Father of Botany, and his two most important surviving works are *Inquiry into Plants* and *Growth of Plants*. Apart from these, his main work was the clarification and development of his teacher Aristotle's concepts.[12]

Notes

1 Homer, *The Iliad*, trans. S. Butler (Chicago: Encyclopedia Britannica Inc., 1952), IV:188, p. 25.
2 Ibid., XVI: 842, p. 81.

3 *Encyclopedia Britannica*, 15th edn (Chicago: Encyclopedia Britannica Inc., 1985).
4 Ibid.
5 *Encyclopedia Britannica*, 15th edn; Avicenne, trans. Henri Jahier and Abdelkader Noureddine, *Poème de la medicine (Urguza Fi 'T-Tibb – Cantica Avicennae)* (Paris: Les Belles Lettres, 1956); and Mazar H. Shah (ed.), Avicenna, *The General Principles of Avicenna's Canon of Medicine* (Karachi: Naveed Clinic, 1966.)
6 *Encyclopedia Britannica*, 15th edn; Avicenna ed. Shah, *The General Principles of Avicenna's Canon of Medicine*; and Hippocrates, *Hippocratic Writings* (Chicago: Encyclopedia Britannica Inc., 1952).
7 *Hippocratic Writings*, p. 131.
8 Ibid., p. xiii.
9 *Encyclopedia Britannica*, 15th edn; Hippocrates, *Hippocratic Writings*; and Aristotle, *The Works of Aristotle*, 2 vols (Chicago: Encyclopedia Britannica Inc., 1952).
10 Ibid.
11 Aristotle, *The Works of Aristotle*.
12 *Encyclopedia Britannica*, 15th edn; and Aristotle, *The Works of Aristotle*.

General information

Jean-Pierre Vernant, *Les Origines de la pensée grecque* (Paris: Presses Universitaires de France, 1962).
Fridolf Kudlien, *Der Beginn des Medizinischen Denkens bei den Griechen von Homer bis Hippokrates* (Zürich: Artemis Verlag, 1967).

5

INDIAN ROUTES

While the western branch of the Indo-European peoples developed their philosophies and their healing crafts, their eastern brethren did the same in India, partly out of the same background material, but with vastly different results. As elsewhere, there was an underlying layer of folk medicine, shamanism and magic, both home-grown by the pre-Aryan inhabitants and a patrimony of the Aryan invaders. Their philosophical base, however, followed a far different path from the Classical one: where the Greeks were ready to apportion separate spheres of influence to the natural and to the supernatural, and therefore created the terrain in which a strictly material interpretation of disease could grow, Hindu philosophy kept the two spheres closely intermingled, giving rise to a medical system in which non-material aspects could have as much, if not more, influence than material ones. This did not mean that the physical aspects were considered unimportant, but that they frequently were and are interpreted on both a material and a non-material plane, and treated accordingly.

The earliest medical writings – and early they were, possibly as far back as the second millennium BC – are found in the *Vedas*, especially in the *Atharavaveda*, traditionally handed down by Brahma to Dhanvantari, the Hindu equivalent of Asklepios. These contain a considerable amount of herbal lore and folk remedies, but the main accent is on magic, religious practices and the exorcism of offending demons. The next major works, the *Charaka Samhita* and the *Susruta Samhita*, are considerably later in date, the former being attributed to between the first and second

46

centuries AD and the latter to between the fourth and seventh centuries AD. They are also works of a completely different nature and quality, showing the development of a complex and effective medical system over the intervening centuries. Attributed to the physician Charaka and to the surgeon Susruta, they contain descriptions of a large number of diseases, instructions covering some highly sophisticated surgery, by far superior to contemporary practices elsewhere, and an advanced system of clinical diagnosis and treatment. All of this was incorporated into an elaborate structure, sometimes with magical and religious overtones, but primarily concerned with a hierarchical classification of entities, in many ways comparable to the Hippocratean Elements, Humours and Temperaments.[1]

Beyond being merely a curative system, Ayurveda, as it is called, covers the entire existence of the individual in both the natural and supernatural spheres, addressing him or her both as a single entity and as a component of the continuous flow of existence, the Hindu Wheel of Life or the Buddhist Path. Diet, hygiene, behaviour and social relations all play a part and are treated to some extent, and the Aristotelian 'macrocosm-microcosm' concept – that events in the natural world mirror to some extent events in the supernatural one – is also present, with direct interconnections between individual and universal wellbeing. As a result we can speak of an 'Art of Life' rather than a medical system, in which the maintenance of health, both physical and spiritual, takes precedence, with the repair skills and facilities seen more as a regrettable backup, required only when the desired equilibrium is disturbed.

The basis of this system is a sophisticated evolutionary classification of spirit and matter, derived from Hindu philosophy and in particular out of the system referred to as *Samkya*. According to it, there are two primary principles, *purusa* and *prakrti*. The former is passive and refers to the spiritual principle, the latter active and represents the primordial matter which gives the phenomenal world its evolutionary direction, and which in itself derives from the three fundamental components of matter – *sattva*, *rajas* and *tamas*, which embody the essences of thought, energy and matter respectively. From this original dyad (which bears more than a passing resemblance to the Chinese Yin-Yang system), emerge *mahat* (or *buddhi*), which can be interpreted as 'intellect', and *ahamkara*, which can be seen as the 'ego consciousness of matter'. Out of this arise firstly those Elements which are at the root of life, from consciousness to physical functions; secondly, the essence of matter itself, first through the subtle Elements (*tanmatras*) – sound, touch, colour, taste and smell – and then out of these the gross Elements. According to the *Panchamahabhuta* concept, these five basic gross Elements are *Prithivi* (Earth), *Apo* (Liquid,

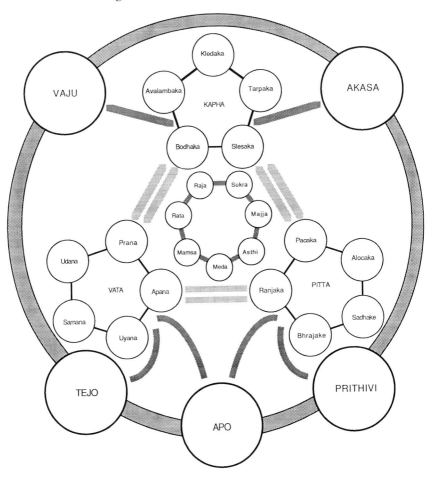

FIGURE 5.1 A graphical summary of Ayurveda's concepts of the body's relationships with the rest of the universe.

Water), *Tejo* (Heat, Light, Fire), *Vayu* (Air) and *Akasa* (Ether); each of these can be perceived through its subtle counterpart. Together, they compose the entirety of matter; each substance contains these elements in varying proportions, but it is classified after the predominant element in each.[2]

Life is regarded as the result of the mutual interaction of body, mind, and soul. While the last two components are open to influences of other kinds, Ayurveda is particularly concerned with the first, and to this purpose a sophisticated logical structure was devised to explain the body's functions. To freely quote P. B. Wanninayaka, Sri Lankan Commissioner for Ayurveda,

> The body of the individual like the other things in the world is composed of *Mahabhutas*. In the human body these are explained in terms of *Dosa*, *Dhatu* and *Mala* and in drugs in terms of *Rasa* (taste), *Guna* (quality), *Virya* (potency), *Vipaka* (the taste that arises after digestion and metabolism of the substance) and *Prabha* (the specific power of a substance).
>
> The human being is a conglomeration of three humours (*Thridosa*), seven basic tissues (*Sapta Dhatu*), and three excretions (*Thrimala*).
>
> The *Thridosa* explain the physio-chemical and phsyiological activities of the body. These are as follows:

1 *Vata* This initiates and promotes the biological activity responsible for all the movements in the body. It is of five types:

Prana Vayu	Controls the functions of salivation, eructation, sneezing, respiration etc.;
Udana Vayu	Controls phonation and speech;
Samana Vayu	Regulates the secretion of gastric juice, the retention of food in the stomach or intestine for the required time and helps in its absorption;
Vyana Vayu	Is responsible for heartbeat and the circulation of blood; and
Apana Vayu	Controls the elimination of semen, urine, faeces etc.

2 *Pitta* This is responsible for the generation of body heat and certain psychological attributes of the individual. In addition, it is responsible for digestion and the body's metabolism and is also divided into five types:

Pacaka Pitta	Responsible for digestion and metabolism;
Ranjaka Pitta	Which converts *rasa* into blood;
Bhrajaka Pitta	Which provides pigment to the hair, skin etc.
Sadhake Pitta	Which is responsible for intelligence and ego; and
Alocaka Pitta	Which has vision and discrimination of colours as its functions.

3 *Kapha (Slesma)*   The main function of *Kapha* is to provide nutrition to the bodily tissues. This again is of five types:

Kledaka	This moistens the ingested food;
Avalambaka	This provides nutrition to the heart;
Bodhaka	Is responsible for taste perception;
Slesaka	This lubricates the joints to facilitate their proper functioning; and
Tarpaka	Nourishes the mental faculties.

These three elements, when they exist in dynamic equilibrium, help to maintain the human body in a healthy condition: then they are termed *dhatus*. Any disturbance in this equilibrium causes malfunction and results in disease, in which event they are called *dosas*. Thus *Vata*, *Pitta* and *Kapha* are alternatively called *dhatu* or *dosa* depending on the effect they have on the functioning of the body. This is called the *Tridhatu* or *Thridosa Siddhanta* and is the fundamental concept of Ayurveda.[3]

From these fundamental Elements, which are more functional than structural, derive the actual anatomical components, namely the *Sapta Dhatus* and the *Thrimala*. The former actually involve the structure of tissues, and there are seven of them, namely *Rasa* (nourishing fluid or plasma), *Rata* (blood), *Mamsa* (muscular tissue), *Meda* (fatty tissue), *Asthi* (bone and connective tissues), *Majja* (bone marrow) and *Sukra* (vital substance). *Mala*, on the other hand, are the different bodily secretions and excretions, in particular the triad of faeces, urine and sweat.[4]

So it was that this theoretical structure, and its further ramifications, formed the skeleton of the medical systems of the Indian subcontinent and of a good part of Southeast Asia. Within it, diet and herbal medicine played the lion's part – Charaka already knew 500 medicinal plants, Susruta 760, and in the relatively more restricted area of Sri Lanka, current pharmaceutical floras mention the use of over 620 species belonging to around

120 families.[5] The tropical vegetation offered a great diversity of materia medica to the village herbalist and to the court physician alike, and they both made full use of it. More significantly, diet and medicines rarely drifted very far apart: aided by strict religious codes, diet found itself studied and codified as much as pharmacy, and treated as an intrinsic part of health maintenance, and the same happened to hygiene. The result was a system of health care which went a long way towards allowing the growth of a complex and densely populated civilization, living under conditions ranging from the high valleys of the Himalays to the moist tropical forests of South India. It was also a cultural medium of exchange, producing ideas which travelled freely between India and the other two great cultural areas with which it was in contact, Persia and the Mediterranean area to the west and China to the east.[6]

Notes

1 *Encyclopedia Britannica*, 15th edn (Chicago: Encyclopedia Britannica Inc., 1985).
2 Gananath Obeyesekere, 'The theory and practice of psychological medicine in the Ayurvedic tradition', *Culture, Medicine and Psychiatry*, 1 (1977), pp. 155–81; and P. B. Wanninayaka, *Ayurveda in Sri Lanka* (Sri Lanka: Ministry of Health, 1982), pp. 3–4.
3 Wanninayaka, *Ayurveda in Sri Lanka*, pp. 3–4.
4 Ibid.
5 D. M. A. Jayaweera, *Medicinal Plants (Indigenous and Exotic) Used in Ceylon*, 5 vols (Colombo: The National Science Council of Sri Lanka, 1981).
6 *Encyclopedia Britannica*, 15th edn.

6

ROMAN CONNECTIONS

Rome, the first city in the world to attain the distinction and the problems of one million inhabitants, in the year 5 BC, had been founded by Romulus 748 years earlier. The settlers of this natural strongpoint, astride seven hills and close to the coast, gradually overcame all neighbouring tribes, eventually conquering the Etruscans to the north and the other Italic tribes as well as the Greek colonies to the south. All the evidence indicates that they not only annexed these peoples but also to a greater or lesser extent their ideas and ideals, including their medical practices. The range of plant materials to which they had access must have been much the same as that available to Greeks, Hebrews, Babylonians and Egyptians before them. However, as their conquests continued apace and their trade routes spread out north, south, east and west, new wonders of the natural world must have flooded into their markets and into the hands of their physicians, both annexed and home-trained.

Communication between Egypt and the Far East, especially India, must have been not infrequent, even though almost completely dependent upon Arab middlemen, since they occupied the eastern side of the Red Sea. On the other hand, signs of some direct contacts have been beautifully described. Charlesworth tells of

a curious farce which has come down to us in papyri fragments, in which some Greek mariners have been wrecked upon a barbarian coast and are being hospitably entertained by the king of the country. He speaks an almost unintelligible language, but as all his phrases are interpreted by one of the Greeks as invitation to drink, the party

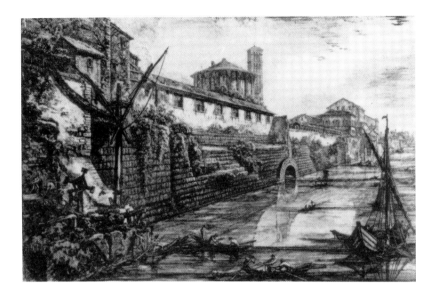

FIGURE 6.1 Rome's public works have enjoyed greater longevity than its medical tradition. Ancient Rome's main sewer, the Cloaca Maxima, shown here in Piranesi's etching *The Tiber at the Mouth of the Cloaca Maxima, formerly called the Bel Lido*, is still extant and at times functional to this day.

proceeds merrily. Recently it has been shown by an Oriental scholar that this language is Canarese, a dialect of Southern India, and we may safely assume that some rough knowledge of these tongues had been picked up by the Greek captains of Alexandria in the course of their voyages. Lastly, in the temple of Redesiya, lying on the desert route to the Red Sea, was discovered a dedication by an Indian to Pan, pointing to a real and direct intercourse between the two people.[1]

As the Roman Empire spread its way across the world, three routes lay open to the rich diversity of plant life and knowledge in the Far East: first, by the Black Sea, along the river valleys of the Caucasus, across the Caspian Sea, up the Oxus, and by northern Bactria – roughly, modern Afghanistan, Tadzhikistan and Kirghizstan – into China and India; second, from Syria down the Euphrates to Nisa and across Persia; and third, by the Red Sea and the Indian Ocean. The first was little known and the second was under

Parthian domination. It is not surprising, therefore, that the third was the one favoured by Rome.[2]

A few decades after Augustus' conquest of Egypt, during the reign of Claudius, an important change took place. Up to then, the trade route to India had been purely coastal, and by and large in the hands of Arab intermediaries. About the middle of the first century AD, a sea captain by name of Hippalus ventured to try the regular monsoon winds, and discovered the direct route across the Indian Ocean. This meant that the round trip was easily possible in less than a year; it also meant that the West was able to control the trade directly, without intermediaries. A huge increase in trade and diplomatic relations followed, which lasted well into Hadrianic times.[3]

Part of this trade must have travelled directly from the ports on the Red Sea, a larger part through Abyssinia, and part through Socotra and Yemen, from which came cinnabar, tortoiseshell, Aloes and myrrh; but further down the coast, in the region roughly corresponding to Somalia, there were trading towns and small factories such as Malao, Mundus, Moselle and Opone, with some contacts as far south as the Ugandan port of Rhapta. Local myrrh, frankincense and other fragrant gums as well as ivory and tortoiseshell were the main exports, but they also acted as go-between ports for rice, ghee, Sesame oil, cotton and sugar, brought there by ships from India.[4]

Considering the rapid increase in geographical knowledge at this period, it can be supposed that the trade with the East was at its height around Hadrian's time. Ptolemy knew about and was able to describe the whole of the coast from Cape Comorin to the Ganges and showed some knowledge of the Malay Peninsula. The most important towns for Roman trade with India were Barygaza, in the north, and Muziris on the Malabar coast, where trade was sufficiently advanced to justify an organized system of pilotage. The harbour of Muziris was the most important for the spice trade, in particular Pepper in bulk, as well as Spikenard, Malabruthum and other commercial stores. Of these, Pepper was by far the most valued. Dioscorides mentions that Ginger was imported to Italy in jars from the port of Muza, presumably in the Yemen; also in his treatise on drugs he mentions especially the Nard of the Ganges

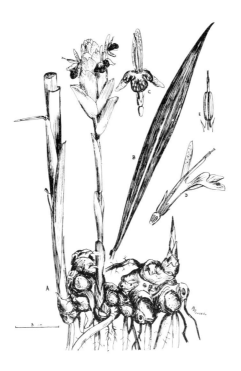

FIGURE 6.2 Ginger (*Zingiber officinalis*), an Asian import already mentioned by
Dioscorides, which has maintained exotic connections until very recently.

and the Indian Pepper. Galen also writes of drugs imported from
India and even quotes a recipe of an Indian physician; it must also
be noted that the Greek terms for Rice, Ginger and Pepper are
derivatives of Tamil words.[5]

Everything points to the fact that the merchants of the Roman
Empire were working their passage steadfastly towards the rising
sun, and finally around AD 160 the inevitable happened; some
daring navigator penetrated the Straits of Malacca and found
himself in direct contact with China, never before accomplished by
sea. Some trade connections were forged, and there are records of
an 'embassy' purportedly sent by Antoninus Pius (An Toun in the
Chinese records) with gifts of ivory, tortoiseshell and the like in
the ninth year of the Yen-Hsi dynasty (*c*.AD 166), which however
was taken less than seriously by the Chinese court. From that time

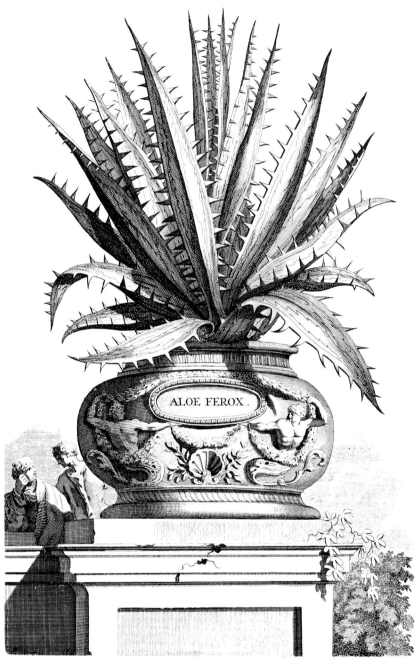

FIGURE 6.3 *Aloe ferox*, Aloes (*Aloe* spp.), part of the Roman Red Sea trade, still widely used as a demulcent and a purgative.

onwards, though, Chinese records include frequent references to the country of Ta-ts'in', Roman Syria. Unfortunately this direct link with China was forged at a time when the Roman Empire was weakening and all trade was flagging. Parthia and the Middle East too were undergoing massive and important changes, and as a result the intermingling of the knowledge and expertise of these two great civilizations was postponed by seventeen centuries or so.

Concerning the overland routes, which though less favoured at the time were nevertheless significant, it is worth mentioning that one important centre of trade was a station called by Ptolemy 'Stone Tower', in the land of the Sacae. This was almost certainly Tashkurgan in Sarikol, a fortified town in the upper Yarkand valley in Bactria, where the Roman traders met with their Chinese counterparts. Here the route from Syria met both with that leading down the Yarkand valley to China, and with that leading to India through the Hindu Kush and the Khyber Pass; here was, therefore, the meeting point of the three great civilizations of the Old World, three civilizations which shared at least some of their secrets and successes in the field of medicine.[6]

Thus we have the beginning of what we have recently begun to call the Global Village, with the gradual interleaving, and at times merging, of the world's cultural streams. But while the Roman contribution to this worldwide mercantile outlook is moderately well known, it certainly did not start with them. Sumerian and Akkadian documents from the third millennium BC show that there was active trade to the Indus valley through Oman (then known as Magan), with a thriving commerce in wood for shipbuilding and spices from India against cloth and grain from Mesopotamia. In the second millennium BC, political changes in India brought abut a change in the trade patterns, and Dilmun (modern Bahrain and its surrounding mainland), always a competitor, took over as the transit port of the Gulf. Certainly the Phoenicians knew about the city of Sur in Oman, whose name is analogous to Tyre, and which Herodotus even suggests as being their place of origin. By the first millennium BC Oman came to the fore once more, thanks to the trade in aromatics with the Mediterranean area. Myrrh and frankincense were exported primarily from the port of Shamar (near modern Taqah), which had been settled by Hadrami colonizers; their trading ventures lasted until the fourth century AD, when the spread of Christianity and the general decline of the Mediterranean economies greatly reduced the demand for such goods.[7]

To a Western audience, firmly taught to believe that all the major trade routes were pioneered by the much later European civilizations, all this may come as something of a shock, but documents and artefacts proving the contrary are now to hand, and many of them had been there all the time for all to see. It must be remembered that the Romans absorbed not only the Greek and Egyptian cultures and scholarship, but the Phoenicians' system of sea trading as well, which besides their eastern and African enterprises included many visits to Cornwall for tin long before Julius Caesar crossed the Channel. It was perhaps through this contact that the people throughout the Celtic fringe built upon the skills and knowledge of their own priest/healers, the Druids, knowledge of more northern plants and beliefs, that we know was passed on to a group of physicians at Myddfai in Wales in the sixth century AD.

By this time Roman influence was draining from Britain as the Christian heritage brought monastic healing into England after AD 597. But the Romans had left their mark on English medicine, and indeed on the English landscape, for they had introduced a number of trees such as Walnut and Sweet Chestnut, and caused the rapid spread of plants like *Plantago major*, aptly named Waybread, along their roads. This became the *Weybroed* of the Anglo-Saxons, one of their nine sacred herbs, and is still one of the commonest and most widespread weeds in Britain, having been recently recorded from all but a few of its 10km grid squares.[8]

The root is something drier than the leaf, but not so cold, it opens stoppages of the Liver, helps the Jaundice, and ulcers of the Reins and Bladder. Dioscorides affirmeth that one root helpeth a Quotidian Ague, three a Tertian and four a Quartan, which though our late Writers hold to be fabulous, yet there may be a greater truth in it than they are aware of, yet I am as loth to make superstition a base to found on, as any of them, let Experience be Judge, and then we weigh not modern Jury-men. A little bit of the root being eaten, instantly slayes the pains in the head, even to admiration.[9]

Other simples used by the Myddfai doctors, who eventually became physicians to the princes of South Wales, were Cleavers (*Galicium aparine*), one of our commonest hedgerow plants and a spring tonic, Wood Betony (*Stachys betonica*), long praised as a panacea, and Vervain (*Verbena officinalis*, a stimulant of the appetite still used in vermouth), amongst at least 172 others which it has been calculated were in regular use. The corpus of their knowledge was written down early in the thirteenth century and handed down in their families, serving them and their patients well for another 500 years.[10]

Notes

1 M. A. Charlesworth, *Trade Routes and Commerce of the Roman Empire* (1926), p. 60.
2 Ibid.
3 Ibid.
4 Ibid.
5 Ibid.
6 Ibid.
7 Ibid.; and Gulbenkian Museum of Oriental Art and Archaeology, Durham University, Co. Durham, *Oman and the Sindbad Project*, expedition pamphlet (1980).
8 John Williams Abithel, *The Physicians of Myddvai* (London, 1891); Barbara Griggs, *Green Pharmacy – A History of Herbal Medicine* (London: Robert Hale, 1981, 1987); and Richard Le Strange, *A History of Herbal Plants* (New York: Arco Publishing Co., 1977).
9 Nicholas Culpeper, *Pharmacopoeia Londinensis or, the London Dispensatory* (London, 1675).
10 Griggs, *Green Pharmacy*; and Abithel, *The Physicians of Myddvai*.

Development

7

Spices of Life

Spices began to be widely used in Western cooking, although mainly in the higher and religious classes, after the sixth century BC. The Greeks, more sober in their tastes and well supplied with aromatic herbs, didn't really adopt them until Byzantine times, some centuries later. The Romans, though they used aromatics in vast amounts – some of which like Cypress, Asafoetida, Rue and Pyrethrum would seem very strange to modern tastes – used spices very little. Apicius, the only Roman chef whose recipe book survives to the present day, considered Pepper as the only really indispensable and highly valued spice – as it remained for hundreds of years to come. When Alaric, king of the Visigoths, entered Rome in 408 AD, part of the ransom he demanded was nearly a ton of Pepper, worth around £30 million in present-day currency.[1]

Pepper was both an item of commerce and of legal standing; rents and feudal tithes could be paid partly or wholly in peppercorns. The monks of Corbie received thirty pounds of Pepper from their tenants from the day of the founding of the abbey. A 'Christmas tax' in Pepper had to be paid by the Jews of Aix-en-Provence to the archbishops Bertrand and Rostaing of Noves, and it played an equally vital part in dowries, tips and bribes.[2]

The word *pimenta* was used for spices in Low Latin: *Aroma*, *aromatica* for aromatics, *condimentaria* for condiments, *pimenta* for pigments. *Species*, a term which even modern taxonomic botany finds easy to use but difficult to define, was in Classical

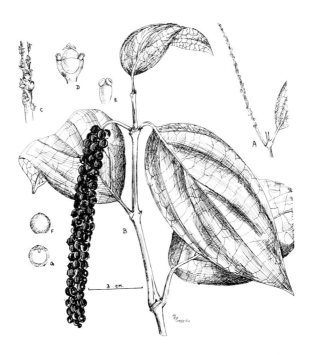

FIGURE 7.1 King's ransom to table condiment: Black Pepper (*Piper nigrum*).

Latin used to indicate both the imaginary and the real aspect of things. Byzantine jurists of the sixth century used *species* to define goods of state, monopoly or importance. Gregory of Tours employed the word both for agricultural goods available for sale and for their monetary value; indeed, he noted both down in the same column of his ledgers. Later the word *piment* (still used in Spanish) appears in the French epic poem, the *Chanson de Roland* (*c.*1100), while at about the same time the more literary *Roman de la Rose* uses the word *espices* in an approximately modern sense. It is interesting to note that at the same time the Chinese ideogram *liao wu*, unencumbered by spelling uncertainties and signifying 'substance/matter', appears with almost the same meaning. Spices were very basic and important things, an old worldwide phenomenon and article of commerce, and so they remained nearly to the present day.

Spices were items of social standing in antiquity, mainly due to their cost. When the Frankish king Chilperic I gave proof of his faith, he endowed the same abbey of Corbie with his entire Cinnamon patrimony – all of three pounds of it, with accompanying deeds of gift and property.[3]

The term *espices* was used for French lawyers' and judges' official and officious remunerations; in fact Louis XI was the first sovereign to insist that these payments should be made in coin of the realm, and it took several centuries more until such orders were fully complied with; like some of the spices before them, some of the rulings took a lot of swallowing.

As up to at least the fourteenth century AD the term Phoenician wares referred to spices, and up until the sixteenth or seventeenth century spices were only known in Europe in their dried and prepared form, it seems right to conclude that at least in Antiquity spices meant aromatic parts of plants of tropical and subtropical origin. What then are they and where did they come from?

Trade

An international trade in spices dates back at least to Sumerian times (4500–1900 BC), for Indus civilization cylinder seals have been found in Mesopotamian excavations of such antiquity. The ancient Egyptians used Myrrh, incense and Cinnamon obtained from the Land of Punt (Ethiopia), to which Queen Hatshepsut sent an expedition of five ships in 1491 BC. It is also recorded that King Solomon built a fleet with the help of King Hiram of Tyre for trade in the Red Sea, especially with the Hadramut and its queen, Sheba.[4]

As mentioned in chapter 6, trade between the Roman worlds and South Asia was carried on long before the Christian era, mainly via Arabian middlemen who evidently did their best to guard their trade secrets. For example, Herodotus (*c.*484–430 BC) believed that Cinnamon grew in shallow lakes defended by monstrous bats. According to the *Periplus Maris Erythraei*, a navigational manual of unknown authorship written some time after Pliny, Roman merchants could obtain a regular supply of silk and furs from Barbaricon and Barygaza in north-western India. A plant and an animal, the silkworm/mulberry combination from China, also played an important part in the story. It is known that around 111 BC, when the Canton region of China was finally conquered, the Chinese emperors hoped to use the southern route, later known as the 'Burma Road', as a trade link with India. However, their control over the area was never sufficiently firm and so the northern routes through Turkestan and Kokand (just south of Tashkent), which had been in use since antiquity, remained the most important.[5]

Silk flowed out in return for horses from Central Asia and both Lucerne (*Medicago sativa*) and Grape Vines (*Vitis vinifera*). The Emperor Wou Ti saw fit to plant the nitrogen-fixing legume Lucerne throughout his empire; and the Chinese name for the Vine, Pou T'ao, could appear to be a transliteration of the Greek

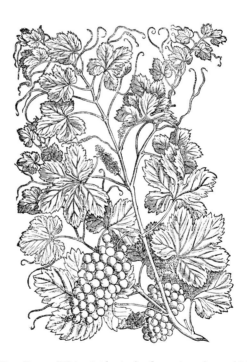

FIGURE 7.2 The Wine Grape (*Vitis vinifera*), the flowering plant which together with its ectomycote became the Western trade counterpart of the Eastern spices.

word for vine, *bodrus* – and at the time it was the hellenicized states which had formed in the wake of Alexander that held sway in western Central Asia. At this time silk was used as a currency medium throughout China, especially for taxation and for government payments. In their efforts to secure their trade sources – and it can be assumed that horses from Turkestan were considered strategic supplies in a period of continuous warfare against the Huns – a Chinese military expedition was sent to besiege Kokand around 102 BC. Apart from having an obvious effect on China's horse bloodstock – the artistic representation of horses in Chinese art changes visibly at about this time – the expedition is noteworthy for the fact that Chinese records speak of 'engineers from Ta ts'in' who worked on the defences of Kokand and on its water supplies: the first recorded encounter between Chinese and Graeco-Romans.[6]

Buddhism too played a part in the cultural interplay between China and Western Asia. It was of great importance both as a medium of communication through the voyages of its pilgrims and as a consumer of luxury goods. Silk, spices and incense by way of gifts and offerings eventually reached such propoportions as to affect the scale and nature of commerce.

Once regular monsoon navigation between the Red Sea and India had been established, three trade routes were available to Chinese goods. The first one was the traditional Central Asian route, which skimmed around the Himalayas from Bactria to Taxila – dangerous and seasonal. The second was the 'Burma Road' leading out of Shetzuan. The third, about which less is known but which might well have been the most important, was the sea route from the South China Sea, through the Malacca Straits or across the Kraa isthmus, across the Bay of Bengal, up to the headwaters of the Ganges, and by land across to the West Indian ports. There is some archaeological evidence that towards the end of the first century AD most of the silk reaching the West came by this route, rather than through Persia. Written evidence is less easy to find – the middlemen kept the source of their trade goods well hidden, as can be seen by the Roman belief that Cinnamon originated in Arabia. Cinnamon, incidentally, was one of the main trade items, reaching (according to Pliny) prices in

Rome of 1500 denarii per pound for the best quality, while Cassia was available at 50 denarii per pound.

The small, fragmented sea trade was profitable, but risky. After the first century AD, a novel situation arose when most of the Eurasian land mass was occupied by four stable powers: Rome, reaching out into Syria; the Parthians, occupying Persia and Mesopotamia; the Kushan Empire covering Afghanistan and North India; and the second Han Dynasty in China. All four had strong commercial policies, and as a result the land route became established.[7]

Intense and regular trade started in the reign of Augustus when envoys from various states of India visited the Roman emperor. The beginning of frequent direct exchanges stemmed from the discovery of the pattern of the monsoons in the Arabian Sea by the sailor Hippalus. Whether Hippalus 'discovered' the monsoons himself or learned about them from the Arabs is unknown, as are his exact dates. The early first century AD is an accurate enough date, linking the economic growth of north and central India with increased trade with Rome. Her traders brought gold and silver coins, silver wares, coral, wine, Sweet Clover (which apparently was manufactured into chaplets in India to be traded back to the Roman Empire) and perhaps some more or less expensive perfume from Italy and other Mediterranean countries, to the two North Indian ports of Barbaricon and Barygaza; glass, clothing and styrax from Egypt and other eastern provinces; more wine, chrysalides, dates, antimony, red orpiment and frankincense from the Persian Gulf and Red Sea; as well as slaves and colourful girdles of no specific origin. From these ports Roman traders carried away indigenous north and west Indian products such as indigo, ivory, cloth, onyx stones, Myrrh and Long Pepper. Other products came from the 'Upper Land': cloth, perfumery products such as bdellium, lycium and Spikenard native to the Himalayas and Costus from Kashmir, turquoise from the Hindu Kush and lapis lazuli from Badakhshan.[8]

Other plant products traded were Pepper (15 denarii per pound on the Rome market), whose consumption had become so important as to warrant its exemption from duty at Rome's gates; vegetable dyes such as red lacquer (carmine), indigo and vegetable cinnabar; Dragon's Blood; pharmaceutical products such as sandalwood, palm oil and cane sugar; and cosmetics such as the bdellium, Costus and lycium already mentioned. It is interesting that several of the products were attempts at substituting for the traditional Arab 'spices' – frankincense and Myrrh – which might well have been approaching over-exploitation at the peak of Roman power, when they were in increasing demand by every temple and every socialite in the Empire. Incense in particular was a carefully controlled commodity, collected only by the Sabaean tribe in the Hadramut and selling in Rome at between 3 and 6 denarii per pound. As it has been estimated that its cost in Gaza or Petra must have been around 1 denarius per pound, one can speak of a sizeable markup, but in no way as big as that applied on those products coming from India or beyond.[9]

The first recorded 'embassy' from Rome – the *Heu Huan Chou* (History of the second Han, *c*.430 AD) – gives a date of 166 AD and the name of the Roman emperor as An Toun, almost certainly Antoninus Pius. It arrived by sea, through the Indochinese province of Je Nan. In connection with this, an interesting find was the discovery in 1944 of the archaeological site of Oc-Eo, in the then Indochinese province of Transbassac, some twenty kilometres from the Gulf of Thailand coast; here, amongst objects of Chinese and Indian origin, were discovered a large number of items of jewellery and carved stones either of Roman origin or modelled on Roman designs, together with medals and coins of the period of Antoninus Pius. No follow-up work has been done so far, but the find opens intriguing possibilities – a stranded embassy with no return ticket, or the first evidence of 'Far Eastern copying'?[10]

As far as the Chinese side of the trade is concerned, Xinru Liu points out that the trade from the ports of western India was not interrupted by the destruction of the Kushan Empire by the Hephtalite Huns in the fourth and fifth centuries, and that according to Hsuang Tsang, the seaports on the west coast were still flourishing in the early seventh century, in other words in the full Gupta age.[11]

There are some items, such as incense, which appear in literary sources as trade goods from India but which leave no traces for the archaeologist. Perfume and incense traded in western Indian ports also appear in Chinese literature from the later Han onwards. By the second or third century AD not only were items such as Styrax and frankincense, brought by Roman ships, sold in China, but so too were many Indian products, which were also shipped to the Roman Empire. Bdellium, native to the dry region of Western India, was imported into China under the name of An hsi hsiang, i.e. fragrance from Arsaces or Persia. Costus, a product of Kashmir, was also mentioned as a Persian product in the official history of northern Wei. Another Indian product, Myrrh, was imported to China through Central Asian routes. These Indian products were obviously desired by both Roman and Chinese markets. Another such substance was red coral from the western Mediterranean and the Red Sea. Since the period of the Former Han dynasty coral had been an extremely valuable commodity, and it had become one of the major items shipped to the East from the time of the *Periplus*. The histories of the Later Han, the Three Kingdoms and the Chin mention coral as a product of Ta ts'in, i.e. the Roman Empire.[12]

Again to quote Xinru Liu:

The strength of long-distance trade in non-subsistence goods is sporadically evident in world history. Eurasian trade in the first few centuries AD which did not supply food, daily necessities, or tools for production nevertheless sustained many caravan cities and seaports from the Mediterranean to East Asia. The shift of trade routes caused the rise and fall of these cities as much as did warfare or other political crises. In North Arabia caravan cities derived their livelihood entirely from long distance trade. . . . In South Arabia ancient kingdoms gradually collapsed because of political, social and economic conditions in the Mediterranean affecting the incense route. The fabulous states in the desert of Yemen once constructed magnificent buildings with imported alabaster, marble and limestone, and built vast irrigation systems. The Roman trade directly with India and Africa from the first century AD struck a blow at this civilization. The shrinking market for frankincense and myrrh, due to the opposition of the early puritanical Christians to what they saw as pagan fragrances in the third century, abruptly terminated trade with the cities, and thereby the prosperity of the cities as well as the irrigation system which surrounded them. In this case only the profit from the lucrative trade made agriculture in the desert possible. . . .

the survival of a few cities along the trade routes of Northern India and North China despite the general urban decline after the third century probably also depended on the persistent long-distance trade in luxury goods.[13]

The *Pei Che* (History of the Northern Dynasties, written around AD 650 and referring to the previous three centuries) mentions four routes to the West, two of which are the northern and the southern routes from the Jade Gate (Yu Men Kuang) around the Lob Nor desert, the others being their continuations leading from the upper Yarkand valley (where Ptolemy's 'Stone Tower' must have stood) to Bactria and to the mouth of the Indus respectively.[14]

Around this time China received from the West the Pomegranate and Myrrh (*mou yao* in Chinese – 'mou herb' – Myrrh is *mor* in Persian and Hebrew) and started importing textiles from the West, in particular Persian brocades. It is also estimated that around AD 420, the main trade secrets of the age were exchanged: the Chinese learned the art of glassmaking, and the secrets of silk production left China and started diffusing throughout Central Asia. Incidentally, Coriander was also introduced from Persia into China, though probably at an earlier stage, and it must have had some special significance, as it is one of the five legumes forbidden to Taoist geomanticians and monks.[15]

By the ninth century, a limited but significant trade between China and the West (of which admittedly only the smallest part actually reached the Mediterranean) had returned to the sea route, mainly in the hands of Arab, Persian and Jewish traders. Camphor and Aloes were part of the known trading stock, and at this time we find the first Western references to Tea and porcelain. The scale of the trade can be estimated by the documented fact that, during the usurper Huang Tch'ao's destruction in AD 878 of Khanfu (approximately Canton, at that time the main export trade port), 120,000 Muslims, Christians, Jews and Mazdeans were killed – figures noted in the Chinese tax records. Cantonese trade ceased at this point, and Sumatra and Malaya (then in the form of the Sri Vijaya Empire) became the main entrepôt for the southern Far Eastern trade, while North China regained the supremacy of trade with its traditional land routes. The geographer Al-Masudi mentions Camphor, Aloes, Cloves, Sandalwood, Nutmeg, Cardomom and Cubeb as products available in Sumatra to Arab merchants; Pepper and further spices would have been acquired in India, on the return leg of the journey. Unfortunately for us, the fine details of the trade will probably remain hazy: with scant exceptions, the Arab travellers of the Islamic Golden Age were traders, not scholars; as a result, even though their testimonies are of great interest, they are just as likely to spin tall tales as to deliberately obfuscate matters where trade secrets are concerned. Around the eleventh century, following the first crusade, the Mediterranean end of the spice trade slipped into the hands of the Italian maritime republics, in particular Venice, Genoa and Pisa, thanks to their protected enclaves in the Levant and elsewhere.[16]

The rise in importance of the Caucasian trade route, eventually controlled at its Mediterranean end by the Genoese trading posts in Crimea and Georgia, was also due to the Mongol expansion, which at its height produced a single non-denominational state reaching from Korea to the Black Sea – a novel attraction to both missionary and trader. In addition, the successors of Genghis Khan in China continued to be friendly to foreigners and to employ them in the public administration, as can be seen from Marco Polo's career there. In this they were an exception, and such favourable conditions did not survive the Ming restoration in 1368. The Caucasian trade route remained important until the fall of Constantinople in 1453 – but by then Europe was in turmoil anyway, regaining its feet after the Black Death which had travelled along the same route two centuries earlier, and the period of Atlantic exploration had begun.[17]

It was this new world of exploration and trade which opened up new spicy possibilities, such as Pimentos, Chili and Cayenne Peppers and Vanilla from South and Central America; spiced further, it must be added, by the addition of Tobacco and the full gamut of the New World hallucinogens, the likes of which had by and large been little known in Europe and Asia. Opium had been known as a useful anti-dysenteric in China at least since the Tang dynasty, and in Europe since Pliny the Elder (AD 23–79), who mentions it in his *Historia*. Yet the first edict mentioning it and prohibiting it as a dangerous drug dates from 1729, well after the East India Company had begun to trade.

The Arab traveller Al-Tastush's amazement at the availability of oriental spices in the Rhineland markets of the tenth century AD indicates the sheer volume of trade then centring on the Republic of Venice.[18] The main cargoes were spices. They were all there: Pepper, Cinnamon, Nutmeg and Cloves; the cargoes also included Camphor, Aloe, musk from Tibet, Rhubarb, Arabian incense, Lybian dates, balsam, Sandalwood and gum. With so much profit to be made and so many risks to take en route, competition became the order of the trading routes: middlemen were always a thorn in everyone's side and their elimination often meant exactly that. So the period from the fourteenth to eighteenth centuries could be aptly called the Spice Wars.

Spices as medicaments

From food additives to pharmaceutics or from medicine to food, this is the real spice route which we will probably never be able to untangle.

There is no getting away from the fact that both to the importer and to the end user spices were precious and foreign substances, welcome to the gods, encapsulating miraculous odour and taste in minimal packages. As such it would have been natural to attribute to them magical (and therefore curative) properties – properties which could be used for the benefit of people. Experience later would prove their beneficial properties in a more material sense. What is more, many of the travelling traders and middlemen must have fallen ill en route. Some may well have been cured by local physicians and so learned from first hand, for example that Cloves can ease the pain of toothache, Cinnamon is a good stopping-upper and Pepper can stop bleeding. Turmeric, the colour of bile, is good when you are feeling liverish, and to make your stay from home a bit more bearable Ginger was a good aphrodisiac and kept you warm into the bargain. Apart from the aphrodisiac properties of the latter, the medicinal uses of all these spices are still employed today, while even the Abbess Hildegard of Bingen (1098–1179) prescribed Ginger against cold and loss of vigour, though with some reservations on the grounds of modesty.[19]

As to the original discovery of the values of these plant products by the local herbalist, one can only guess. The logic of the matter would appear to be thus: spice adds taste to a variety of primary food products, especially when in storage they have begun to go rancid. Miraculously, certain spices, being insecticidal, ward off insect pests and, being bactericidal, help them to keep longer. Under the stress of illness and disease the patients are fed with the best, most tempting food to hand, perhaps more strongly spiced to stimulate the juices or to mask the odours of the sickroom. Many patients respond to the treatment; *quod erat demonstrandum*.

Ginger has been considered an aphrodisiac since earliest time, and became widely used for this purpose in Europe in the Middle Ages. It was prescribed in the *Regimen Sanitatis Salerno* as a 'hot' drug – according to the humoral theory – against 'cold' ailments and loss of vigour. Nutmeg was used in the Middle Ages as a perfume and medicinal, primarily as an aphrodisiac and a local analgesic. During the Renaissance, an astringent paste of Nutmeg and dung was used to make breasts firmer. Saffron was mentioned in Egyptian papyri as a component of *kuphi*, a portentous cure for ailments not further defined, consisting of Saffron, honey, Juniper, Mint and Sage. Considered as both an aphrodisiac and a remedy against drunkenness by the Romans, it was also a component of the famous panacea of the Byzantine doctor Alexander of Tralle, the 'Cynoglossal Pills', consisting of Saffron and minced dogs' tongues. Only in the seventeenth century did it enter widespread gastronomic usage. Pimentos (Chili Peppers) are and have been used by Africans and Amerindians against stomach disorders and intestinal parasites, and its smoke is used as a defence against mosquitoes. It is also interesting to note that scurvy was practically unknown in America up to the St Lawrence river, the northern boundary of the Pepper's distribution.[20]

Notes

1 Paul and Bernard Corcellet *et al.*, *La via delle spezie* (Milan: RCS Rizzoli Libri S.p.A., and Singapore: Times Editions, 1987, 1988).
2 Ibid.

3 Ibid.
4 L. Boulinois, *La Route de la soie* (Paris: Arthaud, 1963).
5 Ibid.
6 Ibid.
7 Xinru Liu, *Ancient India and Ancient China – Trade and Religious Exchanges AD 1–600* (Delhi: Oxford University Press, 1988).
8 Ibid.
9 Boulinois, *La Route de la soie*.
10 Ibid.
11 Xinru Liu, *Ancient India and Ancient China*.
12 Ibid.
13 Xinru Liu, *Ancient India and Ancient China*, p. 178.
14 Boulinois, *La Route de la soi*.
15 Ibid.
16 Ibid.
17 Ibid.
18 C. Diehl, *La République de Venise* (Paris: Flammarion, 1985).
19 Corcellet *et al.*, *La via delle spezie*.
20 Ibid.

8

GOD OR MANDRAKE?

During the period of the supremacy of Rome, Europe had its focal point in the Hellenistic and Graeco-Roman culture, and its political power in Rome. This structure began to crack after the fourth century and 250 years later was non-existent. This demise set in motion the cultures of the eastern Mediterranean – the Byzantine civilization and, later, Islam. The new dominating factor in medieval Europe was the rule not of Rome but of Christianity.

The beginning of the period called the Dark Ages is generally reckoned to be AD 476 with the dismissal of the last Roman Emperor of the West, Romolus Augustulus, their end with the crowning of Charlemagne as emperor of the newly refounded Holy Roman Empire in AD 800. Practically all our evidence of medicine throughout this time comes from the writings then available in the monasteries, the last havens of what had been Classical knowledge in most of Europe. These consisted of:

(a) Greek texts in their Latin translations
Dioscorides (*c.*60), *De Materia Medica*
Galen (130–200), sundry works, mainly fragments
Oribasius (325–403), *De Parabilibus Medicamentis ad Eunapium*
Alexander of Tralles (525–605), *Therapeutica*
Paulus Aegineta (625–690), Book VII of the *Epitomae Medicae*

(b) Latin texts
Pseudo-Apuleius, *De Herbis* (fourth century)

Sextus Placitus Papyriensis, *De Medicina ex Animalibus* (fourth century?)

Pseudo-Hippocratic *Epistles* (fourth century?)

Marcellus Empiricus of Bordeaux: *De Medicamentis* (first half of the fifth century)

Pseudo-Dioscorides, *De Herbis Feminis* (sixth century?)

(c) Pliny's *Natural History*, probably the most widely read non-ecclesiastical author throughout the Dark Ages.[1]

The evolving Christian ethic regarded illness and disease as a punishment sent by God, but the alleviation of such suffering as an act of piety. The Christian influence spread across the length and breadth of Europe, and all the good men and women of the ecclesiastical establishments must have laboured in pastures new far north of the distribution of the plants described in the Greek and Latin literature. They must have scratched their heads at the plethora of plants to hand which fitted none of the descriptions of Dioscorides and Galen and taken heart from the success of the simples used by the local wise women and healers.

Throughout this time (and not only then), anything which was considered important or superior ran the risk of being given magical properties. For example, Quintus Serenus Sammonicus, a Latin physician of the third century, suggested the placing of the fourth book of the *Iliad* under the patient's head against quartan ague.[2] Such exotic magical formulae were still very much in use 300 years later, as the confession of an English judge tells us:

> It is told of Justice Holt (1642–1710) that he led a wild youth, and that on one occasion, finding himself near Oxford and without money, he procured a week's lodging by pretending to charm away an ague from which his landlady's daughter was suffering. He scribbled a few works of Greek on a scrap of parchment that had been used as a label and, rolling it up, directed that it should be bound to the girl's wrist and left there till she was well. Many years after, an old woman was brought before him charged with sorcery. The evidence showed that she professed to cure the fever-stricken by the application of a magic bit of parchment. Justice Holt examined the fragment and found it to be the very piece with which he had worked his miraculous cure many years before, for his own Greek

words were still legible upon it. His lordship confessed and the woman, who was acquitted, was one of the last to be tried for witchcraft in this country.[3]

It is little wonder, then, that wonderful plants should figure high in wonderful tales – and none more wonderfully than the Mandrake, native of Persia.

Merdomgia was the Persian name for this plant, which has perhaps become the epitome of all herbal mumbo jumbo. The beliefs in its magical properties started to accrue in Greek times, partly due to its narcotic effects and partly to its mannikin root. In particular, the legend that it would kill whoever uprooted it and therefore had to be extirpated by a dog should be seen in terms of appeasing a resident spirit or demon. Throughout the Old World, similar stories have attached themselves to other plants with man-like (or phallus-like) roots, for example Bryony. The also common legend that it grows under the gallows might well have originated from the classical myth that it arose from Prometheus' dripping ichor, as told by Apollonius Rhodius. Hippocrates (*c.*400 BC) had already recognized its properties, saying that 'a small dose in wine, less than would occasion delirium, will relieve the deepest depression and anxiety'. It was also mentioned by Aristotle in *De somnis* as a soporific, together with Poppy and Darnel.[4]

The most important book on plants of the early Christian era is that written by Pedanius Dioscorides. He was a military surgeon enjoying the Emperor Marcus Aurelius' confidence, who lived between AD 40 and 90 and who travelled extensively throughout the European provinces of the Roman Empire. The results of his investigations into the properties of 600 herbs and plants he met with are described and 394 of them are illustrated in the oldest surviving edition of his works, a remarkable codex transcribed in the sixth century and later preserved in the Imperial Library at Vienna. The codex is known as the 'Anicia Manuscript', as it was transcribed as a gift for the wedding of the Byzantine princess, Juliana Anicia, daughter of Anicius Olybrius, who was Emperor of the West in about 472, and grand-daughter of the Emperor Valentinian III. It is illustrated with a portrait of the princess, seven full-page miniatures and 394 well-executed drawings in colour by an unknown Byzantine artist dating from about 512.

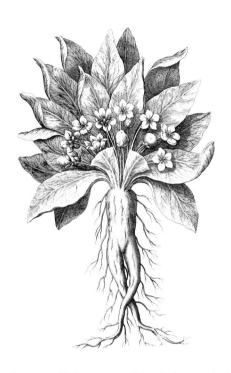

FIGURE 8.1 *Mandragora officinarum*, the Mandrake, magical plant and early anaesthetic, as engraved by the artist Matthaeus Merian in the early eighteenth century.

The work was translated into Latin and printed in the sixteenth century, and continued to be the most popular treatise on plants and their medicinal properties for centuries. Between the years 1652 and 1655, an English interlinear translation was made by John Goodyer, which later graced the library of Magdalen College, Oxford.[5]

Dioscorides appears to have shown considerable interest in the Mandrake, and the legends associated with it evidently appealed to the imagination of the artist, for he devotes two of the full-page miniatures to the plant. One represents Euresis, goddess of discovery, offering Dioscorides a Mandrake root, and shows the dog which has succumbed to its gathering; in the other, the artist is depicted making a drawing of the root. Goodyer's translation of Dioscorides' description is quoted at length by C. J. S. Thompson in *The Mystic Mandrake*:

79

'Mandragoras which some call Antimelon, some call it Dircaea, some Circaea, some Circaeum, some Xeranthe, some Antimnion, some Bombochylon, some Minon, ye Egyptians Apemum, Pythagoras Anthropomorphon, some Aloiton, some Thridacian, some Cammaron, Zoroastres Diamonon or Archinen, ye Magi Hermionous, some Gonogeonas, ye Romans Mala Canina some Mala Terrestria.

'Since that the root seems to be a maker of love-medicines. There is one sort that is Foemall which is black, called Thridacias, having narrow and longer leaves than lettuce, of a poisonous and heavy scent to ye smell, scattered upon the ground and amongst ye apples like Service berries, pale, of a sweet scent in which ye seed as of a pear; ye roots two or three of a good bigness wrapped within one another, black according to outward appearance, within white and of a thick bark but it bears no stalk.

'But of ye male and white which some have called Norion, ye leaves are greater, white, broad, smooth as of the beet, but ye apples twice as big, drawing to saffron in ye colour, sweet smelling with a certain strongness which also ye shepherds eating are in a manner made asleep, but ye root is like to that before it, yet greater and whiter and this also is without stalk. Ye bark of ye root is juiced being beaten when it is new and set under a press.

'But it will behove ye beaters after it is stirred about, to lay it up in an earthen vessel, and ye apples also are juiced in like manner. But ye juice of them becomes remiss.

'And ye bark of the root being peeled off and done through with a thread is hanged up for store. And some do seethe the roots in wine to thirds and straining it, set it up. Using a cyathus of it for such as cannot sleep or are grievously pained and upon whom being cut or cauterized they wish to make a not-feeling pain. Ye juice being drank ye muchness of ye quantity of 2 oboli with Melicrate doth expel upward Phlegm and black choler, as Ellebore doth, but being too much drank it drives out ye life. And it is mixed with eye-medicine and Anodynas and mollifying Pessums but being put to of itself as much as half an Obolus, it expels the menstrua and ye embryo and being put up ye seat for a suppository it causeth sleep.

'But ye root is said also to soften Ivory when sodden together with it for six hours and to make it ready to be formed into what fashion a man will. But ye new leaves are good both for ye inflammation of ye eyes and those upon ulcers, being laid on with Polenta, and they dissolve also all hardness and Apostumes, Strumas and Tumors and being rubbed on gently for 5 or 6 days it will deface scars without exulcerating. Ye leaves preserved in brine are laid up for ye same uses.

'The root being beated small with acetum doth heal ye Erysipelata, but for ye strokes of serpents with honey or oil, and with water it disperseth ye strumas and tumors and assuageth ye pains of ye joints with Polenta. Ye wine of ye bark is prepared without seething but you must caste in 3 pounds into a Metreta of sweet wine and that there be given of it 3 cyathi [a cyathus is roughly equivalent to an ounce] to such as shall be cut or cauterized as is aforesaid. For they do not apprehend the pain because they [are] overborn with dead sleep, but the apples being smelled to or eaten are soporiferous and ye juice that is of them. But used too much they make men speechless.

'The seed of the apples being drank purgeth ye matrix and given as a pessum with brimstone that never felt ye fire, it stays ye red flux. It is juiced, ye root being scarified about divers ways and that which runs out being gathered into a concavity, but ye juice is more effectual than ye liquor.

'But ye roots do not bear liquor in every place. Experience doth show as much.

'They give out also, that there is another sort called Morion growing in shady places and about dens having leaves like to ye white Mandrake but less, as it were a span long, white, lying round about ye root, it being tender and white by a little longer than a span, ye thickness of ye great finger which they say being drank as much as a dragm or eaten with Polenta in Placetum or Obsonium it doth infatuate. For a man sleeps in the same fashionas when he ate it, sensible of nothing for 3 or 4 hours from ye time that it is brought to him.

'And Physitians also use this when they are about to cut or cauterize. And they say also that ye root being drank with Solanum that is called Manicum, is an antidot.'

Dioscorides thus describes three varieties of *Mandragora*. The last named, Morion, was apparently the most powerful and corresponds to the *Mandragora officinalis* with its narrow leaves. The variety he calls the 'male and white', and on the other hand, was probably the *Mandragora vernalis*, but the absence of any description of the flowers renders identification uncertain.[6]

So here amongst the experiment, the mystery and the imagination we have the first account of the use of both local and general anaesthesia. The main problems must have been dose rate and side effects. Pliny, the other widespread Classical source, mentions its toxic effects:

> Persons ignorant of its properties are apt to be struck dumb by the odour of this plant when in excess, and too strong a dose of the juice is productive of fatal results.
>
> Administered in doses proportioned to the strength of the patient this juice has a narcotic effect, a middling dose being a cyathus. It is given, too, for injuries inflicted by serpents and before incisions or punctures are made in the body, in order to ensure insensibility to the pain. Indeed, for this last purpose, with some persons the odour of it is quite sufficient to induce sleep.
>
> The juice is taken also as a substitute for hellebore in doses of two oboli in honied wine. Hellebore, however, is more efficacious as an emetic and as evacuant of black bile.[7]

Pliny's source too is clearly Dioscorides, and some of his comments refer to the ritual of the magic circle when uprooting the plant and the dangers this presents to the gatherer, even though he does not mention the practice of using a dog for the purpose.[8] Further accounts of the medicinal uses of Mandrake by the Romans appear in the works of Aulus Cornelius Celsus, who flourished under the reigns of the emperors Augustus and Tiberius. In his treatise on medicine he alludes to Mandrake as a soporific:

> There is another, more efficacious way for producing sleep. It is made from Mandrake with opium seed and seed of Henbane bruised up with wine.
>
> In headache, ulcerations, lipitude, toothaches, dyspnoea, ileus, inflammation of the womb, pains of the hip, or liver or spleen or side, or in case of any female falling into a fit of hysteria and losing her speech, a bolus like that which follows, aided by repose, remedies the evil.
>
> Of Silis, acorns, wild Rue seed of each a drachm. Castor, Cinnamon of each 2 drachms, of Opium, root of panacea, dried Mandrake apples, flowers of round Cyperus of each 3 drachms and Pepper 56 grains. These having beeen separately powdered are again rubbed all together, passum being from time to time dropped in till the consistence being that of sordes. A small quantity is either taken as a bolus or diluted with water and given in the form of a draught.[9]

In C. J. S. Thompson's work on the Mandrake we find a rich trove of tales concerning its powers. For example, Hannibal, the Carthaginian general, is stated to have captured or slain a large army of African rebels by simulating a retreat, leaving behind him on the battlefield a number of jars of wine in which *Mandragora* has been infused. The rebels drank the wine, which reduced them to a condition of stupor, and when the Carthaginians returned soon afterwards they gained an easy victory over the helpless foes. A similar trick was also apparently played by young Caesar on the Cilician pirates by whom he was captured. Owing to its reputed aphrodisiac properties *Mandragora* was used by the Romans as an ingredient in their love-philtres, and its hallucinogenic properties doubtless contributed to their effects.

It was observed later that the deep and heavy stupor which could be induced by the Mandrake rendered the person to whom it had been given insensible to pain, and so it became the first anaesthetic to be used before surgical operations. Dioscorides is again the first to mention its use for this purpose, when he recommends 'wine of *Mandragora* to be given to such as shall be cut or cauterized'. He further describes another variety of *Mandragora* which was apparently more powerful still, for he says: 'a man sleeps in the same fashion as when he ate it, sensible of nothing for three or four hours from ye time that it is brought to him. And physicans also use this when they are about to cut or cauterise.'[10] This plant he calls *morion*, the leaves of which from his description appear to resemble the *Mandragora officinarum*, but smaller and growing in a cluster about the root. Again, 'The cyathi of the wine were given to persons about to be cut or cauterised, which on account of the ensuing stupor they would not feel pain.'[11]

Another *morion* was the wine also known as 'death wine', said to have been given in Roman times to those subjected to torture or to prolonged or painful death. For this purpose the wine of *Mandragora* was usually made either by boiling down the roots to a third in wine and allowing the liquor obtained to thicken, or by stripping off the bark, hanging it on strings and letting them down into a vessel containing sweet wine and leaving it to stand thus for three months. With regard to this, Richardson remarks that:

At the time when crucifixion was one of the Roman punishments, it was the custom of the women of the Grand Sanhedrin to visit the prisoners upon the cross and to administer to them a sponge charged with morion. Their sufferings allayed by the drug, the victims passed into a death-like sleep. After removal from the cross, recovery took place so frequently that the Roman soldiers were commanded to mutilate the bodies of all crucified before permitting them to be removed by their friends for burial.[12]

Could this 'death wine' in which *Mandragora* and Myrrh formed ingredients, be the same as that described as being offered to Christ during his agonies on the Cross?

From allusions made to the use of *Mandragora* wine in the works of early writers, it is evident that its use as an anaesthetic was general. Thus, in *De Viribus Herbarum*, a manuscript written in the fifth century, it is said: 'If anyone is to have a member amputated, cauterized or sawed, let him drink an ounce and a half in wine; he will sleep until the member is taken off.'[13] Isidorus, in the sixth or seventh century, also says: 'Its bark [*Mandragora*] is given in wine to those who are about to be surgically operated upon that they may fall into a stupor and may not feel the pain.'[14] And Serapion, a Syrian writing in the ninth century, says: 'A measure of four obols is given to drink to a person when it is necessary to cauterize or cut. He will not feel the cauterizing or cutting because of the stupor which ensues. Surgeons administer it when they wish to cut or burn a member.'[15]

Similar comments are made by Avicenna, the famous Arab physician active between the years 980 and 1037, who also advises its administration to anyone who wishes his members cut, and in an early Persian work entitled *Ihliyant Bade*, the statement occurs that the taking of *Mandragora* inwardly renders one insensible to the pain of even cutting off a limb. Paulus Aegineta (625–690) refers to the heavy sleep and stupor caused by Mandrake, and Apuleius in an eleventh-century manuscript of an earlier compilation claimed that half an ounce of the wine was sufficient to make a person insensible to the pain of amputation.[16]

Hugo of Lucca, chief of a successful Tuscan school of surgeons in the fifteenth century, according to his son Theodoric devised in 1490 a preparation which by means of smelling alone could put his patients to sleep before an operation. A sponge was impregnated with the mixture and was called the *spongia somnifera* or 'sleeping sponge'. The preparation was made by mixing opium, unripe Mulberry juice, Henbane, Hemlock and juice of the leaves of *Mandragora*, Wood Ivy and Forest Mulberry, together with the seeds of Lettuce, Dock and Water Hemlock. A new sponge was placed in this mixture and the whole was boiled until the sponge had absorbed it all. When used, the sponge was steeped in hot water for an hour, and then applied to the nostrils of the patient to be operated on until he fell asleep.[17]

The length of time the narcosis lasted naturally depended on the condition of the patient and the strength of the dose, but apparently was quantifiable; for example, Pierius Valerianus in the fifteenth century tells us that 'after a draft of the wine sleep continues to be very heavy for about four hours so that they feel neither the cautery or the knife.' In Meissner's *Skizzen* (1782) there is a story concerning Weiss, who was surgeon to Augustus, King of Poland and Elector of Saxony, who surreptitiously administered a potion to his royal master and when he was insensible cut off a gangrenous foot.[18]

The traditional aphrodisiac virtues of Mandrake appear to have originated in the story of Rachel in the Old Testament, and to have been elaborated in Greek mythology. Its supposed ability to produce fecundity and inspire passion, a belief still current in Palestine and elsewhere to the present day, led to its use in love-potions. Both Theophrastus and Dioscorides mention its use in love-philtres, but neither gives any account of its action. In a passage in a letter of the Roman Emperor Julian the Apostate to the priestess Callixena, the following allusion is made (Epis. 23): 'Who can prefer in a woman conjugal love to piety without being thought to have taken draughts of *Mandragora*';[19] and in the work called *Physiologus*, probably compiled in the early Christian era, reference is even made to its effect on elephants: 'the female seeks out the so-called *Mandragora* plant and partakes of it and going to the male gives him the plant; he partakes of it and is straightway inflamed.'[20]

The legends concerning the Mandrake's role as a rejuvenator appear to have become cosmopolitan and attached themselves to various plants such as Ginseng (*Panax* spp.) and to Shang-luh (*Phytolacca acinosa*) in China. Yet the plant was used in medicine mainly as an anaesthetic right down to the end of the century in which Justice Holt made his confession, thus saving the last witch from the witchcraft of the law. It may well be that the Mandrake, like for example *Cannabis indica*, varies in power and properties according to its place of growth.

It is probably because of all the mumbo jumbo and magical hype which surrounded this plant – which must have relieved much suffering over many years – that it fell into disrepute and, after being prosaically described by Culpeper as an emetic and purgative, it failed to appear in the first modern Pharmacopoeias. And yet in 1888 Benjamin Ward Richardson confirmed the presence in the plant of water-soluble atropine-like alkaloids, later partly identified as hyoscyamine and scopolamine, which acted both as a potent general anaesthetic when taken internally and as a local anaesthetic when applied externally.[21]

Notes

1 Charles Singer, *From Magic to Science* (London: Ernest Benn, 1928).
2 Ibid.
3 Ibid., p. 136.
4 C. J. S. Thompson, *The Mystic Mandrake* (London: Ryder & Co., 1934).
5 Ibid.
6 Ibid., pp. 77–8.
7 Ibid., p. 100.
8 Thompson, *The Mystic Mandrake*.
9 Ibid., pp. 101–2.
10 Ibid., p. 224.
11 Ibid., p. 225.
12 Sir Benjamin Ward Richardson, *Asclepiad*, vols V–VI (1888), pp. 174, 183, in Thompson, *The Mystic Mandrake* pp. 225–6.
13 Thompson, *The Mystic Mandrake*, p. 226.
14 Ibid.
15 Ibid.
16 Thompson, *The Mystic Mandrake*.
17 Ibid.

18 Ibid.
19 Ibid., p. 229.
20 Ibid.
21 Richardson, *Asclepiad*, vols V–VI, pp. 174, 183, in Thompson, *The Mystic Mandrake*, pp. 225–6.

9

A Light in the East – or, Islamic Medicine

'Arabic' Medicine, primarily known as the vehicle by which Classical knowledge survived through the European Dark Ages, was in itself an important melting pot and a source of novel concepts.

There was obviously a pre-Islamic Arab Folk Medicine, but so far as can be judged it was generally indistinguishable from the run-of-the-mill folk medicine practised in Middle Eastern countries and, like theirs, it was tightly bound up with magic. Apart from the fact that it must have helped and cured tens of thousands of patients, the major historical importance of this pre-Islamic medicine lies in the fact that it was eventually edited, probably by the end of the Umayyad period, together with a number of apocryphal texts, and presented as 'Prophetic Medicine' claimed in some quarters to be actually part of the Prophet's corpus of writings. This was probably done by the more religious elements in opposition to Greek Medicine, which was seen as somehow heathen. Nevertheless, it would appear that in the early Islamic and Umayyad period the majority of the doctors were Greeks, Syrians, Persians and Jews, rather than Arabs; one can assume that these were the same physicians who had been practising before the Arab conquest, and who maintained their schools under the new rulers.[1]

The movement of ideas and knowledge from Greece to the Middle East was conditioned by developments in the late Byzantine Empire around the end of the seventh century. With the Christianization of society the corpus of humanistic ideas, the

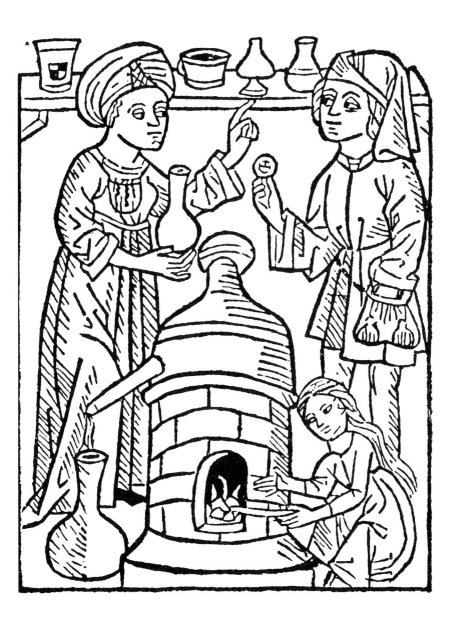

FIGURE 9.1 The still, an early high-tech export from the world of Islam to Europe.

'ethics' of society written in Koine Greek became the preserve of only a limited number of scholars; in contrast, the medical and scientific works of practical utility were to a large extent translated into local languages such as Aramaic and Persian. Thus most of the latter were eventually transmitted to the Arabs, but without the philosophical and literary background in which they had been developed; the neoplatonic works which were to influence Avicenna and Averroes were not translated until between AD 800 and 1000. Before AD 800, the Umayyads simply took over existing institutions – the medical school of Alexandria was still functioning, presumably in Greek, in 719 – but their successors made full use of Greek knowledge and skills, incorporating them into the new Islamic culture.[2]

The main influence was understandably Galen, most of whose works had already been translated into Syriac by the end of the sixth century. From his work derive the doctrine of Humours, the concept of the three digestions and the movement of blood, and the teleological thinking which seeks to recognize and explain each organ and each natural process in terms of its purpose. Hippocrates, known primarily through Galen, played a lesser role, though a significant one: Arab doctors still took the Hippocratic Oath, amended so as to historicize Asklepios as the discoverer of medicine. As in Europe, commentaries on both were far more widespread than the originals. As for Dioscorides, both his original five books and the apocryphal volumes VI and VII on poisonous plants and animals were translated and formed the basis of Arab pharmacology. Significantly, Al-Biruni (d. 1048) commiserated the fact that Dioscorides had not been able to pass judgement on Middle Eastern plants, implying that no Arabic botanist had the skill – or possibly the authority – to do so.[3]

It can also be assumed that by the end of the sixth century the main corpus of Greek medicine had been translated into Persian, and had strongly influenced local practice – the concepts of cold, heat, dryness and wetness were borrowed but polarized according to Zoroastrian dualism: cold and dryness are the evils which the doctor must combat by means of warmth and wet medicaments and diet. The *Pancatantra* and other Indian medical texts were brought to Persia in the sixth century, and by the ninth century

Indian doctors were practising at the Caliph's court. In 850 Ali ibn-Sahl al-Tabari described the Indian medical system in an appendix of his main work concerning Hippocratic and Galenic medicine and Aristotelian philosophy, the *Kitab Firdaws al-Hikma*. His sources were Indian works available in Persian, and he points out the significant differences between the systems. For example, he mentions that the five Elements (air, wind, fire, earth and water) were there understood not as material but as dynamic functional magnitudes; instead of four there were only three Humours (*dosas*): wind, bile and phlegm; and the six elementary substances (*dhatus*) involved in digestion were blood, flesh, fat, bones, marrow and semen.[4]

Arab culture absorbed Greek Classical medicine at its peak and found as little need to improve on it as did the West, but was far more successful at preserving it throughout the period of Western decline. Views alternative to the Galenic tradition (for example, Democritos' atomic theory, or the rebuttal of the Humoral Theory) were known, but only cited as aberrant curiosities: as in the Western scholastic tradition, scholarship by and large involved the preservation of knowledge, not its improvement. An interesting example of this is the importance which gymnastics and exercise were given by many authors, despite the lack of *palestra* and *gymnasia* in which to practise them in the typical Islamic town. Another occasional difficulty was the reconciliation of Classical theory and practice with strict religious observance, for example concerning the use of wine, forbidden by the Koran but described at length in the Arabic translation of Rufus of Ephesus' *Book of Wine*. Even where an Arabic author managed to point out an anatomical mistake in Galen – such as 'Abd-al-Latif al-Baghdadi pointing out that the lower jaw is composed of one bone and not two – the discovery remained buried in an obscure passage in a book about the geography of Egypt and was generally ignored.

Amongst a cohort of skilled and learned physicians, the one who stands out head and shoulders amongst them is Abu'Ali Al-Husayn Ibn 'Abd Allah Ibn Sina, generally known as Ibn Sina, or Avicenna (AD 980–1037). A Persian brought up in an Isma'ili household with its neoplatonic overtones, he became one of, if not the most influential of Arab scholars. Philosopher and physician, his *Canon* became the best known medical text throughout Europe and Western Asia until practically modern times. His material is essentially Hippocrates' and Galen's, but far more lucidly expressed and enriched by his own clinical experience; he was also almost certainly familiar to some extent with Ayurvedic medicine, and there are claims that some of his diagnostic techniques, such as his pulse reading, have some similarity with Traditional Chinese Medicine. At first sight the *Canon* appears rigid and scholastic, with its exact description of characteristics both of the patients and of the remedies, and the schemes according to which they have to be matched. There is, however, a deeper aspect; he defines four orders of Faculties by which medicines can be classified. The first and the second refer to the Hippocratic matching of Humours, and the subtle variations on such matchings using complex remedies of differing strengths and properties. The third, however, refers to those particular properties which a medicine might have, similar to those expected from their humoral nature but sufficiently unique so as to require direct experience for their understanding and use; the fourth, finally, refers specifically to those properties which are not predictable or expected, and which can only be discovered by empirical observation and direct experience. These last two Faculties lift the *Canon* out of Galen's rigid schematics and open the door to new knowledge empirically acquired. The fourth is particularly significant, as through it Avicenna classifies the remedies according to the organs which they affect, laying the foundations both of scientific pharmacology and of the terminology which pharmacist and herbalist have been using since: stomachics, cordials, diuretics, etc. etc.[5]

This novel openness was mainly due to Avicenna's own attitude towards his art. He was primarily a philosopher; medicine was only one of his activities, albeit an important one, and his copious works on a variety of subjects show a much wider outlook than that of his predecessors. Also, regardless of the considerable clinical detail mentioned in the *Canon*, he was very much conscious of the body as a single entity, whose health had to be examined, maintained and restored as a whole. On the other hand, he may have realized that personal experience was not something that is easily taught, and it is worth mentioning that in his *Poem of Medicine* (*'Urguza fi t-Tibb*), a condensed version of the *Canon* in verse form which was extensively used as a teaching text, the Fourth Function is not mentioned: it is possible that it might have been considered a 'higher' form of learning, reserved for those students who showed sufficient promise. Whatever the case, had this aspect of Avicenna's work been given a stronger emphasis, it might well have spurred the development of science much sooner than it did. Unfortunately, this was not the case, and in the hands of the translators and commentators the *Canon* soon became one more rigid text, to be treated as complete and unalterable, both in the East and in the West.[6]

One can assume that, while the courts and the wealthier urban population could enjoy the services of a reasonably qualified class of medical practitioners trained in the Galenic/Hippocratic mould, the vast majority of the population must have made do with traditional healers, whose methods have gone largely unrecorded but were probably a mix of simplified 'Arabic' medicine and traditional folk practices. There is evidence that even in the fifteenth and sixteenth centuries, when Arabic medicine enjoyed its highest reputation in the West, Arab rulers had difficulties in finding suitably qualified practitioners, and on occasions had to resort to European physicians out of need rather than by choice. By the seventeenth century, novel Western ideas such as Paracelsus' Chemical Medicine started appearing in Turkish and Arabic translations; from then on, Western medicine has been seeping into the Islamic lands and establishing itself besides the traditional methods, without replacing them entirely. Classical textbooks (e.g. the Bulaq edition of Avicenna) were published in Egypt as recently as 1877 as practical manuals, and in India, Iran and Pakistan the Classical tradition has remained unbroken through Unani medicine, whose main textbook is and remains the *Canon* of Avicenna and its later minor elaborations.[7]

As mentioned before, possibly the most important effect of Islamic culture on medicine has been the preservation of the Classical heritage through the Dark Ages, and its re-introduction in the West from the eleventh century onwards. The first exponent of this return was Constantinus Afro, a semi-legendary scholar of whom it is told that he was a North African who came to Italy fairly late in his life. He is said to have travelled to Italy when he was forty and, filled with missionary zeal by the miserable status of medicine there, returned to Tunis to study medicine and then returned to Italy to practise it. It is certain that he eventually converted to Christianity and became a Benedictine monk at Monte Cassino, where he died in 1087. Constantinus spent his whole Italian period translating Arabic medical texts into Latin. Even though a lot of his writing is obscure and most of the books he translated were undeservedly circulated under his own name, the eleventh-century revival of the Salernitan medical school certainly owes a good part of its impetus to him.

The next source of the Western revival came through the school of translators active in Toledo in the twelfth century, including amongst others Gerard of Cremona, to whom eventually most of the works whose translator was unknown were assigned. Also worth mentioning is Stephen of Pisa, who carried out translations of medical works in Antioch at the same time, in particular the *Kitab al-Malaki* by 'Ali ibn-al'Abbas al-Majusi, probably the clearest and most widely used medical compendium in the Galenic school available at the time. It was this corpus of eleventh- and twelfth-century translations which was to become the basic literature of medicine throughout the West almost until modern times.[8]

One area of great concern related to pestilence and contagion, for it led to much open discussion rather than blind acceptance of Galen. Camps similar to those of the nineteenth-century 'bacteriologists' and the 'anticontagionists' formed, with one side recognizing the disease as a separate and transmissible entity and the other appealing to fate, divine will and scriptural interpretations. In the field of pharmaceutics, Galen's division between simple and compound remedies was carried through and treated as dogma. Dioscorides was known and considered the supreme authority, and the vast majority of the hundred and more Arabic authors who dealt with medical plants ended up recompiling the same material. An interesting quote on the subject comes from Albertus von Haller (*Bibliotheca botanica*, Zurich 1771): '*Omnes Arabes fratres sunt fraterrimi, ut qui unum eorum de plantis legerit, legerit fere omnes*' – 'All Arab colleagues [brothers] are brothers indeed, and that which one reads, they all read'. In the evaluation of drugs, it also appears that the Galenic criteria were adopted, but it is questionable whether they were actually put into practice to judge medicines unknown to the Greeks, such as those of Indian origin. Here, presumably, the Arabs relied on the experiences of Indian doctors and of tradition.

There was also much concern for what we would call public health education. In the *Kitab al-Malaki*, dietetics is seen to incorporate the patient's lifestyle, his activities and the environment around him. It was this generalized preventive medicine, based on the Classical tradition of moderation and equilibrium, which allowed a schematized and theoretically inaccurate framework such as the Galenic one to function as a complete medical system. The terminology – hot and cold, blood and phlegm, and so on – could be used to describe just about anything, but it was the combination of accurate empirical observations and a series of eminently sensible rules of life involving moderation and basic hygiene which eventually benefited most both the doctor and the patient – facts of life which we are now once again rediscovering in the late twentieth century.[9]

Notes

1 Manfred Ullmann, *Islamic Medicine* (Edinburgh: Edinburgh University Press, 1978), Islamic Surveys II.
2 Ibid.
3 Ibid.
4 Ibid.
5 Avicenne, trans. Henri Jahier and Abdelkader Noureddine, *Poème de la medicine* (*Urguza Fi 'T-Tibb – Cantica Avicennae*) (Paris: Les Belles Lettres, 1956); *Encyclopedia Britannica*, 15th edn (Chicago: Encyclopedia Britannica Inc., 1985); and Mazar H. Shah Avicenna, *The General Principles of Avicenna's Canon of Medicine* (Karachi: Naveed Clinic, 1966).
6 Avicenne, *Poème de la medicine*; Avicenna, ed. Shah *The General Principles of Avicenna's Canon of Medicine*.
7 Ullman, *Islamic Medicine*.
8 Ibid.
9 Ibid.

10

THE MEDICAL SCHOOL OF SALERNO

Salerno in southern Italy was world-famous a thousand years before the bridgehead landings which helped the final phases of the Second World War. It was a place of learning with a famous medical school, more influenced by Greek tradition and culture than by Latin thought. Southern Italy, with its multicultural background and its long history of civic life, gave throughout the Middle Ages greater weight to secular elements as opposed to ecclesiastical ones than did the rest of Europe. The result of this was a greater accent on the naturalistic and the practical than in the medical schools of northern Italy and Europe. Proof of this comes, for example, in a dispute between learned doctors in Paris in the tenth century, which acknowledges Salerno as an independent centre of teaching with its stress on practical knowledge.[1]

Salerno was one of the points of fusion of the four Mediterranean cultures: the Latin, the Greek, the Arabic and the Jewish. One of the earliest influences on the Salernitan School was probably Shabbetai ben Abraham ben Joel (c.913–984), known as Donnolo, a Jew of Otranto in Apulia who had studied Arabic medicine, practising it there and in other parts of southern Italy and travelling widely. We know both from his own statements and from those of his contemporary St Nilus of Rossano that he had travelled among the Latins, which would mean throughout western Europe. His works were written in Hebrew, but in a peculiar Hebrew which contains many Arabic idioms and a few Arabic words. The basis of the treatment detailed in it is in many respects that of the usual Arabic medical works available at the time, ultimately of Greek origin. Of some of the herbs mentioned he gives the Greek form, of others the Latin one, always transliterated into Hebrew.[2]

Several stories have grown up around the Salernitan School, four of which have become legends in their own right: first that it was founded by a Greek, a Latin, an Arab and a Jew; second, that its greatest scholar was Constantinus Afro, responsible for the rediscovery of Classical knowledge; third, that the best-known work originating from it, the *Regimen Sanitatis Salernitanum*, was occasioned by the sojourn in Salerno of the King of England; and finally, that it freely accepted women scholars – indeed one of its main luminaries was a woman.

The first of these legends comes close to the truth in spirit if not in fact: the School was not founded by a Greek, a Latin, an Arab and a Jew, but it is certainly true that the four influences represented by those names were at work in southern Italy in the tenth century. Indeed it was these four cultural influences – Greek, Latin, Hebrew and Arabic – that were welded together in Salerno as the first university in Europe emerged into the light of history.

The second story relates to the most famous of Salerno's doctors, Constantine the African, or Constantinus Afro, already mentioned in chapter 9. Although famous for his translations of Arabic texts into Latin, evidence points to the fact that he was not only a translator, but also a plagiarizer and falsifier of most if not all the works and translations bearing his name, works which have been for the most part attributed to Abu Jakub Ishak Ben Suleiman al Israeli, a respected Jewish physician who practised in Egypt and Kairouan and wrote voluminous Arabic works. Rogue Constantinus may have been, but his writings helped to popularize the wisdom of Classical practical medicine which had thankfully been preserved via the Arabic heritage, thereby providing the West with a much-needed injection of knowledge in the right place and at the right time.[3]

The third legend of Salerno links a king to the most popular medical work ever written, the *Regimen Sanitatis Salernitanum*. Translated into all the European and many Asiatic languages, it has run into hundreds of editions and its verses are quoted rightly or wrongly to this day by doctors, herbalists and quacks the world

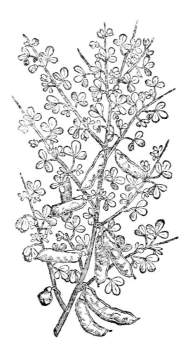

FIGURE 10.1 Broom (*Cytisus scoparius*), the Plantagenets' badge.

over. The king in question was thought to be Robert Plantagenet, Duke of Normandy, eldest son of William the Conqueror and putative heir to the throne. He certainly stayed at Salerno to be cured of a wound on his way home from a crusade in the years 1099–1100; he was evidently cured, but his stay in the Hippocratic city is said to have cost him the English Crown. Be that as it may, the mention of the English king was in all probability just a good piece of advertising on the part of the author – or perhaps the public relations department of the Salernitan School, for other manuscripts of the same text are dedicated to the King of Aragon, the 'King of the Franks' and others to Charlemagne himself. Whichever king or duke it was, the advice given cannot wholly be discredited and has been handed down to the present day in the form of verses such as: 'Joy Temperance and Repose Slam the Door on the Doctor's Nose'. The luckless Robert's stay in Salerno cost him dearly, for it was there he lost his heart to the woman he eventually married – at least proving that women, the object of the fourth legend, were not frowned upon by the Salernitan School.[4]

The fourth legend claims that Salerno was unique amongst all medieval medical institutions for the way in which both women and Jews were admitted to its teachings even in its earliest period. The most famous of these 'Ladies of Selerne' is without doubt Trotula, supposed authoress of the only two books written by Salernitan women that the ages have spared to us. Alas, it appears

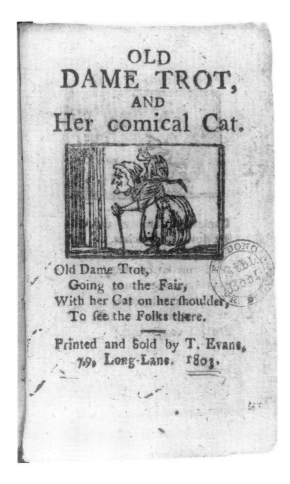

FIGURE 10.2 *Old Dame Trot and Her Comical Cat* (1803) – is this all that remains of the learned Trotula's fame?

that she had no real existence, and the treatises of the so-called Trotula appear to be compilations from much earlier times. The very name Trotula may well signify the compendium of the works of a male doctor called Trottus, spoken of as was the custom of the Italian schools of the day as 'the Trotula'. As these two books dealt with aspects of women's life in a rather intimate fashion they were, perhaps naturally, mothered onto a woman.[5]

Whether a lady professor of medicine did exist in the Salernitan School will always be a matter of gendered debate. There is every reason to believe, however, that throughout the Dark and Middle Ages countless women acted as nurses, midwives and herbalists. Some of them must have been attached to and played very important roles in the medical schools. Perhaps it is this figure of the homely wisdom of a village school teacher, rather than of the first female professor of medicine, which has been handed down in the nursery rhyme figure of Dame Trot.

Notes

1 Brian Lawn, *The Salernitan Questions* (Oxford: Clarendon Press, 1963).
2 Charles Singer, *From Magic to Science* (London: Ernest Benn, 1928).
3 Ibid.
4 Lawn, *The Salernitan Questions*; and Singer, *From Magic to Science*.
5 Singer, *From Magic to Science*.

Middle Age Spread

If Charlemagne's sons had been of equally great stature, the course of history and the eventual spread of the Renaissance might have been very different. However, his genetic lineage was tainted with traits other than those of Christian excellence, as recorded in the nicknames of his line of descent: 'The Simple', 'The Stammerer', 'The Fat' and 'The Child' – and hence the demise of his empire.

Botany, which encompassed the greater part of pharmaceutical science at the time, underwent a similar deterioration in this period throughout the West, and new botanical works were seen more as an adjunct to regurgitations of the encyclopaedic compilations of the past. Another problem in judging European medieval medical works is the scholastic preference of authoritative citation to empirical experience. Added to transcriptional omissions, inaccuracies and unwarranted additions, and to the fact that a considerable number of plants dealt with by the Classical authors were unavailable in central and northern Europe, this means that their claims have to be taken with great caution.

One linking threat throughout Antiquity and the Middle Ages is the development and evolution of the illustrated herbal, which must have done much to advance (and also, as we shall see, to muddle the advance of) botanical medicine. Like organic evolution, that of the herbal depended on replication, with mistakes paving the way to change, and it is no surprise that the mistakes outnumber the successful changes.

The best-known prehistoric representation of a plant is that of a branch with leaves, scratched in Paleolithic times on a piece of reindeer horn from Arcy-sur-Cure, from the Département of Yonne, France (reproduced here as Figure 1.2). As prehistoric paintings were magical in character, often connected with hunting magic, representations of plants are rare: the plant needed no hunting, and its collection was most probably woman's work, and therefore outside the competence of the hunter-magician, while the shaman probably preferred to keep her or his own counsel.[1]

What we may consider the first 'herbal' is probably the bas-relief commemorating Pharaoh Thothmes III's expedition to Syria, which shows the new and strange plants brought back (see Figure 2.1). The inscription runs approximately as follows:

> Year 25 of the King of Upper and Lower Egypt, Living for Ever. Plants which His Majesty found in the country of Syria. All the plants that grow, all goodly flowers that are in the Divine Land [i.e. the country east of Egypt] . . . His Majesty saith, 'As I live, all these plants exist in very truth; there is not a line of falsehood among them. My Majesty hath wrought this to cause them to be before my father Amon, in this great hall for ever and ever.'[2]

Not all the plants are recognizable, but amongst those that are we can see gourds, a heath, a Lotus, two Irises, and a seedling Arum.

In Europe, Greek culture was profoundly centred on man, and the first collection of information about plants came surprisingly late. Diocles of Carystus in Euboea practised in Athens in the fourth century BC and is known to have compiled a book on medical plants, which has unfortunately disappeared without trace. An interesting source of botanical knowledge, of course, were Alexander's campaigns. Fragments of the journal of Nearchus, Alexander's admiral who navigated from the mouth of the Indus to the Persian Gulf, contains good descriptions of the Banyan tree, of Cotton and of Mangroves. There is also some evidence of an expedition at the time to Bahrain with a strong botanical accent. Aristotle's works on plants have disappeared, but parts of them were incorporated in the works of Theophrastus of Eresus and through them became part of the Classical Corpus. By this time there was already a dichotomy between the learned botanist and the herb-gatherer, the 'rhizotomist', and it was one of these, Crateuas, an attendant of Mithradates VI of Parthia, who in the first century BC produced the first illustrated herbal – in other words, a series of plant descriptions with a practical purpose – which again unfortunately did not survive intact, but did pass on some fragmentary knowledge, mainly through the works and citations of Pliny the Elder's immensely popular *Natural History*. As Singer says, 'Pliny is the compiler *par excellence*, the learned collector who will put down anything he is told or can read, without verification.'[3] His stories have so thoroughly permeated European folklore that today's gipsy fortune-teller is still reciting the garbled versions of what Pliny understood to be Hippocrates' and Aristotle's work. In the same way Dioscorides' *De Materia Medica* was also the source of numerous recompilations, and by and large formed the base of most subsequent herbals.[4]

Probably the first Latin herbal was the so-called *Herbal of Apuleius*, translated from the Greek round about AD 400 with highly stylized illustrations. It also contained one of the earliest lists of common names in dialects of the time, an increasing problem with the degradation of Latin as a common tongue. It was this same herbal which was the first to be printed, in Rome in 1474, with little change from the original, prompting the following comment, again from Singer:

> Man is an imitative animal, but we doubt if any better instance of his imitativeness could be found than this constant copying and re-copying, for ever over a thousand years, with enormous labour and technical skill, of a futile work with its unrecognizable figures and its incomprehensible vocabulary.[5]

While still rich in inaccuracies, the poem about herbs of Odo of Meune-sur-Loire, referred to as the *Macer*, the herbal of Mathaeus Platearius referred to as the *Circa instans*, and the *On Plants* of Albertus Magnus, present the great novelty of the twelfth and thirteenth centuries: the arrival of 'Arab' knowledge. From then on, the acquiring of new knowledge, while still carried out in the spirit of recovery of a past glory, at least became a conceivable enterprise.[6]

It is important to realize that the illustrations of these herbals, even when they weren't simply stylized copies of older copies, were usually carried out by a person other than the writer, and frequently in a different place at a different time. Only by the fourteenth and fifteenth centuries do we have the regular appearance of recognizable illustrations. The first such great plant painter was Botticelli (1444–1510), and with Dürer (1452–1519) and Leonardo da Vinci (1471–1528) we finally have artists capable of painting plants recognizable in their finest detail. It was Otto Brunfels (1464–1534) who in the 1530s finally produced a new herbal, the *Herbarum Vivae Eicones*, which owed nothing to previous publications (apart from an unsuccessful attempt at correlating his plants with Dioscorides') and was based entirely on direct observations. Hieronymus Bock (1498–1554) produced a herbal in which for the first time mode and locality of occurrence of the plants was described, and Leonhart Fuchs (1501–1566) produced his *De Historia Stirpium* in 1542; with this, the classical herbals reached their peak: accurately descriptive, with beautiful and exact woodcuts and with no science but observation. By the following year, Vesalius and Copernicus had published their works, and what followed was no longer medieval scholasticism, but early science.

In parallel to the above, a second thread of botanical literature flowed through the Middle Ages, concerned with botany applied rather than purely descriptive. Isidorus Hispanicus (570–636), Bishop of Seville, devoted the seventeenth volume of his *Origines* to plants and agriculture. His criteria were mainly etymological, and confused matters more than clarified them. To him we can ascribe concepts such as *nux a nocendo*, or, that a walnut tree will blight whatever lies in its shade because of the similarity of the two words – a belief generally held for several centuries to follow, and perhaps an unintentional cornerstone to the science of allelopathy, the study of chemical warfare among plants. Nevertheless, Isidorus' list of plants, which more or less covered those species known from Antiquity, remained a standard for a long time. Interestingly, he is the first to mention *Rheum palmatum*, 'reubarbarum', probably from Arabic sources. He also identifies amber as the resin of firs growing on German islands.

The next major author was Hrabanus Maurus, the first German naturalist (784–856). Abbot at Fulda, he retired from his post in 842 to write his *De Universo*, an encyclopaedic treatment derived from Isidorus but seen in a mystic light, finding scriptural and allegorical references for any and all of Nature's works.[7]

It was these texts and their copies which formed the core of scholastic botanical knowledge. On the other hand, the monk tending the monastery's herb garden would have had his own first-hand knowledge and experience, both traditional and novel, to fall back upon, and some of it should have been seeping back into the texts. One problem which had to be faced, for example, was the placing of North European plants which were for purely geographical reasons unknown to the Classical authors. Powerful medicinal plants such as *Digitalis* and *Arcostaphylos uva-ursi* must have been known to the early Germans under their local names, and this knowledge had to be incorporated in the canonical corpus. Both *Digitalis* and *Arcostaphylos uva-ursi*, incidentally, are

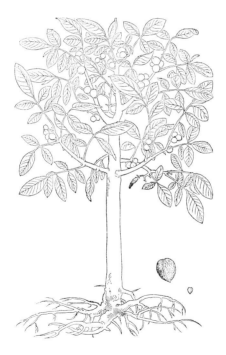

Figure 11.1 *nux a nocendo* . . . According to Isidorus Hispanicus, the similarity between the words meant that the Walnut would blight whatever lives in its shade – yet even here there is a kernel of allelopathic truth.

mentioned in the Welsh Meddygon Myddfai, dating from the thirteenth century, despite the fact that the latter plant is not a native of Wales.

A significant form of learned work, especially in the monastic communities, was the instructional poem, where the subject was put into verses both as a literary accomplishment and as a mnemonic aid. Amongst these, it is interesting to compare the *Hortulus* of Walahfrid Strabo of Reichenau (AD 825) and the *Regimen Sanitatis Salernitanum* (AD 1101).[8]

In Walahfrid's case, we have a recognizable individual naturalist, well versed in the Classical and late Latin literature, producing a poem of high quality concerning the plants in his monastery's garden. His choice is intentionally limited and idiosyncratic, twenty-three plants are covered, and a few more mentioned. In order of appearance they are:

Salvia	(*Salvia officinalis*)
Ruta	(*Ruta graveolens*)
Abrotanum	(*Artemisia abrotanum*)
Melo	(*Cucumis melo*)
Cucurbita	(*Cucurbita* spp.)
Absinthium	(*Artemisia absinthium*)
Marrubium	(*Marrubium vulgare*)
Feniculum	(*Foeniculum capillaceum*)
Gladiola	(*Iris germanica*)
Libysticum	(*Levisticum officinale*)
Cerefolium	(*Anthriscus cereifolium*)
Lilium	(*Lilium candidum*)
Papaver	(*Papaver somniferum*)
Sclarea	(*Salvia sclarea*)
Mentha	(*Mentha viridis*)
Polegium	(*Mentha pulegium*)
Apium	(*Apium graveolens*)
Betonica	(*Betonica officinalis*)
Agrimonia	(*Agrimonia eupatoria*)
Ambrosia	(*Tanacetum vulgare*? or *Chenopodium botrys*?)
Nepeta	(*Nepeta cataria*)
Raphanus	(*Raphanus sativus*)
Rosa	(*Rosa gallica*)

Strabi fuldensis mo

nachi poete suauissimi. quondā Rabani

Mauri auditoris Hortulus nuper apud Hoductios in.S.Galli monasterio repertus.qui Carminis elegantia tam est delectabilis.q̃ doctrine cognoscen= darum quarundam herbarum varietate vtilis. Ad Grymaldū Abbatem.

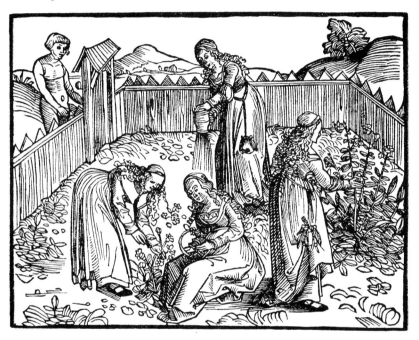

Item Psalmus.41.Sicut ceruus desiderat tc̄. et Psalmus.112.Lau= date pueri tc̄.per Venerabilem Bedam.sono Heroico decātanti.

FIGURE 11.2 The monastic garden, growing pharmacy and vehicle of botanical knowledge: an illustration from a printed edition of Walahfrid Strabo's *Hortulus*.

Significantly, most of the plants on this list are of Mediterranean origin, though nowadays many are garden plants and common weeds throughout Europe. The only two definitely North European plants are *Betonica* and *Agrimonia*, but then these were amongst the most highly considered medicinal plants at the time; indeed,

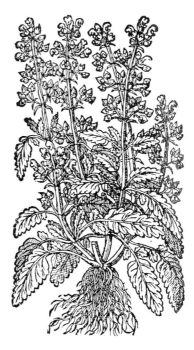

FIGURE 11.3 Water Betony (*Scrophularia aquatica*) was used, as its name suggests, against scrofula and other skin diseases due to its vulnerary properties.

Betonica even had strong occult implications, to the point that during the witch craze a few centuries later the term 'patonyerin' – a wise woman collecting *Betonica* – became a synonym for witch. No wonder that the monks would try to ensure a supply close at hand, regardless of its availability in the field. The descriptions of the plants are accurate, and their properties are generally derived from Dioscorides, with only 'ambrosia' leaving the modern reader in some doubts as to its origin.[9]

The *Regimen Sanitatis Salernitanum*, on the other hand, is a lengthy mnemonic poem in doggerel verse, supposedly dedicated to Robert Plantagenet, Duke of Normandy, in 1101. Regardless of its poor poetical and dubious botanical qualities, it remained a highly considered work – especially as far as dietetics was concerned – up to the nineteenth century, thanks to innumerable re-editions and translations.[10]

The *Subtilitatis Diversarum Naturarum Creaturarum*, which seems to have appeared between 1150 and 1160, is a famous and for a long time highly regarded body of medico-botanical knowledge, the origin of which has been hotly debated. Hildegard (1098–1179), Abbess of the monastery of Bingen in the Rhineland, was known for her mystic visions and speaking in tongues. The *Subtilitatis* is supposed to be the transcript of her visions, in which the secrets of nature and the universe were opened to her. Just how much of the text is actually hers, and how much of it the addition of editors and commentators both before and after her death, remains an open question, and it might be safer to consider the work as a conglomerate of the then contemporary knowledge, reaching from natural history to mysticism. Nevertheless, at the core of it there must have been a scholar or scholars firmly grounded in what knowledge of natural history was available at the time, and probably with a good amount of first-hand experience.

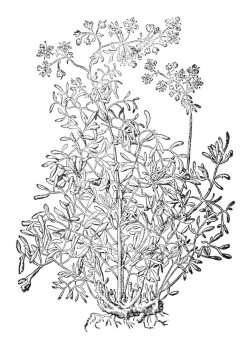

Figure 11.4 Rue (*Ruta graveolens*), an ancient bitter and emmenagogue which appears in spirit bottles to this day.

Plant names and usages known from Galen and Dioscorides are mentioned, and German names are used for those plants which were unknown to the classics. The dietary comments it contains often appear just what an ill person might have considered normal – while the illustrations of her visions, which certainly could not be regarded as normal, have been used by Sacks and other authors as an example of 'fortification images', typical of migraine attacks. She warns the reader of the dangers of eating, amongst other things, eggs, duck, cabbage and raw fruit. Apart from this, the list of plants she describes is considerable for the time, counting amongst others the following exotic medicinal species:[11]

Aloe	(*Aloe socotrina*)
Balsam	(*Commiphora opobalsamum*)
Camphor	(*Cinnamomum camphora*)
Cubeb	(*Piper cubeba*)
Cinnamon	(*Cinnamomum zeylanicum*)
Galang	(*Alpinia galanga*)
Cloves	(*Syzygium aromaticum*)
Ginger	(*Zingiber officinale*)
Liquorice	(*Glycyrrhiza glabra*)
Mandrake	(*Mandragora officinarum*)
Myrrh	(*Balsamodendron myrrha*)
Nutmeg	(*Myristica fragrans*)
Pepper	(*Piper nigrum*)
Styrax	(*Liquidambar orientalis*)
Frankincense	(*Boswellia* spp.)
Sugar cane	(*Saccharum officinarium*)
Cotton	(*Gossypium* spp.)
Lemon	(*Citrus limon*)
Boxwood	(*Buxus sempervirens*)
Cypress	(*Cupressus sempervirens*)
Date	(*Phoenix dactylifera*)
Mastix	(*Pistacia lentiscus*)
Olive	(*Olea europaea*)
Herb Paris	(*Paris quadrifolia*)
Scammony	(*Convolvolus scammonia*)
Nard	(*Nardostachis jatamansi*)

Around this time, too, knowledge of oriental plants was seeping into Europe at a respectable rate, partly through trade, partly through travellers' tales. In Marco Polo's *Il Milione*, for example, we have amongst other wonders identifiable descriptions of *Buxus sempervirens* in Georgia, of Cotton fields in Kurdistan, of Bare Barley (*Hordeum vulgare* var. *nudum*) in Badakhshan, and of Rhubarb in So-schen (incidentally the first description of *Rheum palmatum*'s origin). Cloves, Cinnamon, Camphor and Bamboo are also described, as well as Ebony, Brazilwood, Coconut and the Toddy Palm, *Arenga saccharifera*. We must also remember that such long-distance travels were not the exclusive prerogative of the Western traders – travel in ideas went in all directions. Another important contributor in this way was Dhya en Din Abu Mohammed Abd Allah ben Ahmed, better known as Ibn el Beithar (son of the veterinary), who was born at the end of the twelfth century in Malaga, and died in Damascus in 1248. Throughout his travels throughout North Africa and the Middle East he was intensely active, primarily as a botanist but also as a herbalist and doctor. His main work, the *Djami el Moufridat*, is probably the best and most methodical compilation of edible and medicinal plants which appeared in the flowering of medieval Arabic culture.[12]

Further botanical advances up to about 1500 were mainly recompilations, though with slowly improving nomenclature at the cost of uniformity: species are better differentiated, but local names are used more and more, making the exact identification more problematic. For example, botanical manuscripts appear in England at the time of William the Conqueror (*Tractatus de Herbis, de Aromatibus et Gemmis* of Henry, Archdeacon of Huntington), and multiplied over the next two centuries, but with little variation in content. Beyond the Rhine, the *Dyascorides* – Gothic and later German translations of Dioscorides – were greatly degraded in content due to transcription errors, but with adjuncts concerning newly introduced or at least described plants. The exact identification of the plants mentioned only really became possible after the modern editions of Dioscorides (Berendes 1902, Wellmann 1902) became available. Two medico-botanical dictionaries of the fourteenth century are worthy of note: the *Clavis*

Sanationis of Simon Januensis is a major compilation of Greek and Arabic botanical names, extracted from existing works regardless of claims to originality by the author, and written sometime between 1288 and 1304; Matthaeus Silvaticus' *Pandectae Medicinae* probably dates from the second half of the fourteenth century, and shows more signs of the author's personal experiences and travels, as both plants and their properties are described with some accuracy.[13]

With the strengthening of the burgher classes and the spread of printing, there was an outburst of botanical writing in the fifteenth century. The first printed herbal was the *Herbarius* printed by Peter Schoeffer in Mainz (1484), a compilation especially aimed at the poor and limited to those plants which could be easily found in field and garden (though just how many poor could afford a book in 1484 must have been something else again). This described and illustrated 150 plants, plus assorted medicinal preparations available at the time. Shortly afterwards appeared in close succession, but from different sources, the German and the Latin *Hortus Sanitatis* referred to as small and large, which are dated 1485 and 1491 respectively. The former, also printed by Peter Schoeffer, is again an illustrated compilation of varying worth, where it is clear that the more exotic plants were never seen by either illustrator or describer. Nevertheless, it underwent several re-editions and translations until well into the seventeenth century. The latter, also printed in Mainz, by Jacob Meydenbach, covered 530 plants, 164 quadrupeds, 122 birds, 106 water-dwellers and 144 precious and semiprecious stones, all illustrated and described together with their medicinal properties. Descriptions and illustrations are possibly more artistic than the previous ones, but less rather than more accurate. The properties, on the other hand, show the beginning of a logical structure. It was abundantly copied and translated, amongst others as the *Grete Herball* (London, 1526), the first illustrated work of the sort printed in England. The *Kleine Destillierbuch* of the surgeon Hieronymus Brunschwygk was published in 1500 by Johann Gueninger, concerning medical plants and their distillates. It seems to mark the beginning of the end of the medieval period; while still suffering from the inaccuracies and fanciful illustrations of its predecessors, the author seems to be aware of the problem, and his descriptions of the Central European plants which were available for observation are definitely more accurate; he should be considered the forerunner of the 'Fathers of Botany' of the sixteenth century.[14]

In parallel with the growth of European floristic knowledge, a considerable amount of floristic change took place throughout the European countryside over this period due to the growing and spreading population and the increase in agriculture. It must be kept in mind that at the time most of Europe was still under forest and, at least until the late Middle Ages, broadleaf forest at that; for example, Ammianus Marcellinus mentions in correspondence in the fourth century that Lake Constance was nearly unapproachable due to the impenetrable forest swamps surrounding it. While one can talk of the 'colonization of Eastern Europe' to some extent in earlier times, the main deforestation in Germany took place between the eleventh and thirteenth centuries. Already in 1237 Archbishop Eberhard of Salzburg forbade the agricultural use of cleared forest so as to ensure the supply of wood for his salt mines, thereby anticipating the origins of the United Kingdom Forestry Commission, set up to ensure the supply of pit props during the First World War. In general, oak was more protected than other species because of the importance of acorns as pig fodder. Some medicinal plants seem to have become rarer as well – for example, there is some literary evidence that *Loranthus europaeus* and *Adonis vernalis* became more difficult for herbalists to find.[15]

Another important element must have been the progressive enrichment of the soil due to the increased planting of legumes. Niches for marginal and wasteland species increased, and plants which are considered native weeds nowadays appear in medieval garden lists as cultivated exotics, such as

Birthwort	*Aristolochia clematitis*
Good King Henry	*Chenopodium virgatum*
Horsemint	*Mentha silvestris*
Centaury	*Erythraea centaurium*
Tansy	*Tanacetum vulgare*
Monk's Rhubarb	*Rumex alpinus*

Herb Mercury	*Mercurialis annua*
Black Nightshade	*Solanum nigrum*
Wild Garlic	*Allium scorodoprasum*

and probably also

| Thorn-apple | *Datura stramonium*[16] |

When it comes to food plants and the healthful diet of the times, some interesting points arise. Wheat was probably rare throughout the Middle Ages north of the Alps, and it is still cited as a luxury by Abbot Rumpler von Vorbach in 1500. Einkorn and Emmer gradually decreased in importance throughout this period, while *Triticum spelta* (Dinkel, Spelt) was the staple grain for the so-called Allemannic region – Bavaria, southern Germany and eastern Switzerland. Rye (*Secale cereale*) first appears in the West around AD 400, and is mentioned in documents by AD 800, while Oats (*Avena sativa*) were probably a native; Millet (*Panicum miliaceum*) was probably only of localized importance. The niche now occupied by the Potato was filled at the time by the Field Pea, *Pisum arvense*; one bit of monastic doggerel referring to it ran: *Pisa cum pellibus, dura visceribus, pellibus ablatis bona sunt pisa satis* ('Peas with their shells on, hard guts; remove the shells, and peas are good and filling'), showing its importance as a common staple. As far as fruit was concerned, Apples and Pears had been known since antiquity. Several types of Plum are mentioned by the sixteenth century, while Damsons were probably native. Walnuts, Cherries, Chestnuts and Quinces were probably introduced north of the Alps by the Romans, while the Black Currant (*Ribes* spp.) is probably of oriental origin, as is its name. The main textile fibre was linen; hemp appears in significant quantities only around the eleventh century, while the once widely praised Nettle fibres generally slipped out of use.[17]

Notes

1 Charles Singer, *From Magic to Science* (London: Ernest Benn, 1928).
2 Ibid., p. 171.
3 Ibid., p. 178.

4 Singer, *From Magic to Science.*
5 Ibid., p. 185.
6 Singer, *From Magic to Science.*
7 H. Fischer, *Mittelalterliche Pflanzenkunde* (Munich: Verlag der Münchener Drucke, 1929).
8 Ibid.
9 Fischer, *Mittelalterliche Pflanzenkunde*; and Walahfrid Strabo, *Hortulus* (872; Munich: Verlag Münchner Drucke, 1926).
10 Fischer, *Mittelalterliche Pflanzenkunde.*
11 Fischer, *Mittelalterliche Pflanzenkunde*; and Oliver Sacks, *Migraine: Understanding a Common Disorder* (Berkeley, CA: University of California Press, 1985).
12 Fischer, *Mittelalterliche Pflanzenkunde.*
13 Singer, *From Magic to Science*, and Fischer, *Mittelalterliche Pflanzenkunde.*
14 Singer, *From Magic to Science*, and Fischer, *Mittelalterliche Pflanzenkunde.*
15 Fischer, *Mittelalterliche Pflanzenkunde.*
16 Ibid.
17 Ibid.

General information

R. C. Wren, *Potter's Cyclopedia of Botanical Drugs and Preparations* (London: Potter & Clarke, 1941).
V. H. Heywood (ed.), *Flowering Plants of the World* (Oxford: Oxford University Press, 1978).
K. R. Sporne, *The Morphology of Gymnosperms* (1965; London: Hutchinson University Library, 2nd edn, 1974).

NEW MEDICINES FOR OLD

Christopher Columbus returned to Europe from his three great voyages of discovery bringing back, among other much more useful things, two of the great scourges of mankind. The first of these was tobacco, which for a time was regarded as a herb full of medical virtues, especially as a carminative, and which in less than two centuries encircled the globe, being introduced to the Alaskan Eskimos by way of Russia and Siberia around 1700. The second one was a microorganism which all the doctors, barber-surgeons and herbalists in Christendom found themselves impotent to tackle, and which in all its corkscrew-shaped forms was not to be recognized as the harbinger of syphilis for many centuries. Yet Girolamo Fracastoro (c.1465–1553), a colleague of Copernicus at the University of Padua, had already postulated that contagious diseases, amongst which he included syphilis, were transmitted through minute particles, either by direct contact, through infected objects, or via the air.[1]

Syphilis, though then called French (or whatever nationality the sufferer disliked most) Disease, probably originated in that particularly virulent form in the West Indies from whence it was vectored by the crew of the *Niña* to terrorize Renaissance Europe. It was a truly terrible disease, attacking popes, princes and peasants alike. It can and often does come in three distinct phases or stages, each painful and debilitating, the third often leading to death. Between each stage the symptoms can disappear, thus allowing the patient to think he or she is cured and so unwittingly pass the disease to lovers and loved ones and congenitally to the unborn.

Like the Black Death of 150 years before and in the absence of a better alternative, wise men put it all down to a conjunction of Saturn and Jupiter, itself a bringer of disaster, with hot and dry Mars as a bringer of pestilence. Similarly the physicians, turning to their bibles of reference, Galen and Dioscorides, found little help as they thumbed their voluminous herbals. The roots of Daffodils, one of Galen's stock-in-trade astringents – for it was a plant under the domination of Mars and grew in the cold dampness of spring – was used but to no avail. The professors and practitioners were baffled and the oldest profession of all soldiered and sailored on, spreading what must be regarded – at least in that virulent form – as a new occupational disease, while Europe putrified and waited for a miracle.

There were at the time many self-styled miracle-makers who toiled over furnaces and stills in an attempt to turn the basest of metals into gold and give the basest of people the elixir of life.

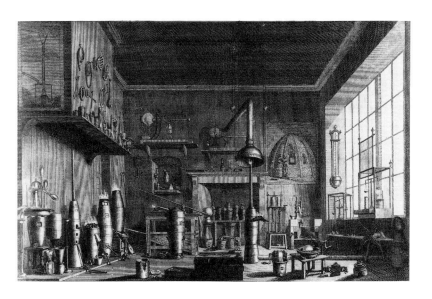

FIGURE 12.1 The alchemist's laboratory, fuelled by fire, earth, water and the hope of the Philosopher's Stone.

They were the alchemists, and alchemy was their discipline. Alchemy, throughout time and human culture, has been the attempt to obtain immortality, wealth and power through 'natural' manipulations and magic. It had been present in some recognizable form throughout Europe and Asia since probably around 300 BC, when metallic mercury, the 'living metal' which plays such an important part in its lore, was discovered. The Chinese alchemists' goal was physical immortality, and hence developed primarily in the fields of pharmacy; their importance was eventually supplanted by Buddhism, with its promise of spiritual immortality. Connections between Indian and Chinese alchemy, while possible, are faint and unclear; Indian and Greek alchemy were doubtless in contact, but it is difficult to say who influenced whom. As in the case of China, Indian alchemy was primarily a quest for the prolongation of life, with the accent on medicines. Greek/Hellenistic alchemy on the other hand grew up in a far more active and inquisitive philosophical environment, and aimed principally at the attainment of spiritual immortality and of material riches; moreover, having to do with material wealth meant that the prescientific discipline which lay at its origin was metallurgy. Thus the concept grew of 'refining' substances; it was believed that they had innate mystical/magical properties, which could be released and intensified by 'purification' and the removal of its material dross; also that such refinement and distillation could render poisonous substances harmless.[2]

Arabic alchemy was even more mystical and astrological in spirit, based very much on the concept that 'That which is above is like to that which is below, and that which is below is like to that which is above.' It was also aimed even more at material enrichment, in particular through the literal transmutation into gold of other – 'baser' – matter. Arab alchemists were more interested in minerals than in plant products, and their line of enquiry resulted in the discovery of significant elements of inorganic chemistry, which reached the Latin world in the eleventh and twelfth centuries together with their medical knowledge. Here alchemy and chemistry became synonymous for a general science of matter. 'Strong Water' (Aqua Fortis) and 'Living Water' (Aqua Vitae) were discovered roughly at the same time, with the introduction of the technique of distillation from the Arab world. Between the two, they greatly boosted the alchemists' activities, as they allowed the production of non-aqueous extracts of plants and aqueous solutions of metals, substances previously unthinkable. The concoction of distillates and elixirs for practical pharmaceutical purposes took shape, and was publicized and diffused by Paracelsus and his followers, of whom more later. By the sixteenth century, medicine was divided between paracelsians, who were willing to use the newly concocted compound medicines, and anti-paracelsians, who insisted on the traditional Galenical simples, and the activities of the more practical alchemists became less and less distinguishable from those of pharmacists. Pure alchemists on the other hand persevered in their search, with varying degrees of honesty and doubtful success. Several workers – for alchemy was The Great Work by definition – claimed to have effected the transmutation of base metals into gold; one of these, Nicholas Flamel (1330–1418), stood out as an example to the hopeful, for his claims were accompanied by a documented, sudden and not otherwise explained improvement in lifestyle.[3]

From the seventeenth century onwards, alchemy abandoned for the most part its material claims, and concentrated on its religious and mystical aspects. These concerned man's relationship with the cosmos and the 'refinement' of his soul, questions which the newly developing scientific disciplines signally failed to answer. Esoteric alchemy, or Hermeticism, has remained a line of mystical philosophical study until the present day, and an offshoot of it, the early seventeenth-century mystical secret society, the Rosicrucian Brotherhood, extended their interests towards the 'refinement' of human society, playing a part in the development of what was to become freemasonry.[4]

So it was that from the dens of the alchemists emerged the quicksilver of hope that was to dominate medical malpractice for the next 400 years, and that in all probability mothered the aphorism 'kill or cure'.

Mercury has without doubt come to the aid of suffering humanity in two ways. First, when used as an inert amalgam to fill the void in aching teeth, second, thanks to its expansive properties, to mark the course of disease when safely sealed in a clinical thermometer. Apart from that, the use of mercury in all its noxious and less noxious forms has produced a sad list of side effects, ranging from foetid breath, stomach cramps, bleeding gums, loss of teeth, renal failure and blindness to debilitation and death. Galen had warned against its use, and yet the barber-surgeons found that the only thing which gave relief from the first stage of syphilis was mercury. So on it went in unguents and creams backed up by all the most expensive ingredients. In many cases it banished fear and symptoms by killing the spirochaetes in the external sore, but did little to combat those within the body, and probably helped the scourge spread even further.

There is one figure which more than any other links together the changes which Renaissance medicine was undergoing; Philippus Aureolus Theophrastus Bombastus von Hohenheim, known as Paracelsus (1493–1541). Son of a Swiss country doctor in Einsiedeln, he studied at the Bergschule in Villach, an early school of mines set up by the Fugger banker family, where he met his first experiences in metallurgy and in the occupational hazards and diseases of miners. He became a goliard, a peripatetic student, at the age of fourteen, generally disappointed by all the universities he visited, as his oft-quoted passage shows: 'The universities do not teach all things . . . So a Doctor must seek out old wives, gipsies, sorcerers, wandering tribes, old robbers, and such outlaws and take lessons from them. A Doctor must be a traveller, . . . Knowledge is experience.'[5] So he travelled widely through Europe and the Orient as an itinerant doctor and military surgeon, during which time he must have tried to deal with many a case of syphilis.

In 1524 Paracelsus became a lecturer at the University of Basel. An iconoclastic rebel who during a student midsummer festival burnt the books of both Galen and Avicenna in a bonfire, he had to leave Basel under a cloud after four years of vigorous teaching and, resuming his travels, he published his magnum opus, *Die grosse Wundartzney*, in 1536. He also wrote a treatise on syphilis and its treatment with mercurials, though throughout he warned against using them too much, for he had seen the miners and the people who lived around the newly opened mercury mines in Slovenia, where even the rats and mice who entered them died of dreadful convulsions. He also was the first to give respectability to the folk belief that 'what makes a man ill cures him', and to connect goitre with mineral intake. He refused astrology, though maintaining a mystical belief in man's power of imagination and creation. He was still firmly attached to the medieval ideas, including alchemy, and his interpretation of 'nature' included its occult and mystical aspects. On the other hand, he was an experimenter willing to modify, and his modifications opened the way to the radical changes which followed him, establishing in the process the role of chemistry in medicine.[6]

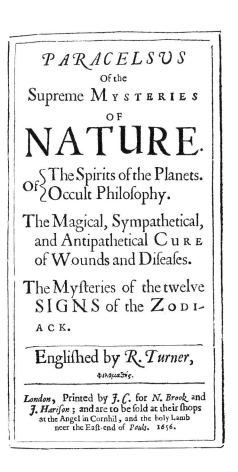

FIGURE 12.2 Title page of one of Paracelsus' works.

The legacy which Paracelsus left the world of medicine is truly amazing. He was indeed the father of the new chemical medicine based on mercury, antimony and the like, which continued to have spectacular results and failures long after his own death – which may well have been due to long exposure to mercury; however, if his followers had taken heed of his warnings about dose rates the whole course of medical history would have been very different. But as Paracelsus pointed out again and again, the iniquities of all practitioners were due to the wish to get visible and rapid results, and to sell as much of the cure as possible, the more complex and hence expensive the better. His disgust can be summarized in a single statement: 'The physician's duty is to heal the sick, not to enrich the apothecary.'[7]

Meanwhile his phenomenal work output continued apace, broadening the horizons of medicine. By pointing out that the specific action of each plant depends on a single active constituent which he and other physicians and alchemists were endeavouring to extract and purify, he opened up the way to modern pharmaceutics. He did, however, emphasize the fact that until such a time as the extracts were prepared, tested and ready, it was best to rely on the well-proven home-grown simples, not upon expensive imports. None of these truisms gained him much respect with his rivals, and intermedicinal war broke out – a classic case of vested interests getting in the way of common sense.

Throughout all this, syphilis raged on unabated. News, however, travelled from the Indies that there the local women herbalists possessed a sure-fire cure for the French Disease – or was it the very similar-looking yaws? Whatever the correct diagnosis, very soon rich syphilitics were on their way to be doctored by the locals. The long emetic sea journey over which Columbus's crew had almost mutinied must have been bad enough, but the Caribbean Cure was not much better than the one being ladled out back home.

In Europe, celibacy, a bland diet and confinement to bed for thirty or more nights covered with an unguentuum of mercury often mixed with irritant herbs like Spurge (*Euphorbia* spp.) and Stavesacre (*Delphinium staphisagria*) appeared to do the trick. Together with a great sweat, the first signs of mercury poisoning

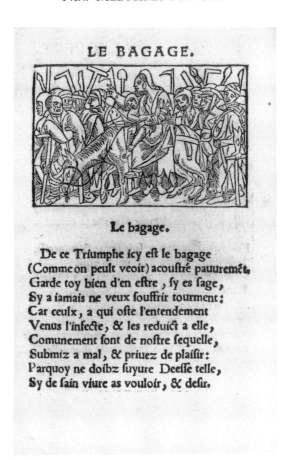

LE BAGAGE.

Le bagage.

De ce Triumphe icy eft le bagage
(Comme on peult veoir) acouftré pauuremét,
Garde toy bien d'en eftre , fy es fage,
Sy a iamais ne veux fouffrir tourment:
Car ceulx , a qui ofte l'entendement
Venus l'infecte , & les reduict a elle,
Comunement font de noftre fequelle,
Submiz a mal , & priuez de plaifir:
Parquoy ne doibz fuyure Deeffe telle,
Sy de fain viure as vouloir, & defir.

FIGURE 12.3 Syphilis riding, surrounded by the poxed and the lame – an allegory
of the first great syphilis epidemic.

made you salivate for days on end: pints and pints of the stuff, cleansing your body of the ill humours of disease, often together with teeth and health in general. In the Caribbean, on the other hand, it was the heat of the tropical sun backed by that from enormous log fires together with celibacy, a bland diet and copious doses of the local plant Guaiac (*Guaiacum officinale*) which drove out the humours! Though unpleasant when taken in its extreme form, the Guaiacum treatment seemed to work, and indeed modern research has shown that if the body temperature is raised

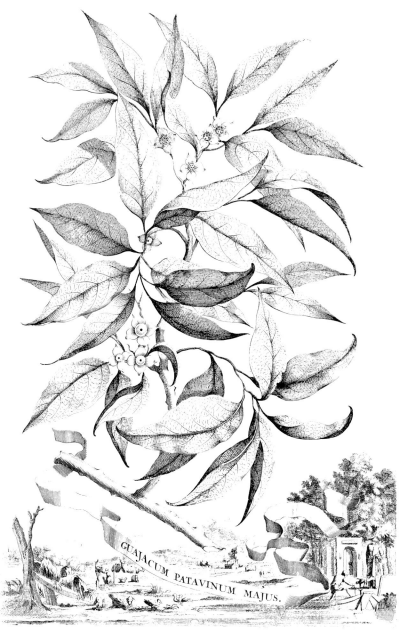

FIGURE 12.4 *Guaiacum officinale*, the great transatlantic hope for pox-ridden Europe.

to 42°C either in a hot room or during the course of a fever, natural or induced, the spirochaetes can be destroyed. As a quick and easy nostrum, though, and this is the form in which European quacks were more than likely to present it, it was as useless as its predecessors. Hope nevertheless opened all doors, and soon enough an enormous international trade in Guaiacum developed: it became available on an open and very lucrative market right across Europe, a market overseen by Messrs Fugger and friends. Little wonder then that they clamped down on the publication of Paracelsus' work, which rubbished the whole Guaiacum boom, advising a little mercury and locally grown cheap herbs.[8]

Somewhere in the voluminous works of Paracelsus was the real answer: the best of the old herbalism, fused together with the essence of the best of the new pharmacy, offered a rational way ahead. Sadly, quick profit and quick relief occupied the minds of too many and the canker of their rivalry has tainted the course of medicine to this day. In their struggle for survival, riches and honour, the physicians and the apothecaries drew up battle lines and the cries of 'Galen' or 'Paracelsus' became the real scourge of the next 300 years. There were of course good men on both sides, but there were zealots too, and as elsewhere throughout the course of history each went to extremes to disprove the other's points in publication, in the courtroom, and in the punishment inflicted on their patients.

Purgation was the *raison d'être* of both camps, and one of the most detailed accounts of the trials and tribulations of a patient patient is to be found in the *Journal de la santé du roi*, which details the day-to-day medicare of Louis XIV of France. The king, God help him, was bled, purged, diaphorized, bled and purged again, again and again from Royal Birth through to Royal Death, all in true Galenical fashion, thanks mainly to Gui Patin. When one reads of the horrors which were being administered by the apothecaries of the day, which ranged from eating whole worms, live spiders, insects, amphibians, and reptiles, through the genitalia and excrements of exotic animals – including unicorns – to urine and choice slices of human cadaver, perhaps regular and spectacular purgation did save a number of lives. However, it all must have made good business for the apothecaries prospered despite and probably because Patin and the Paris medical school railed against them and their excesses. Yet like Paracelsus, whom he reviled, Patin was a good physician at heart and despite his bloodletting extravagancies he prescribed in the main well-tried and tested simples, including a course of purgatives, his favourite being Senna (*Cassia acutifolia*). Patin and his school of practice also had another fight on their hands, against the rival and decidedly paracelsian school of medicine in Montpellier, which advocated the use of the new chemicals in all their forms.[9]

Meanwhile across the Channel in England the publication of the *London Pharmacopoeia* in 1618 marked a truce between all three of these opposing factions. Writing in (just) post-Elizabethan England a surgeon by the name of William Clowes, though an anti-paracelsian by training, wrote:

> If I fynde (eyther by reason or experience) anything that may be to the good of the Patients, and better increase of my knowledge and skil of the Arte of Chirurgery, be it eyther in Galen or Paracelsus, yes Turks, Iewe or any other infidell, I will not refuse it but be thankfull to God for the same.[10]

Clowes was just one of the voices of reason who had the good of their patients at heart. These could now turn to the *London Pharmacopoeia*, for it contained both enough expensive exotics to keep the apothecaries happy and enriched, and a section on the new wonder chemical medicines, including mercury and antimony in all their necromantic forms. This section was written by a Swiss paracelsian called Theodore Turquet de Mayerne, one-time personal physician to Henri IV of France, an appointment which had raised the temperature of the francophone medical debate by many degrees and diplomas. After the assassination of Henri, who had heaped honours galore on Turquet de Mayerne, he was summoned to the bedside of James I of England, an offer which he gladly accepted and for services rendered over the ensuing years was equally well rewarded and honoured. Turquet de Mayerne served three English kings, and although he couldn't save Charles I from the block he was further honoured by the Parliament which beheaded his erstwhile patient. They exempted him from all taxation for the rest of his life and sealed the commendation describing him as 'a man whose extraordinary abilities would make him welcome in any part of Christendom'[11] – thereby also sealing the fate of tens of thousands of patients, condemned to the agonizing side effects of mercury and antimony.

Fortunately the Renaissance was about much more than Galen and Paracelsus, Guaiacum and alchemy. New lights of learning through experimental evaluation of fact began to punch holes in tunnels which stretched back into the Dark Ages. Windows providing hope for a more enlightened future were opened by such as Andreas Vesalius (1514–1564), who wrote the first comprehensive book on anatomy based on first-hand information, demonstrating that Galen's anatomical knowledge was based on extrapolation of animal characteristics, and therefore far from the last word on the subject. His *De Humani Corporis Fabrica* (1543), with woodcuts probably from Titian's school in Venice, was the first real anatomical atlas. His work was the culmination of the Renaissance's revival of humanistic knowledge, and of the new studies in human anatomy which had started tentatively in the fourteenth century when, for example, Leonardo Da Vinci had carried out anatomical studies and had already commented on the homology of organs in animals and man. With Vesalius, medicine becomes a science. Nearly contemporary with Vesalius' work, the first pharmacopoeia appeared in Nuremberg in 1546, as a first attempt at standardizing the composition and dosage of the medicaments used by medical practitioners in the city. The *London Pharmacopoeia*, which appeared three-quarters of a century later, was the first time such a principle was applied on a national scale. By this time, too, the West was well into what has come to be known as the Age of Exploration, and new horizons, geographical as well as intellectual, were opening up. The discovery of the 'Indies' had brought with it novelties – new people, new animals, new plants, new diseases (syphilis amongst them), new medicines, and none of them described by the Classics! In 1552 an illustrated manuscript on Mexican plants was written by the Aztec Martinus de la Cruz and translated into Latin by his colleague Badianus for use in the medical curriculum in the College of Santa Cruz, without however greatly affecting European pharmacy; other similar manuscripts have unfortunately disappeared.[12]

Other plants out of this crop which formed the Guaiac league in an attempt to combat syphilis were China Root (*Smilax china*) and Sarsaparilla (*Smilax aristolochia*), while an admirable new purge with the enematopoeic name of Jalap (*Ipomoea purga*) burst upon the scene. The botanical horizons of the whole New World were beginning to open up more and more local knowledge and more and more paying patients.

Throughout this time, the greater familiarity with plants in general, as opposed to animals, by the majority of physicians and healers meant that botanical knowledge grew out of proportion compared to zoology and anatomy. This growth in botanical interest brought with it major and necessary advances in classification. The alphabetical or geographical lists which had sufficed for the traditional herbals proved unsatisfactory, and scholars searched for a more rational system. Gaspard Bauhin, a Swiss botanist of the late sixteenth and early seventeenth centuries, designated plants by generic and specific binomials, but with no attempt at classification. Only much later did Carolus Linnaeus (Carl von Linné) develop upward classification, describing plants and then grouping them according to their characteristics, and with his *Species Plantarum* (1753) lay the basis of the binomial system still largely in use nowadays.

Probably the most important step in recognizing the human body as a functioning mechanism was William Harvey's (1578–1657) concept of the circulation of the blood, described in his *De Motu Cordis* in 1628. This was validated and completed by the discovery of the capillary system in 1661 by Marcello Malpighi, the first microscopic histologist, and later, in 1775, by Lavoisier's explanation of the role of oxygen.[13]

Notes

1 *Encyclopedia Britannica*, 15th edn (Chicago: Encyclopedia Britannica Inc., 1985); and Harold E. Driver, *Indians of North America* (Chicago: University of Chicago Press, 1969, 2nd edn).

2 *Encyclopedia Britannica*, 15th edn.

3 Ibid.

4 Ibid.
5 Ibid., IX: 134–5.
6 *Encyclopedia Britannica*, 15th edn.
7 Ibid., IX: 134–5.
8 Barbara Griggs, *Green Pharmacy – A History of Herbal Medicine* (London: Robert Hale, 1981, 1987).
9 Ibid.
10 Ibid., p. 73.
11 Ibid., p. 74.
12 *Encyclopedia Britannica*, 15th edn; and Driver, *Indians of North America*.
13 *Encyclopedia Britannica*, 15th edn.

13

SIMPLE ENGLISH

At the same time that Malpighi was looking at the intricate structure of animals in Italy, the same was being done for plants in England. Nehemiah Grew was born in 1628, the son of a clergyman. He studied at Cambridge in England and Leyden in Holland, where he must have come across the work of Anton Van Leeuwenhoek and his microscopes. Probably as a result of this, though graduating as a human physician, he spent his whole life studying the anatomy of plants under the microscope.

All his voluminous works, many of which were presented to the Royal Society, show his prowess as a scientific investigator, using all the then current techniques and technologies of science. One rather strange little volume records experiments in which he tested the effect of a number of chemicals on many things, including the plants then used in medical practice. The following quotation adequately reflects the limitations of the scientific endeavours of that time, the legacy of the Doctrine of Signatures and perhaps the birth of eclectics and of pharmaceutical science.

> *Experiments in Consort of the Luctation arising from the affusion of several Menstruums upon all sorts of Bodies.*
> Exhibited to the Royal Society, April 13th and June 1st, 1676.
>
> Chap. 1 What is to be generally observed upon the affusion of the Menstruum, and what particularly of Vegetable Bodies.
>
> 1 The bodies whereupon I made tryal, were of all kinds, Animal Vegetable and Mineral. Amongst Vegetables, such as these. Date-Stones, Ginger, Colocynthis, Pyrethrum, Hawthorn-stones,

Staphisagna, Euphorbium, the Arenulae of Pears, Semen Mili Solis, Tartar, Spirit of Scurvygrass, Spirit of Wine etc. . . . [1]

4 The liquors which I poured hereupon severally were these. Spirit of Sal Ammoniac, Spirit of Harts-Horn, Spirit of Nitre, Aqua Fortis, Oyl of Salt, Oyl of Sulphur and Oyl of Vitriol, commonly so called.

5 In a mixture of these bodies, two things in general, are all along to be observed, viz. First, which they are, that make any or no Luctation. For, as some which seem to promise it, make none. So many, contrary to expectation make a considerable one.

6 Next, the manner wherein the Luctation is made, being with much variety in the pure sensible Effects.

1 Bullition, where the Bodies mixed produce only a certain quantity of froth or bubbles.
2 Elevation, when like Paste is baking, or Barm in the working of Beer, they swell and huff up.
3 Crepitation, when they make a kind of hissing and sometimes a crackling noise.
4 Effervescence, then only and so properly so called when they produce some degree of heat.
5 Exhalation, when not only fumes but visible steams are produced. . . .

9 Again, although the Luctation which most vegetables and most of their parts make with acids be but small, yet some they make, especially with some acids, as with spirit of Nitre and Aqua fortis. Whence it seemeth plain That there is an Alkaline Salt existent in many Vegetables, even in their natural estate, and it is not made Alkaline but only Liscivial by the fire. Or, there is some quantity of Salt, call it what we will, in the said Bodies, which is so far distant from an Acid, as to make a Luctation therewith. . . .

10 And first of all vegetable Bodies. Date-stones are amongst the least apt to make a Luctation with Acids, if they may be said to make any at all. Hence they are not so potent Nephriticks, as many other Stones which make a more sensible Luctation. [1]

It is of more than passing interest that at that time stones in the kidney were as much one of the great curses of society as they are to this day. The cure of 'being cut for the stone', although developed by the surgeons of the time into a rapid and skilful routine craft, was exceedingly painful – so much that the brother of John Evelyn, a contemporary writer and botanist of great note, died rather than be subjected to the experience. We must remember that although certain herbs such as the Opium Poppy and the Mandrake were in use to deaden pain, the rediscovery of anaesthetics was still 200 agonizing years away.

Herbalists, however, had remedies enough, and most from very common plants which displayed their signature of success even in the towns. Pellitory-of-the-wall, *Parietaria officinalis*, has the strength to grow out of walls, breaking down the stones in full view of physicians and patients alike. Scarlet Pimpernel, *Anagallis arvensis*, also known as the 'Poor man's weather wiser' for its flowers which open in the sun, is a weed of stony places, breaking up the ground and bringing relief to all backaches along with the warm weather. The Horsetails, *Equisetum* spp., which were then sold at market as scouring rushes, were ideal for the job of cleaning pewter and treen thanks to their high content of silica, plant glass; if they could clean the treen, surely they could clear the kidneys. Likewise Butcher's Broom, *Ruscus aculeatus*, another very tough plant whose hard leaf-like stems were used by butchers to scrub their blocks, and by the Romans to scourge their chilblains, found favour as a diuretic and nephritic.

At the same time as Grew in England and Malpighi in Italy were looking inside plants and animals for other virtues, Slaht in Germany was searching for the soul of all things, the inner spark, the ghost in the machine which his mechanistic opponents like Boerhaave in Holland were busy describing. In the meantime the herbalists got on with their job, easing pain and curing some afflictions.

Of all the names associated with herbal medicine one more than any other stands out in the English language, that of Nicholas Culpeper. Culpeper's main claim to fame is his *Pharmacopoeia Londinensis* (1675), the vast majority of which, apart from the names of the simples and compounds, was in English rather than Latin. It also went straight to the heart of the matter, listing illnesses and what could be used to secure relief. As you can guess, the professionals were incensed: here was a member of the College who dared reveal all the secrets by which they made their living, and what is more in the common tongue so that everyone who could read could set up in business or, perish the thought, cure themselves. So they poured scorn on the whole thing, and especially on Culpeper's adherence to what they called astrology.

A similar thing was happening in other countries too, where translations into the vernacular were being made by other working herbalists. Working in the field and gathering their own plants, like Galen and Paracelsus before them, they knew and understood that, like animals and patients, plants react to the environment, to moisture, light and heat. They knew by long experience that time and method of harvest were of great importance if the essence of the simple was to be captured when it was most active, effective and in greatest abundance. Lacking better explanations for such phenomena, they often turned for an explanation to astrology, a lore which at the time was only just beginning to go out of fashion. Arguments they may have caused, but their books became the local bibles, giving great heart to other working herbalists who had also learned through long apprenticeship the simples of their trade, a multitude of unsung heroines and heroes who had carried on the grassroots work of comforting the sick and doing what they could to bring their patients through each and every crisis, on land and at sea. If only the medical profession had taken heed of Culpeper's simple advice for curing the scurvy: 'Water Cresses and Garden Cresses are hot and dry in the fourth degree, cleanse the blood, help the scurvey.'[2]

Likewise seventy-five years earlier Gerard, in one of the most famous herbals of all, had sung the praises of Scurvy Grass, *Cochlearia officinalis* – a plant which grows exactly where it is needed, and in abundance: on the shore line, about docks and ports, advertising its antiscorbutic virtues in deep green leaves and pure (tooth) white flowers. John Woodhall in his *Seagoing Surgeon's Mate* (1617) did the same for the juice of lemons, but to no avail except amongst old sea-dogs who kept their teeth and survived a life at sea. Throughout this time the medical establishment sought reasons for the disease which (though they scorned astrology) ranged from 'a contagious Act of God' to 'a salino-sulphurous

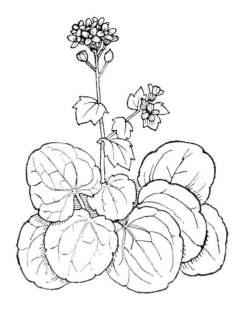

FIGURE 13.1 Scurvy Grass (*Cochlearia officinalis*), a seaside cure and Gerard's recommendation against the disease suffered by so many sailors.

discrasy of the blood' or an 'extraordinary separation of the serous part of the blood from the crassamentum'. In contrast to Culpeper's simples, the great Boerhaave recommended what else but 'the opening of bowels and pores . . .' and the use of a whole complex of antiscorbutics, unfortunately so dried and extracted as to be devoid of any active vitamin C, which would be identified centuries later. He also suggested that in its terminal phase mercurials should be used.[3] And so it was not until 1795 that the might of the British Navy bowed to the evidence which had accumulated over the years and had in fact been tested out with great positive effect by James Lind, ship surgeon on HMS *Salisbury*. From that time on, an ounce of lemon juice was given as a ration from the sixth week at sea onwards. It did the trick and at least put the British ships in line with those of Holland, whose sailors rarely suffered from scurvy thanks to liberal helpings of sauerkraut – cabbage fermented and not cooked. (This, incidentally, had also done good service with Captain Cook on his long voyages of exploration a quarter of a century earlier.)

Perhaps more bewildering than the story of death on the high seas is the high incidence of scurvy in the New World colonies. How many people must have remarked on the shiny white teeth of the local Indians and compared them with the foetid breath and ulcerated toothless gums of the settlers. The locals knew their landscape and the virtues of all the plants it had to offer, there to be eaten, each in due season. Their lives were ruled by the gifts of nature and were ordered by the seasons themselves. Just as the wild animals in winter retreated into the depths of the forest to find fresh green food not covered by frozen snow, so too the Indians ate Fiddle-heads (the lush young leaves of ferns), dug fresh roots and made infusions of the young shoots of the Spruce and Fir trees. All these simple things gave them ample protection against scurvy. Trappers and pioneer families alike soon learned to follow suit, protecting themselves and their families, especially from the harshness of the long winters which were a feature of the northern part of this continental landmass.[4]

The Pilgrim Fathers soon learned from the local Wampanoag people how to use certain local plants – Corn, Beans and Squash – and it is believed that the local Cranberries helped them to celebrate the first Thanksgiving feast in 1621. The first three plants were the staples of the Indian race, disseminated across the length and breadth of America by previous Indian civilizations. The last, of local provenance, was used in many different ways, as a source of dye, in the treatment of wounds infected by poison arrows, and as a vital constituent of one of their favourite dishes, pemmican: the original burger, a fully balanced fast food loaded with proteins, fats, carbohydrates, vitamins and minerals, and which stored well, an attribute of great importance to tribes on the move.

As the paleface settlements grew in size, however, pioneer contacts with the survival skills and healing knowledge of the local people became less and less, and scurvy and other deficiency diseases began to take their toll. At the same time the native inhabitants began dying like flies in the face of simple Old World ills like the common cold, chickenpox and mumps, to which they had no inbuilt resistance – a fact shamefully abused by some unscrupulous landgrabbers, and equally shamefully used by some medical men to denigrate the obvious skills and successes of the shamanic (heathen) medicine men and women. So for the next 150 years medicines were mainly imported from the Old World to the New. In the *New York Gazette* of 3 August 1752, Dr Charles Scham advertised 'a choice Assortment of Medicines quite fresh', arrived in the *Nebuchadnezzar*. One can only hope that they were indeed 'quite fresh', for scurvy was still rampaging throughout the colony.

The herbs and sallets originally grown in the gardens of that first English settlement on the banks of the Snake River amongst the Cranberry Bogs were as follows:

Barberry, Common	*Berberis vulgaris*
Basil, Sweet	*Ocimum basilicum*
Borage	*Borago officinalis*
Bouncing Bet	*Saponaria officinalis*
Catnip	*Nepeta cataria*
Columbine	*Aquilegia vulgaris*
Costmary	*Impatiens* spp.?
Elecampane	*Inula helenium*
Flax	*Linum usitatissimum*
Germander	*Teucrium chamaedrys*
Heartsease	*Viola tricolor*
Lavender Cotton, Grey	*Santolina* spp.
Lavender Cotton, Green	*Santolina* spp.
Marjoram, Sweet Knotted	*Origanum vulgare* (*et* spp.)
Mints, Peppermint, Spearmint	*Mentha* spp.
Mullein	*Verbascum densiflorum*
Mustard, White	*Sinapis alba*
Pot Marigold	*Calendula officinalis*
Rue	*Ruta graveolens*
Sage	*Salvia officinalis*
Sassafras	*Sassafras albidum*
Savory, Summer	*Satureia* spp.?
Savory, Winter	*Satureia* spp.?
Southernwood	*Artemisia abrotanum*
Tansy	*Chrysanthemum vulgare*

| Thyme | *Thymus vulgaris* |
| Wormwood | *Artemisia absinthium*[5] |

All except Sassafras had been brought to the settlement from the Old World, and many if eaten raw and used as advised by Culpeper would have helped ward off scurvy and other then common maladies. However, their use was rapidly supplanted by the import of 'all manner of Chymical and Galenical Medicines' including mercury and antimony in vast amounts, blistering plasters, syringes, clyster pipes, Jalap, Scammony, Bryony, Buckthorn and many others. Scurvy cures included Elixir of Vitriol (sulphuric acid), which must have done wonders to sore gums and decaying teeth alike, though there were some good imports like herbal purges and cathartics, Peruvian Bark against malaria and Chamomile flowers for upset stomachs and upset nights. One medicine to flow in the opposite direction was Cranberries, for, to appease King Charles II's wrath for their coining the Pine Tree Shilling, the settlers sent him, amongst other things, ten barrels of the antiscorbutic berries. Another was American Ginseng, and thereby hangs another royal tale, which will be told in chapter 15.[6]

Notes

1 Nehemiah Grew, *Experiments in Consort of the Luctation arising from the affusion of several Menstruums upon all sorts of Bodies*, Exhibited to the Royal Society of London, April 13th and June 1st, 1676 (1676).
2 Nicholas Culpeper, *Pharmacopoeia Londinensis or, the London Dispensatory* (London, 1675).
3 Barbara Griggs, *Green Pharmacy – A History of Herbal Medicine* (London: Robert Hale, 1981, 1987), p. 129.
4 Griggs, *Green Pharmacy*.
5 M. B. Gordon, Medicine in Colonial New Jersey and Adjacent Areas, *Bulletin of Health and Medicine*, 17 (1945).
6 Ibid.

14

TRADING ON ILL HEALTH

On the last day of the year 1600 Queen Elizabeth of England granted a group of London merchants a charter which permitted the foundation of the East India Company, a charter which entrusted it with the monopoly of trade to the Far East. As Northcote Parkinson succinctly put it:

> How was this East India Company controlled? By the Government. What was its object? To collect taxes. How was this object attained? By a large standing army. What were its employees? Soldiers mostly, the rest civil servants. Where did it trade? China. What did it export from England? Courage. And what did it import from China? Tea.[1]

The tea filled the main and driest part of the holds, and their bilges, as we have been finding from recent excavations of a few of the multitude of wrecks, were filled with china, porcelain and armorial plate, none of which could be spoilt by short or long-term immersion. Then there was the so-called privilege tonnage carried for the personal profit of the captain and the ship's surgeon. It was here that both the export and the import of medicines and other exotica found their main focus, for the East India Company had been founded by that group of London merchants in an attempt to counteract the fact that the Dutch, who had held the monopoly of trade with the East, had suddenly upped the price of pepper from 3s to 8s 6d a pound – a significant step in the Spice Wars which had been waxing and waning for almost 300 years.[2]

On the first of May 1498, Vasco da Gama dropped anchor in

Calicut on the first voyage into the Indian Ocean around the tip of Africa. Asked what they were seeking, the landing party replied: 'Christians and Spices'.[3] By this time the London Guild of Pepperers, who through the twelfth and thirteenth centuries had been separate from the Spicers, had joined forces with them to become the Fraternity of St Anthony – an unholy alliance of the Pepperers, Spicers and Apothecaries. The Spicers, mainly Lombards and Genoese who dealt in spices and in drugs, were widespread through the realm, and by the mid-1400s had come to be known as Grocers; many practised as apothecaries too. The sixteenth century was one of bloodthirsty European expansion, a massive increase in the Spice Trade, and eventually a clash of European powers for its control. In 1552 the first Portuguese ships docked in Antwerp: 500 pounds of Cloves which had cost 2 ducats in the Moluccas eventually made 1600 ducats in London. Others soon followed, though initially with less luck. The first French interlopers were Jean and Raul Parmentier (a name which appears again in the story of plant movements, including the Potato), who visited Sumatra in 1526, but little followed – piracy was more profitable. After them, in 1521, came Magellan's crew, coming from the East.[4]

The Portuguese colonies grew rapidly, and disproportionately to the mother country's resources. Nevertheless, the main possessions – Goa, Dieu, Cananore, Cochin, Malacca and Ceylon – were held firmly until 1580, when the unification of the crowns of Spain and Portugal meant the closure of the Dutch ports to their wares. Great navigators, the Portuguese had proved themselves indifferent traders, and had left most of the actual commerce in the hands of Dutch and Flemish merchants. The changed political situation gave the English and Dutch the incentive they needed to penetrate the Spice Trade on their own account. The first serious Dutch spice trader was Cornelius van Houtman, who sailed in 1595 from Amsterdam for Bantam, and returned with 245 sacks of Pepper and 45 sacks of Cloves, losing 160 men out of a crew of 249. The final blow to Portugal's Eastern power was the reconquest of Hormuz in 1622 by the Shah of Persia, with English help.

Regardless of how good the relations between the English and Dutch in Europe were at the time, their rivalry in the East often had violent overtones; the East India Company generally left the Malay archipelago to the Vereenighde Oostindische Companie, and concentrated on India. As trade rapidly increased, Amsterdam became the centre of the Eastern trade: beyond 'classical' spices, the main goods (apart from manufactured ones) were Turmeric, Tamarind, Cassia, benzoin and indigo. Profits could vary between 50 and 400 per cent. With the establishment of Cape Town in 1652, the Dutch strategic structure was complete: the Eastern trade was controlled at source, and so were the staging-posts to it, cutting out rivals completely. Part of this policy was disinformation, and it is noteworthy that Dutch maps and navigational aids published in this period are rich in deliberate mistakes – usually intended to lead the user to disaster. Also, in the interest of security, the spice plantations became specialized: for example, Nutmeg was grown almost exclusively in Banda, and destroyed almost entirely on other islands such as Ceram. The human cost was high as well: in 1624 the entire male population of Banda was liquidated, and a century later 10,000 Chinese were 'purged' in Batavia. In Ceylon, 'theft' of a single Cinnamon branch was punishable with death. By the mid-eighteenth century, Cinnamon was being cultivated in Ceylon, and production was high enough to warrant stocks being withheld from the market to sustain the price.[5]

In the City of London, the Apothecaries remained a section of the Company of Grocers until 1617, when James I instituted their charter. At first these traders all came from the Hanseatic cities of the East Baltic, whence the name Easterlings by which they were also known. A very lucrative trade it must have been, too, as from that term the word 'sterling' has been derived; and in with the spices and tea came the drugs.

In 1588 only 15 per cent of drugs had come from outside Europe; by 1621 the figure had risen to 48 per cent, and by 1669 it had attained 70 per cent, the majority coming from India and the East Indies, with an import value of £6,000. They were sold on to the London druggists and eventually to the provincial druggists, all part of the Company of Grocers from which they obtained their supplies. Demand, especially for Rhubarb, Cassia and Camphor, soon outstripped supply, and so a so-called 'Drug Concern' was formed in London. Each season the Concern sent out treasure from England to the East, mainly silver bullion and almost $50,000 worth of goods, lead, Cochineal and Prussian Blue. (The latter was used amongst other things for dyeing sub-standard tea leaves, so the Grocers cashed in at all ends of the Drug Concern.)

The following brief account, taken from Denis Leigh's *Medicine, the City and China*, gives a fascinating insight into the times when to be at sea was probably one of the most risky professions to follow, thanks to pirates, shipwreck and scurvy.

What were these drugs which China alone could supply? Searching the records of the cargoes of East Indiamen from 1687 onwards, there are entries regarding Camphor, Rhubarb, China Root, Dragon's Blood, Ginseng, Cambodge, Zingiber, Cassia, Cinnabar, and what are called 'various'. The first mention of drugs from China occurs in the records of the Courteen Association, which had been licensed by Charles I in 1635 to undertake a voyage to Goa, the ports of Malabar, the Coasts of China and Japan, 'there to trade'. The *Dragon, Sunne, Catherine, Planter* and two pinnacles, the *Anne* and the *Discovery*, left the Downs on 14 April 1636, under the command of Captain John Weddell. Their voyage took them to Goa, Malacca, Macao, and past the Bogue up to the First Bar, within fifteen miles of Canton.

After a number of adventures, by 1637 the *Catherine* was loaded with commodities obtained in Canton and Macao, her cargo including 100 piculs of China Root. Fifty years later, in 1687, the *London* and the *Worcester* were despatched to Bombay to Amoy. Amongst the commodities positively ordered on the Company's account were '300 Tubbs of Camphire'. In the log of the *Anson* on her voyage to Whampoa in 1750, kept by the commander, Jonathan Ramsay, is a record of thirteen chests of Rhubarb being shipped home in his privilege tonnage, whilst, in 1764, some of the private trade included the following: Captain John Mitford of the *Northumberland*, 6 boxes of Rhubarb, Captain James Moffat of the *Latham*, 8 Boxes of Rhubarb, Captain John Sandys of the *Norfolk*, 7 boxes of Rhubarb, Captain Richard Hall of the *Worcester*, 10 chests of Rhubarb and 18 chests of Cambojium.[6]

The only real problem in all this was a fact which had been revealed very early on by Sir Robert Hart when he wrote: 'The Chinese have the best food in the world, Rice, the best drink, tea,

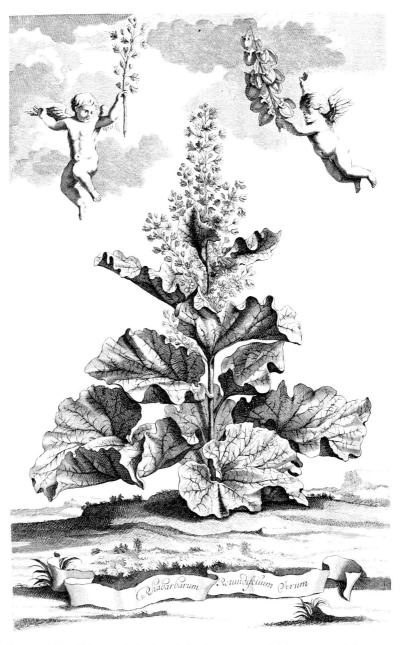

FIGURE 14.1 Chinese Rhubarb (*Rhabarbarum rotundifolium*), one of the prizes of the China trade.

and the best clothing, silk and fur. Possessing these staples and their innumerable native adjuncts, they do not need to buy a penny's worth elsewhere.'[7] The East India Company soon found he was right: the only thing they wanted in exchange for their tea was hard bullion, and there often wasn't enough to go round. Cotton grown in India began to fill part of the trade deficit, and it was soon followed by opium from the same source. It was the iniquitous trade in the latter which finally brought the bullion back to Europe and led to the fall of the Chinese Empire as it was opened up to the new products from European and American industrialization – a particularly sad state of affairs when it is remembered that the emperor Ch'ien Lung had rebuffed the Macartney Embassy which had gone out to trade a variety of articles being made in our manufacturing towns: 'Strange and

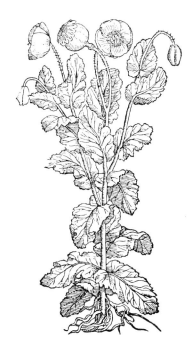

FIGURE 14.2 The Opium Poppy (*Papaver somniferum*): sacred narcotic, mainstay of the East India Company, nemesis of the Chinese Empire and scourge of Western societies.

costly objects do not interest me. As your ambassador can see for himself, we possess all things . . . we have no use for your country's manufacturies.'[8]

If only China had turned her back on opium, which in its alcoholic tincture, Laudanum, was to wreak havoc in Europe, the course of history might well have been very different.

By 1760, huge quantities of opium was being consumed and even larger quantities of spices were burned yearly, both in Amsterdam and in Batavia, to control the supply. With the Anglo-Dutch Wars (1781–2) and the Seven Years' War conditions changed, and England both displaced the French in India and broke Holland's monopoly of the Far East trade. In 1770, the aptly named Pierre Poivre managed to smuggle seedlings of *Myristica* and *Eugenia* from the Moluccas to the Jardin des Pamplemousses in Mauritius. By 1793, the first shipload of seeds and seedlings reached Paris – the first time in the history of the Spice Trade that Europe actually saw the plants from which their precious condiments originated. With this, the concept of production monopoly around which colonial politics had turned over the previous centuries became obsolete, and the fight for the Spice Trade became botanical and commercial rather than military.

Malayan plantations gave good results initially, turning Penang and Singapore into centres of trade, but they were for the most part destroyed by a plant epidemic in 1860. After Malaya, the most important producer of Cloves was and still is Zanzibar.[9] Vanilla production followed a different route – introduced to the French island of Réunion in 1819 from Cayenne as a botanical curiosity, it became of commercial importance only in 1841 when a successful method of artificial pollination was discovered. The first shipment to Paris was in 1848, and by 1898 production was 200 tons. The largest consumer of Cinnamon in the nineteenth century was Spain; it was used both for incense and as a component of chocolate. This latter was defined in the *Diccionario de la Academia Española* as 'a mixture of Cocoa, sugar, and Cinnamon', and was of sufficient social importance that the question of whether or not it broke fast had to be presented to Pope Paul V – who after trying it came out in its favour, declaring: *hoc non frangit jejuneum.*[10]

HEADLAND'S
HOMŒOPATHIC OR DIETETIC COCOA.

Cocoa, as an article of daily diet, is confessedly the most digestive and nutritious ; and being also devoid of the exciting principles of Tea or Coffee, is universally recommended to patients under a course of Homœopathic treatment.

Effectually to meet this desired end, its *purity* must be of the first consideration, and it was with this view that our preparation of Cocoa was first submitted to the Public by Mr. Wm. HEAD-LAND nearly fifty years ago, as being *entirely free* from those unwholesome and deleterious admixtures with which the Cocoa of commerce notoriously abounds.

The general demand which has consequently arisen (from its being the most palatable of its kind) for this preparation of the *pure powder* of the nut, has induced many of the manufacturers and grocers to pass off their common, impure, and indigestible fabrications as the genuine Homœopathic Cocoa, an imposition not only grossly deceptive, but liable to be attended with consequences the most serious to those who, under the impression of partaking of *pure Cocoa*, are in fact imbibing a composition injurious, and altogether incompatible with their successful treatment, and of the Homœopathic remedial agents.

In Packets, 9d. and 1s. 6d.

CONCENTRATED COCOA.

This perfectly pure Cocoa is prepared from the finest beans, carefully selected, and from which a large proportion of fat has been extracted, by improved processes, without injury to quality or flavour. It is guaranteed pure, and particularly recommended to our patrons as an agreeable and nourishing drink for invalids and consumers generally. Being in a very concentrated form, this Cocoa will be found very economical. It is easily prepared, directions for which will be found on each label.

Sold in Tins only, at 1s., 2s., and 3s. 6d. each.

FIGURE 14.3 Cocoa: food, drink and panacea.

Notes

1 Denis Leigh, *Medicine, the City and China*, The Monckton Copeman Lecture, given at the Apothecaries' Hall on 31 January 1973; *Medical History*, 18 (1974), pp. 51–67; p. 52.
2 Leigh, *Medicine, the City and China*.
3 Paul and Bernard Corcellet, *et al. La via delle spezie* (Milan: RCS Rizzoli Libri S.p.A., and Singapore: Times Editions, 1987, 1988).
4 Ibid.
5 Ibid.
6 Leigh, *Medicine, the City and China*, p. 55.
7 Ibid., p. 51.
8 Ibid., p. 52.
9 Corcellet *et al.*, *La via delle spezie*.
10 Ibid.

15

GINSENG AND THE
ROYAL SOCIETY CONNECTION

The Royal Society of London was founded on 15 July 1662 under the patronage of Charles II, some 3,310 years after the Yellow Emperor of China mentioned Ginseng in his Herbal and only five years after tea, 'that excellent and by all Physicians approved China drink', was first publicly sold at Garways Coffee House in London. The Society became a centre of discussion concerning this root, which is doubtless the best known, though hardly the best understood, Chinese medicinal plant in the West.[1]

In the first volume (1665) of the *Philosophical Transactions* of that learned society, which has as one of its aims 'the further promoting by the authority of experiments the sciences of natural things and useful arts', there is a brief mention of Ginseng, highly prized by Chinese doctors 'as an extraordinary Restorative and Cordiall, recovering frequently with it agonizing persons'. In 1679 Sir Thomas Browne, already a great experimenter in natural medicine, wrote the following to his son Edward, who had been able to put the letters FRS – Fellow of the Royal Society – after his name since 1667: 'You did well to observe Ginseng. All exotick rarities & especially of the East, the East India trade having increased, are brought into England the best profits made thereof.'[2] On 26 June in the same year, a Dr Andrew Clench, with Sir Christopher Wren as vice-president in the chair, presented the Society with 'a certain root lately brought from China, called Ginseng, of great esteem in China for its virtue in restoring consumptive persons, and those emaciated with long sickness to their former health and strength. It was valued in China at thrice its weight in silver.'[3]

Dr Clench was elected a Fellow of the Royal Society and of the Royal College of Physicians in 1680, and his specimen of Ginseng was described by Nehemiah Grew as 'like a yellow parsnip and divided in the same way as the mandrake into two legs. Not known to grow [wild] anywhere but in the Kingdom of Corea. In which place, also in Tunquin, China and Japan, it is much used, and relied upon in Epilepsy, Fevers, and both Chronick and Acute Diseases.'[4]

In the same vein John Ray, one of the fathers of English natural history, includes a very similar description in the second volume of his *Historia plantarum* (1688). It would, however, appear that both based themselves on Gulielmus Piso's work, published in Amsterdam thirty years earlier. Nevertheless, it was enough to further stimulate the interest of the Fellows in the wonder plant Ginseng. Dr Robert Whittle, a medical practitioner first of Hull, then York, then London, relates his own experiments with Ginseng to the Royal Society in a letter to Daniel Colwall. Pointing out that

> Cardan, physician to King Edward VI, was 'reported by some famous Divines' to be in Hell for his refusal 'to tell the World a secret with which he wrought great cures', he says he is resolved not to be censured in the same way and will freely communicate 'this Noble and Excellent Medicine'. Despite his hatred for all 'Pretences to Secrets' and 'Printed Bills of Quacks who pretend to Nostrums', he considers that 'if any Man can communicate a good Medicine, he shews himself a lover of the Country more than himself and deserves Thanks of Mankind.'[5]

Having covered himself from every direction, Whittle goes on to record that having been given a packet of Ginseng while practising in Hull, he used it with wonderful success, particularly on his relative Andrew Marvell, the celebrated poet and satirist, who was

> much emaciated, and reduced into a pefect Skeleton a mere Bag of Bones by a long Hectick Fever, joyned with an Ulcer of the Lungs. Being despaired of by all his Friends, I was resolved to try what the Tincture of the Root could doe, which I gave every morning in Red

Cows Milk, warm from her Duggs. And I found his Flesh to come again like that of a Child, and his lost Appetite restored, and his naturel Rudely Complexion revived in his cheeks, to the amazement of his desponding Relations, that he was called 'Lazarus the Second'.[6]

He cites half a dozen other cases in which the tincture, spirit and extract made from Ginseng root had proved 'a known, safe and experimented remedy' for young and old patients suffering from consumptive and respiratory illnesses. Referring to Gulielmus Piso's high regard for Ginseng, he says:

Public Fame saith that the Popes of Rome, who are chosen to that Office when they are very Old, do make great use of this Root, to preserve their Radical Moysture and natural Heat, that they may the longer enjoy their Comfortable Preferment.[7]

Finally, he also states that Robert Boyle (whose law every science pupil has learned in Physics) once told him 'that he thought it was a Medicine sent from Heaven to save the Lives of Thousands of Men, Women and Children'. Whether Boyle ever did experiment with Ginseng is not known, though being a director of the East India Company he must have had ready access to supplies.[8]

Meanwhile Andrew Cleyer, a chemist with a medical degree and chief of the Dutch East India Company's factory at Deshima in Japan, wrote the article *De Radice Ginsingh*, which was published by the German Scientific Society, Academiae Naturae Curiosorum, founded in 1652, in their *Miscellanea Curiosa*, a publication which was regularly read and discussed along with the *Philosophical Transactions* of the Royal Society. The account of Ginseng came to the attention of Engelbert Kaempfer, Germany's leading explorer and natural historian of the Baroque period, for he makes mention of it in his widely acclaimed *The History of Japan*. This was translated into English by J. G. Scheuchzer, librarian to Sir Hans Sloane, patron of London's first Physic Garden in Chelsea. On the death of Kaempfer in 1716, Sloane purchased all his drawings, manuscripts and collections. Among these, and still present in the Sloane Herbarium, is a Japanese Ginseng plant with several leaves and seeds. Sloane was elected to the Royal Society on 21 January 1685, at a time when there was a great upsurge of critical interest and practical experimentation on the plant, and there are no less than twelve other specimens of Ginseng in the Sloane Collection.[9]

The Royal Society played an important part in the popularization of Ginseng by publishing in 1713 a translation of an account of the Tartarian plant written by Pierre Jartoux, a French Jesuit missionary in Peking. Jartoux, a mathematician, was ordered along with other Jesuits to compile an accurate atlas for the Emperor K'ang Hsi. While surveying on the Chinese border with Korea, a Mandarin brought the Jesuits four Ginseng roots he had found growing in the area. Jartoux tested the plant himself, recording: 'In an hour after I found my Pulse much fresher and quicker. I had an Appetite, and found myself much more vigorous, and could bear Labour much better and easier than before.'[10] A scientist at heart, he tried the root under a variety of conditions and always found that it lived up to its reputation as an excellent restorative. Extolling its virtues to the Procurator-General of his Order, he stated that it would 'prove an excellent Medicine in the Hands of any European who understands Pharmacy, if we had but a sufficient quantity of it to examine the Nature of it Chymically and to apply it in a proper quantity according to the Nature of the Disease for which it may be beneficial.'[11]

Here too for the first time the Western world of science and medicine has an accurate description of the plant, of its preparation as a medicine, and of its habitat and geographical location, the latter appended by what must be regarded as a prophetic suggestion, that it might well be found growing in a parallel environment in Canada. And indeed it was found growing in Canada at 45°31′N and 74°45′E, between Montreal and Ottawa, by Joseph François Lafitau, another Jesuit missionary who had read of Jartoux's prediction in his Order's publications. His description of Canadian Ginseng was published in Paris in 1718 long before the idea of continental drift used the 800 species of the Aralia family as proof positive that the floras of the now far separated parts of the New World and the Old World were once one and the same. That Canadian and Tartarian Ginseng were one and the same species appeared to be borne out by their appearance and by the fact that the local Iroquois Indians used the root as a stimulant and pick-me-up, especially in extreme exhaustion; so it soon had its advocates on both sides of the Atlantic.[12]

One of these, William Byrd Jr, who called it the King of Plants, also found it of great help while on survey work when he led a commission in 1728 to settle a long-standing border dispute between Virginia and North Carolina: 'Though Practice will soon make a man of tolerable Vigour an able Footman, yet as a Help to bear Fatigue, I us'd to chew a Root of Ginseng as I Walk't along. This kept up my Spirits, and made me trip away as nimbly in my Jack-Boots as younger men cou'd in their Shoes.'[13] Pointing out that Ginseng 'grows also on the northern continent of America, but as sparingly as Truth and Public Spirit', he summarizes the properties of American Ginseng as seen at the time:

> Its vertues are, that it gives an uncommon Warmth and Vigour to the Blood, and frisks the Spirit, beyond any other cordial. It cheers the Heart even of a Man that has a bad Wife, and makes him look down with great Composure on the crosses of the World. It promotes insensible perspiration, dissolves all Phlegmatick and Viscous Humours, that are apt to obstruct the Narrow Channels of the Nerves. It helps the Memory, and would quicken even Helvetian dullness. 'Tis friendly to the Lungs, much more than Scolding itself. It comforts the Stomach, and Strengthens the Bowels preventing Colicks and Fluxes. In one Word, it will make a Man live a great while, and very well while he does live.[14]

Quaker botanists, both English and American, were amongst the many people who actively promoted the discovery and knowledge of American Ginseng. Chief amongst them were Peter Collinson, FRS, eminent English naturalist and antiquarian, and John Bartram, the first native-born American botanist and in Linnaeus' view the greatest 'natural botanist' in the world. It must be remembered that at the time the whole of the North American continent was opening up its botanical treasures, not the least of which was Ginseng, to an Old World Europe which was then finding it more and more difficult to discover new species for description. Bartram pioneered America's earliest botanical garden in his home near Philadelphia, where both Benjamin Franklin and George Washington came to rest and philosophize.

Bartram's discovery of Ginseng on the banks of the Susquhanna River was announced in the *Pennsylvania Gazette* on 27 July 1738. On 7 December, Peter Collinson showed members of the Royal Society two specimens of North American Ginseng which he had been sent by Bartram. By 1740 Collinson had the plant growing in Peckham in Surrey, where it flowered in June 1743 and set fruit in the autumn. References to Ginseng both Canadian, American and Chinese proliferated in the records of the Society and the minds of its Fellows. Although some of their thoughts revolved around the exact identity of the three plants, many turned to their more lucrative aspects.[15]

An important scientific event in the tale of Ginseng took place in 1753 when Linnaeus gave it the first systematic description, calling the genus to which the plant belongs *Panax*. Yet it would take another eighty-nine years of thought and investigation before the Russian botanist C. A. Meyer differentiated clearly between the species, naming the one from China *Panax ginseng*, that from North America *Panax quinquefolium* and that which strays over the border and grows in Canada *Panax trifoliata*. Helping this research on its way, Dr John Amman, FRS, another former librarian of Sir Hans Sloane and founder of the Russian Academy's Botanical Garden, wrote to Sloane from St Petersburg with a request for some 'true Ginseng' lately found in Pennsylvania.

From this point on, trade in Ginseng increased sharply, for it had become a valuable commodity and the Quaker botanists played an ever active part, so much so that Collinson, using his worldwide contacts as a merchant, informed Bartram in 1739 that: 'I sent some Ginseng roots to China. If they sell well, a profitable trade may be carried on. In the mean time, sow the seed and make a stock to furnish my friend when he returns.' A fortnight later he repeated the plea, adding:

> I have compared yours with the Chinese, and found them in all respect the same. Your proprietor was kind enough to send me a considerable parcel, and I have trusted a particular friend with it, to carry to China, to see how they approve of it, and to find what price it bears, but my friend is under promise not to discover that it is American, for if they know that, they are so fanciful, it may not be so good as their own . . .[16]

They evidently found a good use for it, especially as their own root was so rare that they were willing to buy imported Ginseng at exorbitant prices. Nevertheless, they did not confuse it with the 'real thing', and recognized it as a separate plant with differing tonic properties, just as they did for Korean and Japanese Ginseng. *Panax quinquefolium* is still considered a 'cold' drug, energizing and relaxing, as opposed to the 'hot' *Panax ginseng*, which is energizing and invigorating. Leung, for example, mentions a first-hand case where American Ginseng was successfully used to reduce scarlet fever; he also mentions that Russian workers have in recent years found distinct chemical differences between the two species. The Chinese interpretation, incidentally, mirrors the some-what sporadic use to which American Ginseng was put by Amerindian tribes.[17]

In 1750 Dr John Fothergill, FRS, informed Charles Alston, Lecturer on Materia Medica and Superintendent of the Royal Botanic Garden in Edinburgh, that: 'We now begin to receive considerable quantities of Ginseng from America, it is not yet much used, but I have one very singular instance of its good effects in the case of impotency.'[18] By 1753 trade in Ginseng was proving so lucrative that the *Gentleman's Magazine* states that profits would have been even greater had the root been collected at the right season and cured in the Chinese manner. So much so that Peter Collinson, who must have made a lot of money in the early days of the trade, wrote concerning the trade in American Ginseng to China, where it was sold at great profit:

> From this intelligence a rage after Ginseng commenced. I call it so because all the mountains and uncultivated country was ransacked for this valuable root, and imported hither by hogsheads full, and the market in China glutted with this root, which had been artfully concealed and prepared by the Chinese, and sold under great secrecy to the people for True Chinese Ginseng, but its great plenty soon discovered the cheat, and then it sank to nothing. The Americans were great losers when this became known, and great quantities were re-exported for the sake of getting the bounty, had this been managed wisely, it would have been an article of profit, it was first sold here for a guinea a pound, afterwards for twelve shillings, but now forgot.[19]

Notwithstanding Collinson's remarks, both the trade and the Royal Society's interest in Ginseng continued and indeed flourished while Sir Joseph Banks, founder of the Royal Botanic Gardens at Kew, was its president. In 1786 Banks wrote to Humphry Marshall in Pennsylvania for a very large supply of Ginseng, explaining that he would use it to 'try some experiments upon curing the root of Ginseng which, if they succeed, may become important both to your country and mine'[20] – two countries now divided by the American Colonies' Declaration of Independence ten years earlier. Whether Banks or those who attended the Boston Tea Party had taken any notice of an *Essay on the Virtues and Properties of the Ginseng Tea*, published by a Count Belchingen in 1786 and subtitled *Observations on the Pernicious Effects of Drinking Tea in General* is not known. However, in his reply seven months later, Marshall informed Banks that his nephew had travelled about 200 miles west of Chester County through the mountains, and 'as the Ginseng is either dug up for sale or rooted up by hogs so much, that it begins to grow scarce in the inhabited parts.'[21]

There is no record of Banks having received the hundredweight of roots despatched from Pennsylvania, yet we know that it was grown at Kew, for in William Woodville's authoritative *Medical Botany* (1790–3) there is an illustration of American Ginseng drawn from a specimen growing at the Royal Botanic Gardens. So ended years of interest in Ginseng by the members of the Royal Society, to be rekindled in recent years by the publication of a paper by John H. Appleby entitled 'Ginseng and the Royal Society' in 1983 – the same year that a Ginseng Centre was opened in London.[22]

This was by no means the only attention Ginseng has attracted in recent times. Some Western (and Western-trained Oriental) scientists have been trying to fit Ginseng into some sort of recognizable category of Western pharmacology throughout the twentieth century, usually with scant results and even less recognition. The identification and naming of the supposed active ingredients – glycosides such as panaquilon, which influences the endocrine secretion mechanism and raises the amount of hormones in the blood, and panaxin, which stimulates the brain, improves muscular tone and acts as a tonic for the cardiovascular system, and saponins such as the groups referred to as ginsenosides by Japanese workers and as panaxosides by Russian ones, may drop some hints of the plant's properties, but hardly explains its purported 'whole body' effects. While a better answer may arise out of current research trying to connect Traditional Chinese Medicine with the more recent discoveries concerning the immune system, probably the best approach yet has been that of the Russian workers who have coined the term 'adaptogen' for *Panax* and its related tonics. By this, they mean a substance which measurably increases the body's resistance to external stresses of various kinds, acting on the whole body rather than on single organs or tissues, and helping it in maintaining its normal function – which is more or less what Chinese doctors have been saying all along.[23]

The very names of the plant allude to its high reputation, *Panax* comes from the Greek *pan* 'all' and *akos* 'cure', that is all-healing, a panacea, which is in turn derived from the repute of the plant in China, where the specific and in this case the international common name Ginseng is a romanization of the sound of two Chinese characters, *gin*, which stands for 'man', and *seng*, which is the equivalent of 'essence', the substance that underlies all outward manifestations. According to a conventional Chinese belief, Ginseng is the crystallization of the essence of the Earth in the form of 'man'. Already in the Shennong Herbal (*c.*200 BC) Ginseng was considered to 'vitalise the five organs, calm the nerves, stop palpitation due to fright, brighten vision, increase intellect, and, with long term use, prolong life and make one feel young'.[24]

Ginseng is not, however, regarded or employed as a panacea in Chinese medical practice, indeed its use is very specific and restricted, mainly during convalescence or through long-term use in preventive medicine. As Shiu Ying Hu points out in his authoritative account of Ginseng in Chinese medicine, only the well-to-do can afford to observe a period of convalescence, and together with the generally high price of the substance this means that probably more than 90 per cent of the population have never tasted Ginseng; in all likelihood, this has been true throughout the ages. Also interesting are the contra-indications concerning it that frequently crop up in the literature. For example, one should never mix Ginseng with any of the elements of *Veratrum nigrum* or *Veratrum maackii* (presumably due to the veratrine alkaloids they contain), nor should Tea and Turnips be taken during an intense Ginseng treatment.[25]

Apart from *Panax ginseng*, four other Chinese species of *Panax* are used in Traditional Chinese Medicine, of which *Panax pseudoginseng* (San-ch'i, 'Three Seven') is a pain reliever and haemostatic, prescribed for cancer, boils, swellings, bleeding, bruises, internal bleeding and irregular periods, while *Panax japonicum* (Chu-chieh Seng, 'Bamboo Ginseng'), *Panax bipinnati-fidum* (Yu-yeh Chu-chieh, 'Feather leaf Bamboo Ginseng') and *Panax major* (Ta-yeh San-ch'i, 'Big leaf San-ch'i') are used primarily in folk medicine and by ethnic minority groups. Incidentally, *Panax pseudoginseng* is also the main constituent of Yun Nan Bai Yao, also referred to as Jin bu huan, 'gold no trade'; this powerful haemostatic, now again available, disappeared from the open market in the 1970s: the entire production was being devoted to the first aid kits of the North Vietnamese army. Within each type, the roots are classified commercially according to provenance, quality and method of preparation. For true *Panax ginseng*, the main classifications are first between Wild Ginseng (Ye-shan-seng) and Cultivated Ginseng (Yuan-seng), then by preparation, namely Raw Sun-dried Ginseng (Sheng-sai-seng), Red Ginseng (Hung-seng), which is steamed and dried, Sugared Ginseng (T'ang-seng) and Loose Rind Ginseng (T'ao-p'i-seng), which is first sugared, then repeatedly leached and dried;) there are further subclassifications according to size and appearance.[26]

There is some irony in the fact that only after three and a half centuries of scientific study and commercial exploitation is the West starting to take a serious interest in *Panax* for its actual medicinal and tonic properties.

Notes

1 John H. Appleby, 'Ginseng and the Royal Society', *Notes and Records of the Royal Society of London*, 37 (1983), no. 2.
2 Ibid., p. 122.
3 Ibid.
4 Ibid., pp. 123–4.
5 Ibid., pp. 124–5.
6 Ibid.. pp. 125.
7 Ibid.
8 Ibid.
9 Appleby, 'Ginseng and the Royal Society'.
10 Ibid., p. 127.
11 Ibid.
12 Appleby, 'Ginseng and the Royal Society'.
13 Ibid., p. 130.
14 Ibid., pp. 130–1.
15 Appleby, 'Ginseng and the Royal Society'.
16 Ibid., pp. 133–4.
17 Albert Y. Leung, *Chinese Herbal Remedies* (London: Wildwood House, 1985).
18 Appleby, 'Ginseng and the Royal Society', p. 135.
19 Ibid., pp. 137–8.
20 Ibid., p. 141.
21 Ibid.
22 Appleby, 'Ginseng and the Royal Society'.
23 Daniel P. Reid, *Chinese Medicine* (Wellingborough, Northants: CWF Publications, Thorsons, 1987); Ron Teeguarden and Caroline Davies, *Chinese Tonic Herbs* (Tokyo: Japan Publications Inc., 1984); and Shiu Ying Hu, 'The genus *Panax* (Ginseng) in Chinese medicine', *Economic Botany*, 30, (January–March, 1976), pp. 11–28.
24 Leung, *Chinese Herbal Remedies*; and Shiu Yiing Hu, 'The genus *Panax* (Ginseng) in Chinese medicines'. Quotation from Shiu Yin Hu.
25 Leung, (1985), *Chinese Herbal Remedies*; Reid, *Chinese Medicine*; and Shiu Ying Hu, 'The genus *Panax* (Ginseng) in Chinese medicine'.
26 Reid, *Chinese Medicine*; Shiu Ying Hu, 'The genus *Panax* (Ginseng) in Chinese medicine'; and Jake Fratkin, *Chinese Herbal Patent Formulas* (Institute of Traditional Medicine and Preventive Health Care, 2442 SE Sherman St, Portland, Oregon 97214, 1986).

16

VIRTUES OLD AND NEW

Despite the fact that Charles II of England was the founding patron of the Royal Society, which was to advance scientific experiment and reasoning by leaps and bounds, his surgeon Robert Wisemann could still affirm that the 'Royal Touch' was the appropriate cure for scrofula.

Such belief was part of the so-called vitalistic school of thought, or vitalism, which though originating in Aristotle still held sway in the seventeenth century. At its root lay the belief in a vital force peculiar to living organisms and differing from all other forces outside living organisms. Those who opposed the vitalists at the time maintained that life could be fully explained in terms of the known physical laws; considering the extent to which these were then known, despite the publication of Newton's *Principia* in 1687, such an explanation was understandably difficult. An early clash was that between the so-called iatrochemists and their counterparts, the iatrophysicists; while the latter based themselves on Descartian mechanism, attempting to interpret living things as 'perfect mechanisms', the former carried the heritage of alchemy and the links between the transformation of substances and the mystical sphere that it implied. A significant figure amongst these was Jan Baptist van Helmont (1580–1644), who may be taken as the link between the traditional alchemists and the chemists of the modern age: a careful experimenter and observer, in contact with Galileo and Harvey, and yet devoted to the search for the Philosopher's Stone.[1]

While all this high science and, in the case of Ginseng and other saleable commodities, high finance, were going on the world was changing rapidly. Human lifestyles were becoming more and more removed from any real contact with the land, let alone with nature. Throughout this time, as before and indeed to this day, trained medical practitioners and apothecaries were few, and in most places, especially in the colonies, far between. The fields were thus open and ready for harvest by all manner of charlatans and quacks. What is more, when a member of a profession, a guild member or craftsperson is placed under increasing pressure (and there can be no greater pressure than living surrounded by sick and dying people), he or she may well pay less attention to detail and more to rapid and spectacular results. For such practitioners, the most important authority of the time was Boerhaave, who had opened what was in reality the first teaching hospital in Europe at Leyden in Holland. There he taught multitudes of students at his patients' bedsides, and there in effect he turned the teachings of Galen and Paracelsus into medicine by numbers. These are the symptoms, 'no keyhole physick' here; these are the treatments, bleeding, blistering and good well-tried simples, evacuants and vomits. There is no getting away from the fact that a three-year period of hands-on training like this advanced the course of medicine much more than mere book-learning at a university. There is also no getting away from the fact that the patients paid the price both in blood, chime and motions, and in gold. If they couldn't afford the money or found the cure more distasteful than the complaint, they could at least turn either to the seething band of quacks or to the local herbalist.

In the wake of Culpeper, and to meet the growing need as people moved from the countryside towards the maddening crowds of the growing industrial towns, new revolutionaries appeared on the scene. John Wesley added to his soul-saving tracts of evangelism a small treatise called *Primitive Physic; or, An Easy and Natural Method of Curing Most Diseases*. The vital power of God was there, for he stressed that, if man led a good life, nature would supply all that he needed for good health; however, prayer and praise and the use of Primitive Physic could set the lost sheep back on the road towards it. The spreading of Methodist chapels across the length and breadth of the land speaks of his success, just as the gravestones which record truncated lives speak not only of the corruptibility of man but the failure of all types of physic. Prices were rising, times were hard and no one was going to make a decent living by selling hedgerow plants and homespun cures. So the new-wave druggists maintained their links with the grocers, selling their healing wares alongside mops and buckets, while the professions poured scorn on Primitive Physic and Primitive Methodists alike.[2]

Wesley's little book is full of good country sense, and the wisdom of well-tried herbs. His own favourite was Tar Water, from the resin of the North American pines which were also used in the construction of so many of his chapel pews. He had

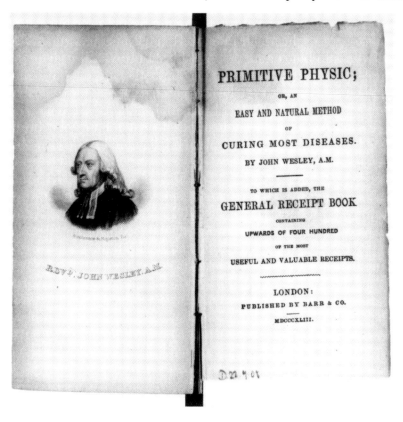

FIGURE 16.1 Frontispiece and title page from John Wesley's *Primitive Physic, or, an Easy and Natural Method of Curing Most Diseases* (1843).

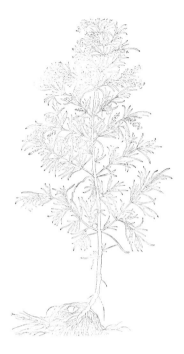

FIGURE 16.2 Rosemary (*Rosmarinus officinalis*): tonic, astringent, diaphoretic,
stomachic, nervine, and a good hair tonic into the bargain!

probably learned of this Indian remedy while preaching in
Georgia, where he had been impressed not only by the broad white
smiles but by the rugged healthful lifestyles of the Indians,
lifestyles which commendably included hard work and regular
immersions in cold water. If Wesley's belief in Primitive Physic and
its Indian antecedents fell on deaf ears amongst the professionals
and would-be professionals in England, there was no immediate
rush to accept them back in their home country. By all accounts,
all the members of the Amerindian tribes living in their natural
state maintained reasonable health. They lived active outdoor lives
in small communities, had a satisfactory and balanced diet and
were tended in sickness and in health by their beliefs and the
knowledge and skills of their shamans. It must be remembered
that between AD 1000 and 1500 great Amerindian civilizations
had formed and in places even urbanized the land. The Anasazi,

Hohokams, Mogollons, Hopwellians and Mississipians came, had their day and passed on, leaving their mounds, irrigation systems, rose-pink cities and stockades to tell of their lifestyles. There is no evidence of catastrophic war, nor of pestilence, but if the latter had come about there is no doubt that the more crowded 'urban' societies would have suffered most. Whatever the reason, the lands of the Anasazi or of any of the other urban cultures were not left fallow for long, for when the Europeans came to the New World they found not an empty land but one overflowing with a diversity of peoples: some 287 principal tribes of Indians in all, hunting, gathering, fishing and many still planting Corn, Beans and Squash; each tribe making the most of everything their particular bit of real estate had to offer, which included the whole armamentarium of local herbal remedies.[3]

Although the New World-trained medics were in great demand and grossly overworked, there were some who took heed of the local cures, for like many of the doctors back home they had been brought up with a good grounding in materia medica, an interest which some developed further, to become doctor-botanists. One of these, Cadwallader Colden, a Scot at one time raised to the elevated position of mayor of New York, was certainly at the periphery of the Ginseng saga. He acted as a staging-post through which colleagues all over the expanding states sent accounts, seeds and cuttings of promising local remedies. These included Cherokee Pinkroot (*Spigelia marilandica*), an excellent vermifuge, Pokeroot (*Phytolacca americana*), only now being reinvestigated as a cure for skin cancer, Wild Geranium (*Geranium maculatum*) for dysentery, and *Lobelia*, which was shown to cure English soldiers of syphilis within a week and therefore gained the specific name of *syphilitica*. Seneca Snakeroot (*Polygala seneca*) had long been employed by the settlers to ease and cure pleurisy and Colden sang its praises as well.[4]

Unfortunately, as already stated, most of the establishment did their best to ignore this 'folk' knowledge and continued to import most of their business. This again left room for the quacks, and in they came, further dragging the claims of Indian physic into disrepute. Their escapades and calamities have now become part of the legends of those pioneer days, though they must have been far less entertaining to their patients at the time. Amongst the baddies there were also goodies like William Byrd (the same that sent Ginseng to Banks), who became a legend in his own right. Byrd was one of the richest landowners in Virginia, who did much to pioneer real Indian Physic by using it not only on himself but on the valuable slaves who kept his plantations and bank balance growing. He believed in the efficiency of Indian knowledge, like James Adair, a successful trader with the Southern Cherokees, who wrote: 'They as well as all other Indian nations, have a great knowledge of specific virtues in simples, applying herbs and plants, on the most dangerous occasions, and seldom if ever fail to

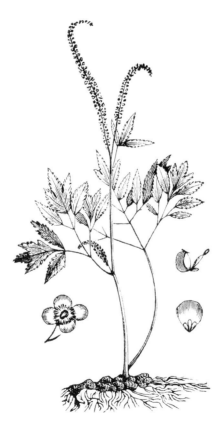

FIGURE 16.3 Seneca Snakeroot (*Polygala seneca*), the American settlers' diaphoretic.

163

effect a thorough cure.'[5] Along with the requested Ginseng, Byrd had sent the excellent vermifuge Jerusalem Oak (*Chenopodium ambrosoides*) to England with news of his two favourites, Indian Physic (*Porteranthrus trifoliatus*) for dysentery and Dogwood Bark (*Cornus florida*), which he used on his many expeditions to cure malaria when they ran out of imported Peruvian Bark.[6]

It wasn't just in the New World that discoveries, or rather re-discoveries, were being made and none were at that time more important than the hidden virtues of one of England's commonest wayside plants, the Foxglove (*Digitalis purpurea*). No mention of the plant is found in Culpeper, and Gerard states: 'The Fox-gloves in that they are bitter are hot and dry with a certaine kind of clensing qualitie joined therewith, yet they are no use, neither have they any place among medicines according to the Antients.'[7] Yet when researched by William Withering for his book *A Botanical*

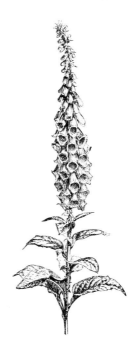

FIGURE 16.4 William Withering's re-discovery, the Foxglove (*Digitalis purpurea*).

164

Arrangement of All the Vegetables Naturally Growing in Great Britain with Descriptions of the Genera and Species according to Linnaeus he had found the contrary, namely that in his native Shropshire this very poisonous plant was used as a diuretic in the treatment of dropsy. He went on and followed his own advice as recorded in the book: 'It is certainly a very active medicine and merits more attention than modern practice bestows on it.'[8] He found backing for its use against dropsy in Yorkshire in Leonhart Fuchs's *De Historia Stirpium* (1542) and discovered that it was used against tuberculosis in the west of England. We must wonder whether he asked why, since it was such an effective and violent purge, it was not in more regular use. Perhaps the answer came in his experiments on turkeys, which demonstrated just how lethal it could be. His painstaking research continued and showed just how right Culpeper had been concerning the harvesting of simples at the correct time and state of development of the plant. Withering found different degrees of activity in the leaves collected at different times of the year. He limited his gathering to the most active period, which he determined was just before seed set; in this way he was able to produce a dried and powdered preparation which allowed for quantifiable dose rates. Once safe in the knowledge of quality control, he went on with great success to treat his patients for oedema and all the other symptoms which made dropsy one of the most uncomfortable diseases of the eighteenth century.

Withering's *Account of the Foxglove* was published in 1785 and is today a highly valued classic of medical history – an honour it richly deserves, for there amongst all the excellent research, case histories, side effects, successes and failures he points firmly in the direction in which research into materia medica should have gone, suggesting 'that the virtues of plants might be learned from the recognition of empirical usages and experience – regardless of the source from which it springs'.[9] Unfortunately few if any took notice of this visionary plea, and many who killed their patients by using large doses of Foxglove as the powerful emetic it was, blamed its folk origin rather than their own Boerhaavian arrogance. Just how many hearts were stimulated back to health, cleansing bodies and minds of the bloat of dropsy, we shall never know;

nevertheless, the world has much to thank William Withering's first patient for. It was she, Helena née Cooke, amateur botanist and botanical artist, who won his heart away from the 'disagreeable ideas' he 'formed of the study of botany' while a student at Edinburgh, then the world's foremost medical school[10] – a medical school well steeped in Boerhaave and echoing the vitalist *vs.* mechanist deliberations of the day. To cite just one of the more memorable debates, we may mention those surrounding John Brown (1735–1780), three times president of the Royal Medical Society of Edinburgh, who defined life as the effect of external stimuli on organisms, diseases either as 'sthenic' if the result of overstimulation, or 'asthenic' if the result of understimulation. His treatments consisted almost exclusively of stimulation, generally with alcohol, or sedation as a rule with opium, and using massive dosages in either case. Even though he eventually died in poverty in London, apparently by his own medicine, his ideas found considerable popularity, to the point of being the subject of a two-day brawl between Brunonians and Anti-Brunonians in Göttingen in 1802.[11]

Notes

1 *Encyclopedia Britannica*, 15th edn (Chicago: Encyclopedia Britannica Inc., 1985).

2 John Wesley, *Primitive Physic, or an Easy and Natural Method of Curing Most Diseases* (London, 1781), in Barbara Griggs, *Green Pharmacy – A History of Herbal Medicine* (London: Robert Hale, 1981, 1987).

3 David J. Bellamy, *Bellamy's New World* (London: British Broadcasting Corporation, 1983); and Harold E. Driver, *Indians of North America* (Chicago: University of Chicago Press, 1969, 2nd edn).

4 Griggs, *Green Pharmacy*.

5 Ibid., p. 138.

6 Griggs, *Green Pharmacy*.

7 Marcus Woodward, *Gerard's Herball – The Essences Thereof Distilled* [from 1636 edition] (1927; London: Spring Books, 1964).

8 Griggs, *Green Pharmacy* p. 144.

9 Ibid., p. 146.

10 Ibid., p. 143.
11 Griggs, *Green Pharmacy.*

General information

Richard Le Strange, *A History of Herbal Plants* (New York: Arco Publishing Co., 1977).

17

Botanical Medicine

Throughout the nineteenth century herbal or, as it came to be known, Botanical Medicine flowered in popularity, thanks to some vociferous, articulate and forthright champions. In America there was Samuel Thomson, son of a poor New Hampshire farmer who learned the basics of his herbal lore from the widow Benson, the local healer. The farm and surrounding wilderness, still peopled with those remnants of local Indian tribes who had survived the onslaught of introduced Old World diseases, became his university and laboratory. One of his own major discoveries was *Lobelia inflata*, a remarkable expectorant, emetic and in the right doses, a pick-you-up. Thomson had learned a healthy distrust of the methods of the professionals, mainly blistering, bleeding and calomel, by the bitter experience of the pain, suffering and death it had failed to alleviate within his and his neighbours' families. After nursing one of his own children back to health when the local doctor had almost given up, he set out on what became a life-long crusade to put Botanic Medicine on the rapidly expanding map of America. It was not an easy road; the profession ridiculed him, trumped up charges against him, took him to court and even had state laws passed to curb his success.

Thomson soldiered on with some triumphs, such as the time when an epidemic of an unknown disease, probably of yellow fever, swept through New Hampshire towns. All his patients survived; many of those treated by the opposition died. The Thomsonian good news spread and his successes finally culminated in his patenting of the 'Improved System of Botanic Practice of

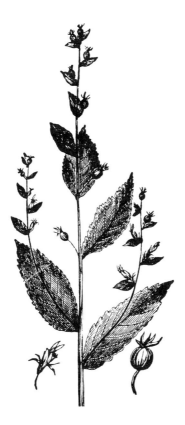

FIGURE 17.1 The favourite of Cadwallader Colden and Dr Thomson – the emetic, expectorant and antispasmodic *Lobelia inflata* (*syphilitica*).

Medicine', a masterful move on his part. His dream was of a countrywide system of trained agents, each with the knowledge and the skill to sell 'Family Rights' (in a country whose very ethic was a Bill of Rights, it was a very saleable word) for twenty dollars. This provided each subscribing family with membership of the Friendly Botanical Society, which allowed him to prepare and use the Thomsonian methods and medicines. The agents took a commission and Thomson kept them well supplied with literature and materia medica from a central warehouse.[1]

You can imagine the outrage of the professionals: teaching uneducated people to kill themselves! We paid good money for our sons to go to medical school and even more good money for our bleeding and our calomel! A countrywide network of commissioned agents, a monopoly of supply and demand! A money-making quacket!

If Thomson had come along at any other time in American history he could well have remained a local herbal doctor. But his was pioneer, self-help medicine, and those were pioneer, self-help times when self-discipline and family ties and rights were all-important. So despite all the 'professional' hullabaloo, by 1839 Thomson had three million faithful followers, all of whom must

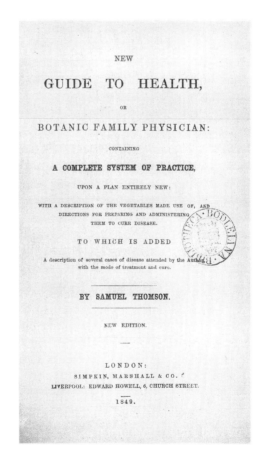

FIGURE 17.2 Title page from Thomson's *New Guide to Health* (1849).

have been or known satisfied customers. What is more, all were able to read and re-read all the stories of success in the *Thomsonian Recorder*.

Success, based on the use of the steam from a hot bath and well-tried herbal remedies which were administered in large doses, brought its own problems, and profligate advertising began to weaken the cause. But the acrimonious attacks of the establishment were muted, at least in part, when many states began to repeal the laws they had passed protecting the same establishment against Thomsonian success.[2]

Others took up the call and likewise began to work wonders. Charles Whitlaw, a landscape gardener from Scotland on a study course at Philadelphia's then, and now, deservedly famous botanic gardens, turned his attentions to Botanic Medicine and soon became an up-market Thomson. He was a scholar and an ardent student of Carl von Linné, the Swedish naturalist whose peripatetic teachings and voluminous publications under his latinized name of Carolus Linnaeus firmly established the binomial (twin Latin name) system, turning the study of natural history into a family of sciences. It was a life-long study, in which he was always fascinated and frustrated by the way in which the good and the bad, the virtuous and the poisonous properties of plants varied from species to species within genera, let alone families. Charles Whitlaw also learned much from the local herbal Indian doctors about plants which Linnaeus had never seen and about their methods of applying the plants' virtues to treat all manner of illness: 'A few heated stones, in the first instance are heaped together, round which something like a soldier's tent is erected. The person or persons to receive the bath are sealed round the stones upon which are thrown herbs, and water sprinkled with the hand.'[3]

From such notes and detailed research, using various herbs found in the Colonies, Whitlaw triumphed first in London and later in many other fashionable English towns, so much so that by 1830 his Vapour Bath Institutions could claim success on a whole range of diseases tackled at all stages in some 60,000 patients. The fact that he patented his methods, used imported American herbs and that his institutions were run by agents and committees showed that he had gleaned much from Thomson, although he never mentioned him in his writings. Thomson steamed and dosed the poor, Whitlaw steamed and suffused the rich. If only they had got together to present a unified botanic front, perhaps they would have been able to convince the profession of the virtue of their ways. Unfortunately, this was not to be.

Another aspiring branch of the alternative line was the so-called Eclectic Medicine. This linked the best of the old with the best of the new, the latter being resinous extracts and concentrates of what were supposedly the plants' active principles. It was the brainchild of one Wooster Beach, who decided to go down the more formal road by creating medical schools and producing graduates who produced more and more concentrates.

Concentrated medicine appealed to the masses, who disliked the immense Thomsonian doses almost as much as they disliked bleeding and mercury. So for a time Eclectic Medicine was the in thing, with drug houses taking up the challenge and the profit. Unfortunately many of these concentrated medicines didn't work, which not only sent the patients back to the crude herbs, but set the ranks of both Thomsonians, the Physico-Medicals – that is Thomson with a pinch of Eclecticism – and the Eclectics on a war which was uncivil in the extreme.[4]

Likewise with homoeopathy, the life-work of one Christian Friedrich Samuel Hahnemann (1755–1843). A largely self-taught polymath in his youth, he later studied and qualified as a physician. For the first half of his life, he alternated periods of medical practice with work as a translator of scientific and literary works, including most of the materia medica available in his day. Profoundly and personally involved in a search for *the* concept of healing, he must have been significantly influenced both by the vitalist traditions which preceded him – the debate concerning which was still raging in his day – and by the scientific developments which he was witnessing in his own lifetime. He was a competent and compassionate physician, whose early ideas on hygiene and patient care were well in advance of what was the norm at the time, and who in daily practice tried to be guided more by empirical and practical principles than by any doctrinal idea. Nevertheless, when he finally formulated his theories and published his fundamental work, the *Organon der rationelle*

Heilkunde, in 1810 – and regardless of how much inspiration he obtained from the Classics, from Paracelsus or from alchemy, the synthesis which resulted was his and exclusively his: it was both a radical departure from anything the healing arts had come up with before – a doctrine rich in mystical connotations, having an uncompromising coherence which made it totally unamenable to adaptation without loss of integrity – and the basis of a healing craft about which the only scientifically verifiable characteristic was the sizeable number of satisfied patients it could boast of.

It is difficult to say exactly what led him to his ideas. It might well have been the realization of the miserable state of that medical science to which he had devoted his life. It might have been the conclusions drawn from the large number of clinical observations he accumulated, or from the numerous pharmacological experiments which he was wont to carry out on himself. It might have been the end result of the exposure to the dozens of theories which were floating around him, most of which were unverifiable and unexplainable with the scientific knowledge available at the time. Whatever he was, Hahnemann was *not* an 'alternative practitioner', but a mainstream physician developing his own methodology at a time when almost all medicine was experimental. Whatever formed his theories, homoeopathy, as he named his method, became one of the significant medical movements in the Western world until the end of the twentieth century, and has yet to be placed in some form of satisfactory perspective.

In spirit, homoeopathy is closer to the hermetic 'science' of the alchemists than to any form of conventional medicine. At its core lies the concept that diseases – or, taken to the extreme, The Disease – are as much a spiritual as a material entity, and as such unobservable and unknowable. What can be observed are the symptoms, not so much of the disease as of the body's reaction to it, a reaction which, far from being predictable and specific to its cause, is uniquely specific to the patient in that particular state in which he finds himself at the time of the diagnosis. This reaction is also the best possible response that the body can offer at the time to the miasma attacking it on the three planes: the physical, the emotional and the mental. Because of this, any attempt at inhibiting the reaction, in other words of suppressing the symptom (which a conventional, or 'allopathic', doctor would describe as curing the specific disease), will only force the body to respond in a less than optimal manner, producing a different, deeper-seated and eventually more damaging symptom, which an allopathic practitioner would erroneously recognize as an entirely different and unconnected ailment. Any pathogen involved is not so much a cause, but an occasion for the body to choose a particular form of reaction over another, and therefore just as much an effect of the disease as any functional tissue damage or metabolic dysfunction that might occur.

What help the homoeopathic practitioner has to offer is that of aiding the body into resolving its diseased status, easing the passage from one morbid state to its 'natural' successor until the disease is either expelled entirely or at least relegated to a lesser chronic symptom, the unavoidable residuum of an irresolvable internal conflict. To this end, the patient is given a remedy which would produce his same symptoms in a healthy individual, with the intent of first intensifying the present phase, and then carrying it through to its necessary conclusion. At this point, a different pathology will appear, and a new treatment suited to it will be applied, the process being repeated every time the symptoms show some significant change. The remedies chosen suit the illness, but in terms of some indefinable vital force rather than through any material effect.

It is this effectively 'spiritual' nature of the remedies that lies behind the most publicized feature of homoeopathy – the extreme dilution of the substances used. To prepare a medicine, the active substance, chosen for its capacity of inducing the relevant symptoms in a healthy subject, is progressively diluted in a neutral medium, and the higher the dilution, the greater the potency. In terms of conventional chemistry, such cures have nothing behind them – literally. Already at the lowest potencies only faint traces of the substance are left in the medicament, and by the relatively modest twelfth centesimal dilution the concentration has fallen below Avogadro's Number – the number of molecules present in a gram molecular weight of a substance, 6.0225×10^{-23}. From this point onwards, whether or not a patient actually encounters a molecule of the active component during his cure becomes matter of statistics, not of pharmaceutical certainty; and yet, dilutions of one-hundred-thousandth centesimal and higher might be prescribed in the most serious and chronic of cases.

In terms of hermetic 'science', on the other hand, the process makes sense. Just as the alchemist hoped to liberate the quintessential spiritual power of a substance by freeing it from the material dross imprisoning it, so the homoeopathic pharmacist can claim to intensify the non-material effects of a remedy by removing the material components affecting it. It is worth mentioning that conventional practitioners of medical systems which have kept a spiritual dimension, for example Ayurveda, are far readier to consider homoeopathy's claims than their Western counterparts.

The implications of such concepts are considerable. First of all, homoeopathy separates itself from any other form of medical practice, whatever its nature, and classifies it by definition as malpractice, for any attempt by doctor or healer to improve the patient's perceivable condition can only by the purest chance avoid being injurious. Second, it makes homoeopathy totally uncompromisable: the distance between it and allopathic medicine is such that any attempt at bridging it will invariably lead to the loss of its basic tenets. It is no wonder, therefore, that homoeopathy has at different times become the focus of acrimonious debates.[5]

As mentioned above, Hahnemann was first a physician and then a homoeopath. The theory arose out of his experiences and grew with them. Compared to the usual treatments of his day, his technique was a spectacular improvement, and spread rapidly in Europe and, even more, in the United States. The good homoeopathic practitioner had to be a good hygienist and a first-class diagnostician, and had to follow his patients closely over lengthy periods of time; it is nor surprising that the patients preferred him to a fast purveyor of purges and cathartics. At the time, Asiatic cholera was sweeping America, and its progress seemed only alleviated by a homoeopathic remedy, Camphor, to be taken in one-drop doses every five minutes in the first stages of diarrhoea and collapse. No wonder the public sat up and took notice; and so did even some members of the medical profession, who began to return to their botanical roots, making use once more of the curative properties of their native herbs.[6]

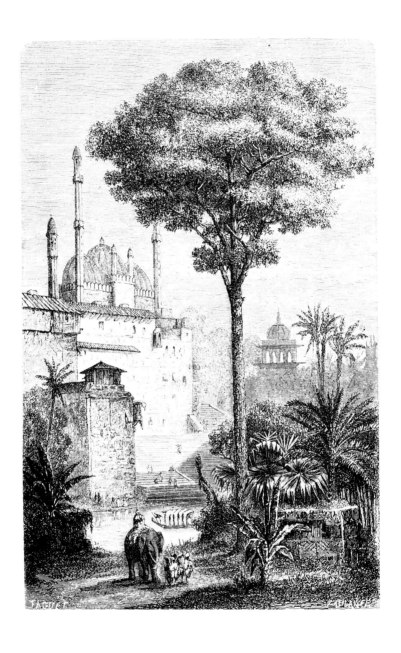

Figure 17.3 The Camphor tree (*Cinnamomum camphora*), ancient spice and one of homoeopathy's answers to cholera.

Homoeopathy took such a hold that as early as 1835 a regular physician by the name of Dr John Bigelar came up with the idea that most diseases are self-limiting and that given a chance they go away of their own accord. It was his way of denigrating the efficacy of the homoeopath's minuscule doses. It probably did exactly the opposite, for society was learning that botanic medicine in all its forms gave the diseased a much better chance than the regular medical practitioners. Success spread an epidemic of jealousy, and contempt spread throughout the whole medical junket: those with the most to lose shouted abuse the loudest. If only Thomson had not been blighted with the failings of human nature, the black bile of melancholy might not have spilled over and the course of the history of botanical and the nascent alternative medicine could have been very different. If only homoeopathy had continued in vogue a little longer, perhaps the whole process of immunization and the understanding of the immunological system might have progressed much faster. Sadly, a botanical canker set in against which even *Lobelia inflata* was not effective, a canker which the medical profession did everything to advance in the public eye.

Unfortunately, homoeopathy carried the seed of its own demise as well. The orthodox practitioner could only try to develop the technique along the intellectual lines which Hahnemann laid down, and while such arguments were defensible at the end of the eighteenth century, they became less and less respectable as the scientific developments of the late nineteenth and early twentieth centuries unfolded; as a result 'pure' homoeopaths found themselves further and further relegated to the ranks of the spiritualist cranks. The eclectic practitioner, who tried to combine homoeopathy with the novel insights in medicine and biology as they became available, had sooner or later, explicitly or implicitly, to deny the philosophy which lay behind the very methods he was trying to keep relevant, regardless of the plethora of inconclusive experiments attempting to find some scientific explanation of their claims – experiments which themselves are to be considered heresy in Hahnemann's terms. In addition, a self-service brand of homoeo-pathy, in which the patient could treat himself 'by numbers', following lists and keys of symptoms, grew enormously in

(a)

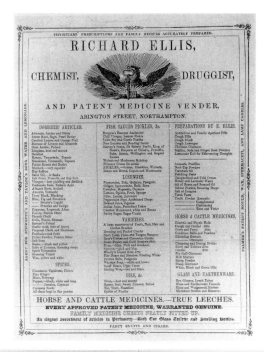

(b)

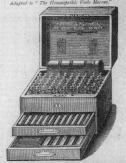

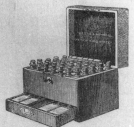

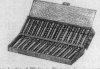

popularity, again especially in the United States. As this dispensed with the most important component of the method, the experienced healer, it helped considerably towards bringing homoeopathy into disrepute. In the middle of the nineteenth century, homoeopathy was one of the most important medical systems in the West. By the beginning of the twentieth, under the attack of the medical profession and the pharmaceutical industry, and unable either to evolve or to justify its existence in scientific terms, it had become a marginal minority interest, classed as a belief rather than as a science. Today, even though it is undergoing a renewed burst of popularity, it remains as before a strange and unexplained craft whose every claim remains unproven, except for the crucial one: that its patients do seem to benefit from it.[7]

Whether homoeopathy is 'right' or 'wrong', whether or not it is still defensible nowadays, or indeed if some of its tenets could be used in a novel synthesis, goes beyond the scope of this book. What is worth pointing out is the resemblance between its concepts and those developed a century and a half later by the various psychoanalytical schools. The idea of a suppressed core malady wrapped in layers of variable symptoms seems like a vague predecessor of the concept of the layers of consciousness; the idea of an intrinsic, non-material property of substances capable of influencing the material world sounds like a precursor of Jung's archetypes. Could it be that Hahnemann, working at a time when the role of the mind as distinct from an essentially religious soul was even more confused than it is at present, was attempting to answer the same questions which later Freud and Jung were faced with, but with tools of his own day which were not adequate to stand the test of time? In this case, as the knowledge of the interactions between mind and body grows, there may well be lessons to be learnt from his legacy.[8]

FIGURE 17.4 (a) Homoeopathic poster: Richard Ellis tradecard; (b) homoeopathy by numbers in a handsome mahogany chest – but Hahnemann would have turned in his grave.

Notes

1 Barbara Griggs, *Green Pharmacy – A History of Herbal Medicine* (London: Robert Hale, 1981, 1987).
2 Ibid.
3 Ibid., p. 195.
4 Griggs, *Green Pharmacy.*
5 *Encyclopedia Britannica*, 15th edn (Chicago: Encyclopedia Britannica Inc., 1985); and Richard Grossinger, *Planet Medicine: From Stone Age Shamanism to Post-industrial Healing* (Boulder, CO, and London: Shambhala, 1982).
6 Griggs, *Green Pharmacy.*
7 Ibid.
8 *Encyclopedia Britannica*, 15th edn; Grossinger, *Planet Medicine*; and R. Ornstein and David Sobel, *The Healing Brain* (London: Macmillan, 1988).

18

URBAN SPRAWL

If it was the pioneer spirit and situation which saw the successful incubation of Botanical Medicine in the New World, it was exactly the opposite environment which did the same in Europe.

At the start of the nineteenth century, about 20 per cent of the people of England and Wales lived in towns of over 5,000 inhabitants. One hundred years later the figure was nearer 80 per cent. Urbanization: was it to be the only hope for servicing the needs of an exploding population, or was it the scourge of humanity? Whatever the answer, it had come to stay and by the end of this sad century it will be the lot of more than 60 per cent of the world's people.

The problems were then as they still remain: the supply of an adequate healthful diet, of potable water and the disposal of human waste, which back in the 1800s meant faeces and urine, for society as a whole was not rich enough to disown rubbish. At one end of the problem great institutions like Covent Garden and Smithfield market did their best, while ships of many lines scoured the Empire for food and its seabird colonies for fertilizer. At the other end of the line (about 36 feet of it in the case of a grown man) rivers like the Thames became open sewers, dangerous to live, let alone govern, beside. In the big stinks of the 1850s blankets soaked in phenol were hung up at the windows of the Palace of Westminster to keep the hot air in and the foetid air out. The most readily available water supply was thus rendered unfit for any consumption; some of it was so ripe, charged with organic matter, that it could be brewed into Wapping Beer.[1]

It wasn't just human waste either; animal excrement added its own colour and texture to street life, when wet a knee-deep quagmire, when dry a potent snuff. It is estimated that in 1830, three million tons of horse exhaust cascaded onto the streets of English towns; by the turn of the century those same streets were composting under ten million tons of the stuff each year. Added to that were the semi-liquid assets of the stock exchange, cow slurry, sheep droppings and the blood and unwanted guts from neighbourhood abattoirs, while in some places pigs vied with human living space in a ratio of three to one. Victorians liked their dogs and their free range eggs just as much as their modern-day counterparts, all adding their bit to the stinking pile. Then there were the coal-fired, multistoreyed tenements, gas works and gas lights, coal-driven manufactories and sweat shops, dust-filled cotton mills, potteries, cutleries and the New Age chemical works, all thrown up in double quick time. All in all, a recipe for disaster, and it came in the form of disease. Streetwise language included tuberculosis, dysentery, pneumonia, scarlet fever, diphtheria, cholera and death in its vocabulary.[2]

There must have been many good men and true within the medical establishment who did their best against the rising tide of urban disease. The truth of the matter was, however, that there weren't enough medics and there wasn't enough knowledge; what is more, the message was plainly written on the mortuary wall: they came, they purged, they bled again and again from birth through to premature death. So it was that the new urban fields were ripe for botanical medicine, and it came via France in the guise of one of Thomson's pupils with the unlikely and highly ridiculable name of Dr Albert Isiah Coffin. A youthful and promising apprentice to the local doctor back in America, he had fallen victim to consumption, tuberculosis or something like it. He was on the point of death, or so his oft-told story went, when he was cured by an old woman from the local Seneca Indian tribe, who by that time had been reduced to a gipsy-like lifestyle. Forsaking mainstream medicine he, in his own words, 'threw in my lot with these roving tribes . . . imbibed their tastes and habits and gleaned from them all I could regarding the herbs, barks etc. with which they were acquainted.'[3]

Coffin later met and learned from Samuel Thomson, recording his many successes in the *Thomsonian Recorder*; then, full of zeal, he set off to heal Europe. Having limited success in France and in London owing to the stranglehold of mainstream medical practice and malpractice, he turned his attention and his considerable energy and power of rhetoric to the pains of the growing towns of industrial England.[4]

There he found instant succes in a Victorian setting in which family and teetotalism were the cornerstones of an evolving, hard-working society which still had its roots in the countryside to which many returned if they could at the weekends and holidays – a countryside which still insinuated itself into the erupting urban sprawl. Unofficial green space, accessible and full of weeds of virtue like Goosegrass (*Galicium aparine*, Pellitory-on-the-wall (*Parietaria officinalis*), Jack-by-the-hedge (*Alliaria petiolata*), Pile-wort (*Ranunculus ficaria*), Lungwort (*Pulmonaria officinalis*), Nipplewort (*Lapsana communis*), Birthwort (*Aristolochia* spp.) and many more. Coffin learned rapidly, seizing every local opportunity and, set against statistics which showed it was healthier to live in the countryside and to be rich, he just had to win. Home-grown simples were backed up by huge imports of New World materia medica, mainly grown on Shaker farms, showing how well the movement was doing back in the homeland. In true Thomsonian fashion he taught the locals once more to make use of their home-grown herbs, recruiting a growing band of male and female practitioners at family parties where ladies served tea and light refreshments. In Dr Coffin's hands, health once more became a family affair.[5]

The establishment hated his every move and trained all their guns on him, but they were on the losing side: the Coffinites were filling the widening gap of health care with more humane treatments and remedies at more humane prices, and on many occasions they were seen to work. The advice he gave also made sense: don't purge the newborn with castor oil, let alone calomel; don't lance gums to ease the natural process of teething; feed them with breast milk, it's nature's way; when constipated, regulate your diet and eat rye bread; corsets and drugs are no good for rickets, let the children have fresh air, good food and take plenty of exercise in the open air. These were the basic tenets of Coffinism, rammed home at every opportunity in lecture, pamphlet and journal, and few people would disagree with any of them today. He also took up the cry against the use of laudanum, which was at that time being sold for all manner of things from all manner of outlets. It found a special use in keeping babies quiet – I well remember gripe water and that only contained alcohol. In Nottingham one member of the town council sold 400 gallons of laudanum a year; no wonder they were called 'druggists'. Opium by any other name would be as addictive, and yet it was so widely used that Mrs Beeton gave advice for dealing with overdoses in many editions of her famous book on household management.[6]

No wonder infant mortality rose to 67 per cent in some towns, where working mothers clubbed together to employ communal wet-nurses to mind their children so that they could return to the loom immediately after giving birth. Women, men and children worked in appalling conditions, their new-born next generation of workers crèched into crowded rooms, dark lives touched rarely by the sun. No wonder that exhausted baby-minders and parents alike turned to the soporific effect of opium to quell the cries of their sick children so they could obtain a good night's sleep or midday nap.[7]

The babies became addicts and died. They died for this and many other reasons and burial was a costly business, so infant burial clubs flourished in every town, and for as little as a penny a week you could insure each frail life so that in the event of early death the bills could be paid. The only problem was that the unscrupulous could make a handsome profit, especially if they subscribed to a number of such clubs: it was an odds-on game in some towns. The Friendly Societies Act of 1846 banned the insurance of any child under the age of six and yet the practice continued apace; by the end of the century 80 per cent of all the nation's children were insured. The companies had hedged their bets. Cot, or at least family bed, deaths were the scandal of the time and 'smothering' or 'overlaying' was the prime cause. As the vast majority occurred on Saturday nights, the reason was probably a mixture of drunken parents and addicted babies, not murder with parental forethought. Dr Coffin was one strong voice

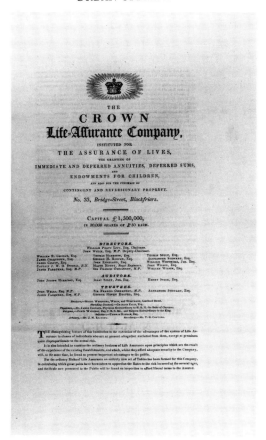

Figure 18.1 Child endowment policies formed a substantial part of the life
assurance companies' trade in Victorian England.

among many who railed against the inadequacies of the law, and
in 1868 the Pharmacy Act was passed, which allowed opium to be
sold only by qualified pharmacists.[8]

Unfortunately for the cause of herbalism, Albert Isiah Coffin
succumbed to the same problems of human nature which afflicted
his never-mentioned mentor. Quarrelling among his supporters
and among the new breeds of botanical medics who burgeoned in
the wake of his immense success opened wounds in the armour of
all their arguments: wounds which the establishment blistered and
bled to their hearts' content.

Yes, there were quacks, and of the worst sort, within the ranks of the herbalists, but Botanical Medicine should have survived in much better heart, for many strong voices within the profession were warning of the problems of the excesses of calomel and bloodletting. Florence Nightingale spoke of the common sight of

> a great grandmother who was a tower of physical vigour, descending into a grandmother perhaps a little less vigorous but sound as a bell and healthy to the core, into a mother languid and confined to her carriage and house, and lastly into a daughter sickly and confined to her bed.[9]

In America Dr Worthington Hooker in a widely publicized prize-winning essay on Rational Therapeutics stated that

> The deliverance from the suffering that formerly came from fruitless medication is of itself no small gain. The amount of life saved would be seen to be very small if only we could obtain correct statistics.[10]

Or to put it in Barbara Griggs's words:

> much of Heroic Medicine had been a ghastly mistake, and that the modern doctor, simply by doing less, achieved more for his patients.[11]

Again, in the more forthright words of Oliver Wendell Holmes to the Massachusetts Medical Society in 1860,

> I honestly believe that [apart from opium and a small number of specific drugs] if the whole materia medica as now used could be sunk to the bottom of the sea, it would be all the better for mankind – and all the worse for the fishes.[12]

The medical profession just had to pull its socks up and tone their dose rate down. They began to do just that, and for example by 1870 the *Buffalo Medical and Surgical Journal* could state that 'Men of high reputation in the profession . . . rely mostly on nature and hygiene.' The good men had probably always been there, but the quacks both Regular and Botanical carried on their war of non-dependence which led eventually to the relegation of herbal medicine to back-street shops. Yet it was probably hygiene in the guise of Victorian civil engineering which did most to change the whole course of medical practice.[13]

Victorian society, for all its faults, and drawing on the immense resources of an Empire upon which the anti-rickettsian sun never set, slowly at first and then majestically began to solve the problem. They made and installed flush toilets, they dug and laid cathedral-like trunk sewers with branches out to every stool of potential corruption. They built vast works which collected and discharged the sewage out into rivers and estuaries below the towns' water intakes. These stupendous feats of civil and civilizing engineering, though out of sight and so out of mind, deserve world heritage status just as much as the pyramids of Egypt or the cities on the spice routes of the past – as does the handle of the pump in Broadwick Street, London W1.

The cholera epidemics of the early 1800s which swept the urbanizing world found the medical profession entirely wanting: bleeding and purgation simply exacerbated the dire symptoms. Here again the botanical medicorps had to come to their aid. In America the homoeopathic use of camphor by the hourly drop was such a success that, though ridiculed at first, the medical profession had eventually to admit to a Convention of the American Medical Association 'That camphor had been one of the most valuable remedies used in the treatment of cholera';[14] while in England Coffin published daily accounts of his successes and others' failures in his *Bulletin of Health*. In fact, he eventually had to cure himself, and did so using *Lobelia*, composition powders, stomachic bitters and much Cayenne Pepper.[15]

It was, however, the brilliant detective work of Dr John Snow which traced the source of what, thanks to him, became London's last cholera epidemic. Though others scoffed at the absurd idea of such a virulent disease being carried by water, Snow removed the handle from the offending Broadwick Street pump and the scourge of cholera was conquered. From that momentous day on, it was up to the civil engineers and scientists, who turned their awesome powers to the problem and solved it by using simple sand filters backed up by steam pumps, housed in brick and marble palaces of cleanliness. The first modern national health systems were thus gradually put in place and the disease and death rate began to fall away. The decline in tuberculosis in the second half of the century was entirely due to the improvements in hygiene, which also accounted for about half the total decline in the death rate over that period. All this despite the fact that, for example, in 1901 in Finsbury it was estimated that 10 per cent of all the milk cows produced tubercular milk and in 1903, 32 per cent of the milk on sale contained pus and 40 per cent dirt. There was still a long way to go, for at the outbreak of the First World War probably one-third of all wage earners in England and Wales were below Rowntree's poverty line, or to put it in his words, they lived in 'a state of bare physical efficiency'.[16]

Thomas Malthus in his famous *Essay on Population* published in 1798 had casually included great towns amongst the positive checks to population, along with wars, plagues, famines, extreme poverty and other miseries – a gamut of inequalities which are today the only thing slowing down the population explosion in the so-called Third World, where even the World Health Organization admits that when sanitary conditions are rudimentary and disease endemic, diet, or lack of it, may be the crucial factor in infection. It is perhaps little wonder that it is in these backwaters of human endeavour that Botanic Medicine still flourishes today.

Notes

1 Anthony S. Wohl, *Endangered Lives – Public Health in Victorian Britain* (London: Dent, 1983).
2 Ibid.
3 Barbara Griggs, *Green Pharmacy – A History of Herbal Medicine* (London: Robert Hale, 1981, 1987), p. 200.
4 Griggs, *Green Pharmacy*.
5 Ibid.
6 Wohl, *Endangered Lives*; and Griggs, *Green Pharmacy*.
7 Griggs, *Green Pharmacy*.
8 Ibid.
9 Ibid., p. 237.
10 Ibid., pp. 237–8.
11 Ibid.
12 Ibid.
13 Ibid., p. 238.
14 Ibid., p. 229.
15 Griggs, *Green Pharmacy*.
16 Wohl, *Endangered Lives*, p. 45.

19

Survival, and the Unfit

Throughout the latter part of the nineteenth century, apart from sanitation and public hygiene, one other factor appeared to be making major inroads into the death toll due to disease: it was called immunization. Thanks to the pioneer work of Louis Pasteur, which culminated in the acceptance of the germ theory of disease, the sciences of bacteriology, virology and immunology were born.

In 1798 the first vaccine was produced by Edward Jenner, a British physician who noticed that the virus of cowpox (called *Vaccinia*) when inoculated into humans could provide lasting protection from one of our own most ancient and disfiguring diseases, smallpox. The arguments both for and against immunization have waxed and waned ever since and will continue so to do for a long time yet. In the early years one of its most vociferous and without doubt scientifically competent opponents was Alfred Russel Wallace.

Wallace was born the year after Pasteur and like him spent a lifetime accurately observing the detail of things natural. He shared the honour, along with Charles Darwin, of opening the world's eyes to the concept of evolution by natural selection, and despite the fact that he and all his family were vaccinated, in his later years he took up the cause of the anti-vaccination lobby. All around him he saw the basically Malthusian relationship between the environmental conditions in which the poor existed and the incidence of the killer smallpox. Indeed, it was the writings of Thomas Malthus which had inspired both Darwin and Wallace in

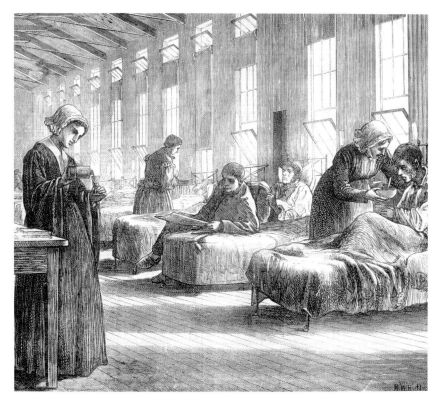

FIGURE 19.1 A nineteenth-century hospital isolation ward. It was against the scourge of epidemics that Western health care won its finest battle, through improvements in hygiene and sanitation and through vaccination.

their formative years. Wallace observed that other diseases like cholera, typhus and leprosy had already been greatly reduced in the West, and he could see no reason why other forms of disease would not die out if living and hygienic conditions were improved.

Why, he asked, take the risks involved in spreading a disease by inoculating practically every person who might in the ordinary course of life have escaped from it? By 1853 nobody could escape from vaccination for it had become compulsory by law, and in 1867 legislation made non-compliance subject to prosecution. Lacking, as he readily admitted, medical knowledge, Wallace turned his attention to the published statistics of success and safety, where he discovered both falsification and rank exaggeration. His indignation culminated in the following statement which he made after giving evidence to the Royal Commission on Vaccination set up in 1890 to investigate the many allegations of serious side effects and the accruing evidence that long-term protection was not ensured. He pointed out that more than half the Commission were doctors and wrote that they were

> so ignorant of statistics and statistical methods that one great doctor held out a diagram, showing the same facts as one of mine, and asked me almost triumphantly how it was that mine was so different. After comparing the two diagrams for a few moments I replied that they were drawn on different scales, but with that exception I could see no difference between them. The other diagram was on a greatly exaggerated vertical scale, so that the line showing each year's death rate went up and down with tremendous peaks and chasms, while mine approximated more in a very regular curve. But my questioner could not see this simple point; and later he recurred to it a second time, and asked if I really meant to tell him that those two diagrams were both accurate; when I said that, though on different scales, both represented the same facts, he looked up at the ceiling in an air which plainly said: 'If you will say that you will say anything.'[1]

Despite his standing in Victorian scientific circles, Wallace's stance alongside the anti-vaccination lobby labelled him as a crank. The only satisfaction he got from all his efforts was that nobody could seriously challenge his figures. Would that Wallace had lived to read the review in the *British Medical Journal* in 1964, cited by his biographer Harry Clements:

> . . . *The British Medical Journal*, 28th November 1964, an editorial appearing under the heading *Neurological Complications of Smallpox Vaccinations*, and after a detailed review of the various illnesses which might follow vaccination special emphasis was laid on the neurological complications. That these serious nervous disorders complicated the vaccination procedure was frankly admitted, as also was the fact that medical men have been aware of these dangerous complications for a great many years. And the more recent cases were also discussed: 'In January 1962 smallpox became epidemic in South Wales. Forty-five cases were reported, with seventeen deaths. Mass vaccination of 800,000 people took place, and thirty-nine patients with neurological complications were seen.' All these cases were carefully assessed by two doctors, and the journal in summing up made this significant statement: 'These authors draw attention to

the paucity of accurate and up-to-date information on neurological sequelae of Jennerian vaccination.'

In further comment on the changing opinions about the vaccination the journal went on: 'The decision to postpone primary vaccination from the first year of life to the second and subsequent years is a sound move for a number of reasons. It should reduce the risk from post-vaccinal encephalitis; it should eliminate virtually all deaths and most of the severe reactions due to generalised vaccinia.' With equal emphasis it stated: 'Smallpox vaccine does not give lifelong protection, as is often supposed . . . '[2]

This story perhaps encapsulates the arguments for and against the in-vogue claims both of regular orthodox medicine and of herbal traditional medicine. Vested interests, despite Hippocratic Oaths and age-old traditions, will justify or vilify the means long before any end is in sight. The end of the smallpox saga came in 1979 when the World Health Organization could officially back statements to the effect that since smallpox was no longer endemic, routine vaccination (with all its problems) was no longer necessary. The combined attack of better living conditions and a worldwide programme of vaccination has banished one of the oldest enemies of humankind to the culture flask, if not to the wall of extinction.

The fact that today, at least in the Western world, most children are vaccinated against diphtheria, rubella, whooping cough, measles and polio speaks of the public acceptance of the process. Likewise, the fact that all high-risk itinerant travellers have yellow pages appended to their passports which record vaccinations against yellow fever, cholera, typhoid, paratyphoid and in an increasing number of cases hepatitis, speaks against the fears of Wallace and the anti-vaccination lobby for the claims of the medical profession. However, it must also be borne in mind that at that time from both without and within the profession there was a good deal of controversy about the use of drugs in the treatment of illness. Joining in the criticism, Wallace had written: 'Our orthodox medical men are profoundly ignorant of the subtle differences of the human body in health and disease, and can thus in many cases do nothing which nature could not cure if assisted by the proper conditions.'[3]

Wallace had himself been cured of bronchial asthma by adherence to a high-protein diet, the so-called Salisbury Diet, which to this day helps many sufferers. It must also be realized that Wallace believed that there is nothing in nature which is not useful.

> On his principle the purpose and use of all parasitic diseases including those associated with pathogenic germs, is to seize on the less adapted and less healthy individuals – those who are slowly dying and are no longer of value in the preservation of the species and therefore to a certain extent inferiors to the race by requiring food and occupying space needed for the fit.[4]

Rough justice indeed for those deemed less fit; and so the medical profession strove within the new horizons of allopathy to find what came to be known as 'magic bullets', which would cure with the least amount of killing, and to hang with the evolution of the perfect organism.

It was during this time that Jesse Boot gave up the presidency of the Eclectic, Botanic, Medical and Phrenological Institute of Derby and started to set up his own empire of Boots Cash Chemists. In his own words, penned later, 'I thought the public would welcome new chemists' shops in which a greater and a better variety of pharmaceutical articles could be bought at cheaper prices.'[5] Whether he was inspired by the arguments of splinter groups within the herbal movement, by the increasing cost of importing the eclectic concentrates from America, or by the pressure of the new chemotherapeutics is not clear, but Sir Jesse brought modern pharmaceutics to the high street. In September 1911 he and his wife declined their invitation to the opening of the British Herbal Association School.

The human organism, being far from perfect in both the physical and the moral sense, was open to all sorts of infections both acute and chronic, and there was then still none more worrying than syphilis. Mercury had worked and was still working for some and causing havoc for others, so it was not surprising when the latest wonder drug, an arsenical called Salvarsan, soon showed its side effects: jaundice, kidney disease, optic atrophy, anaphylactic shock and arsenical dermatitis, which could skin the bloated patient alive. The pleas of the National Association of Medical Herbalists that they had successfully cured thousands of cases in all its stages went unheeded, as on the syphilis front of the First World War legislation made it illegal for any but medical practitioners to treat the disease. Meanwhile pneumonia, puerperal fever and meningitis were raging through the desperate clientele on both sides of the argument. The only difference was that if they died under the care of a regular physician, few questions would be asked, except perhaps by the physician; while if they died while under the care of a medical herbalist, questions might well be asked at a very expensive Crown Inquest.

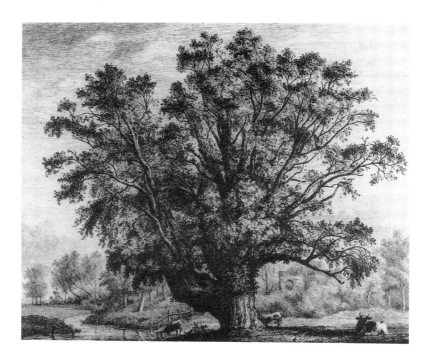

FIGURE 19.2 The Willow (*Salix* spp.), whose decoction had long been known to give relief from the fevers arising from the damp places in which it grew, has given its name to the main component of aspirin and its related febrifuges, salicylic acid.

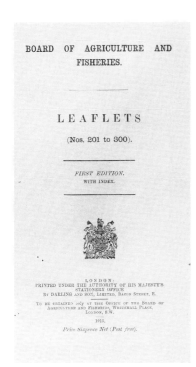

Leaflet No. 288.

BOARD OF AGRICULTURE AND FISHERIES.

LEAFLETS

(Nos. 201 to 300).

FIRST EDITION.
WITH INDEX.

LONDON:
PRINTED UNDER THE AUTHORITY OF HIS MAJESTY'S
STATIONERY OFFICE
BY DARLING AND SON, LIMITED, BACON STREET, E.

TO BE OBTAINED only AT THE OFFICE OF THE BOARD OF
AGRICULTURE AND FISHERIES, WHITEHALL PLACE,
LONDON, S.W.

1915.

Price Sixpence Net (Post free).

BOARD OF AGRICULTURE AND FISHERIES.

The Cultivation and Collection of Medicinal
Plants in England.

Medicinal herbs have been cultivated in this country for centuries, and in the middle ages were grown in kitchen gardens attached to monastic establishments and the mansions of noblemen. At the present day materia medica (or drug) farms exist at Mitcham, Carshalton, Hitchin, Ampthill, Long Melford, Steppingley, Market Deeping, and Wisbech, but for many years the main source of British drugs has been Mid-Europe, particularly Germany and Austria-Hungary.

During recent years the acreage devoted to drug cultivation in Britain has been more and more restricted by competition with wild foreign products, and the result has been a slow but sure ousting of British grown drugs from the market. The advent of a European war has completely changed the situation, and an effort on the part of growers and drug merchants may largely secure for England the collection and cultivation for the future of medicinal plants which can for the present no longer be imported from central Europe. Supplies of drugs, especially of Belladonna leaves and root, are much in demand, but in the case of other Continental drugs grown in England the shortage is not so serious.

The price of Belladonna has risen seriously (more than 100 per cent.) since the outbreak of war (*see* p. 5), and as it takes at least two years to grow this drug in quantity the drug grown next year is likely to realize high prices. This applies in lesser degree to chamomiles, dill, dandelion, and valerian. The prices of colchicum, digitalis, fennel, henbane, stramonium, and " botanical herbs " must also be considerably affected.

The limited outlet for most drugs makes overloading the market a comparatively easy matter, and any grower who proposes to devote attention to the cultivation of medicinal plants should give the matter careful consideration before embarking on it to any serious extent. For a number of growers, however, who can successfully raise good crops, handsome profits should be made in the near future.

Co-operation. — The most important drug industry—cinchona bark production—has witnessed quite recently the fruits of co-operation between producer and manufacturer in restricting the output within reasonable limits. So far, consumers appear to be unaffected, while all other handlers

FIGURE 19.3 Under pressure of war, some prejudices started to break down: this 1914 Board of Agriculture leaflet aimed to encourage the growth and collection of medicinal plants.

It seems strange that this should have been so when it is realized that at the outbreak of war in 1914 the then Board of Agriculture and Fisheries had issued a pamphlet on *The Cultivation of Medical Plants in England*. Despite the fact that the Association had not been consulted, the public response had been enormous and the booklet certainly helped fill the gap of materia medica which had been in the main imported from the Continent. One particularly important product of this herbal home front was onions, to be used as an antiseptic for suppurating wounds. In 1916 the government urgently asked for tons of them, and offered the munificent price of 1s a pound, so highly were they prized by the front-line surgeons. Those odoriferous bulbs were used to great effect, along with the adsorptive and healing power of Sphagnum Moss, which was collected wherever it grew in abundance from Scotland to British Columbia (in the latter region it had long been employed as diapers for Indian babies, who rarely suffered from nappy rash). Another herb which found favour on the front where gas attacks had occurred was Lily-of-the-valley (*Convallaria majalis*). It was used as a cardiac tonic, for it not only had that smell of garden corners which will be forever England, but also a digitalis-like action for which today's serviceman's atropine syrette (the self-injection device all armed forces issue against poison gas) is intended.

Thanks to these stories of success, and to two stalwart ladies, Maud Grieve and Hilda Leyel, and many others, the public interest in herbal remedies outlasted the war effort. The end result was the setting up in 1927 of the Society of Herbalists in its headquarters, Culpeper House, Runton St, London W1. In those days herbalists' shops like that of Potter and Clarke's in Farringdon Road – presided over not by Dame Trot but by a Miss Oakley, as Barbara Griggs so fragrantly records – attracted a wide cross-section of customers:

> Office girls anxious to lose weight came in to have made for them a mixture containing Bladderwrack (*Fucus vesiculosus*) – that black rubbery seaweed with the round pod-shaped bubbles which children love to pop – believed to counter obesity by stimulating the thyroid gland. Tired businessmen dropped in for a tonic made out of Kola (*Cola* spp.) – as stimulating as caffeine – and Damiana (*Turnera diffusa* var. *aphrodisiaca*) which, as its official name suggests, is believed in Mexico to be especially good for tired businessmen.[6]

However, throughout this time both the herbalists and the regular practitioners had more to worry about than tired businessmen and inquests on the deaths of patients. All, and especially the latter, were open to infection from their own patients. A prick or scratch could bring the terror of systemic

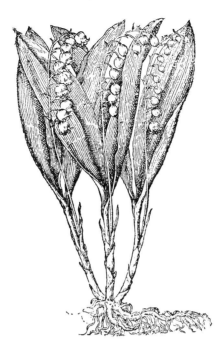

FIGURE 19.4 Lily-of-the-valley (*Convallaria majalis*), conscripted to the trenches as a remedy against gas attacks.

infection and even of gas gangrene raging through their own bodies. Some turned to Onions, perhaps even backed up by a handful of blowfly maggots, which had been used with success in the trenches to clean up wounds. Others turned to the new rage – specific serums and vaccines produced *de novo* as new infections turned up on the scene. Some of these worked, but many failed miserably, so much so that in *The Practitioner* in 1936 a pharmacologist described them as 'one of the greatest delusions of a generation' and further stated 'few now regard them as anything but a danger in the treatment of acute and generalised infections.'[7]

As I myself (DJB) write, I am aware of a scar on my left arm where for three agonizing weeks drainage tubes protruded from a persistent abscess. Then Dad came home from the shop with 'May & Baker 693', one of the then new sulphonamide-containing wonder drugs. Twenty-four hours later – no more tubes, no more lancets, no more hot fomentations – my arm was on the mend. I (DJB) was born in 1933 in Queen Charlotte's Hospital in London, where the first sulphonamide, Prontosil Red (researched and developed by the brilliant young Swiss biochemist Paul Ehrlich) had reduced the death rate from puerperal fever from 20 to 5 per cent. My mother, who had suffered fron anaemia during her pregnancy, had been fed on raw liver, a cure recently discovered, along with the role of pancreatic insulin in diabetes. 1928 had seen Fleming's miraculous discovery of penicillin and my brother, three years my senior, had been taken to meet one of my father's night school friends, Lewis Holt, who was working in Fleming's laboratory at St Mary's hospital in Paddington.

These were heady times for medicine, and especially for the pharmaceutical industries. Allopathy and its 'magic bullets' appeared to hold the key to universal health and to multinational wealth. Botanical Medicine and herbalists all of a sudden began to take on a folksy and outdated appearance, except perhaps in Germany where despite a very lucrative drug industry Adolf Hitler aided the passing of a law which gave naturopaths and herbalists almost equal status with doctors and surgeons; in France, too, the *herboristes* (herbalists) found increasing national support. In beleaguered Britain, though, things herbal went from bad to worse. The 1941 Pharmacy and Medicines Act removed the right of the National Association of Medical Herbalists to do what they were set up to do: they could no longer legally supply their patients with herbal medicines. They took their complaints to the highest authorities but to no avail. More pressing matters overtook the government, for the Second World War demanded the manufacture of penicillin on a massive scale, and thanks to the work of Howard Florey, Ernest Chain and their colleagues, the pharmaceutical industry came up with the goods. They grew *Penicillium chryso-genium* successfully in deep culture, and so the Allied armies marched in to save Europe – some, fittingly, through Salerno – almost immune from the effects of venereal disease. There were deaths and debilitating side effects, but this was war against an age-old enemy. Moral codes were redrafted as the age of antibiotics opened the door to Streptomycin, isolated from soil, and with a stream of new biosynthetic (i.e. formed by bacterial fermentation manipulated by controlling the growth medium) and semi-synthetic (produced by chemically altering the structure of 6-amino-penicillic acid) chemicals, bespoke antibiotics were upon us.

New-rage pharmacists and old-style herbalists alike forgot that these were in the main natural products which had been employed back in Classical times, as recorded in the Ebers Papyrus; likewise 2,500 years ago the Chinese healers had used mouldy Soya Bean curds to treat skin infections. Of all the twentieth-century developments, antibiotics more than any other should have forged links between herbalism and modern medicine, not produced new rifts and divisions. So indeed should immunization, which can be regarded as no more than an extension of the natural process of passive immunization, the way by which primate and rodent foetuses via the placenta and hoofed animals via the colostrum gain immunity from their mothers at least for the first vital months of their lives.

If only these things, which must have been known, had been put to creative use then perhaps Aneurin Bevan, visionary statesman that he was, when drafting plans for the National Health Service would have included herbalists within its remit. The fact that he didn't is particularly hard to understand, since in the post-war years there was good news on the herbal medicine front. Many of the pharmaceutical companies appeared to be turning away from the magic bullets of chemotherapy towards reinvestigating at least some of those 'impure' whole plants.

Notes

1 A. R. Wallace, *Vaccination – A Delusion; Its Penal Enforcement – A Crime* (1898) in Harry Clements, *Alfred Russel Wallace* (London: Hutchinson, 1983).
2 Clements, *Alfred Russel Wallace*, pp. 140–1.
3 Ibid., pp. 147–8.
4 Ibid., pp. 146–7.
5 Stanley Chapman, *Jesse Boot of Boots the Chemist* (London, 1974), in

Barbara Griggs, *Green Pharmacy – A History of Herbal Medicine* (London: Robert Hale, 1981, 1987), p. 243.
6 Griggs, *Green Pharmacy*, p. 268.
7 Linnel 'Further examples of the misuse of common remedies', *The Practitioner* (1936), p. 212.

20

IATROGENICS AND GERIATRICS

Chemotherapeutics supposedly began when Mithridates IV, king of Pontus on the Black Sea (120–63 BC), out of fear of being poisoned, experimented with animal and vegetal poisons and tried to immunize himself by taking increasing but sublethal dosages of the poisons he had tested on his slaves. The whole affair backfired when, defeated repeatedly by Rome and under siege by his own mutinous troops led by his son, he tried to commit suicide by poisoning – and failed miserably, so that he had to order one of his mercenaries to kill him.[1]

Apologies, we are digressing; it is almost the end of the story.

Chemotherapeutics really began with Paul Ehrlich (1854–1915), who involved himself early in his career in studies in immunity, and developed the theory that it depended on specifically adapted molecular side-chains on proteins. He also showed that immunity to toxic substances in mice could be increased to thousands of times its normal value by slowly increasing exposure to them. He eventually developed an organic arsenical for combating the spirochaetes of syphilis and yaws. Salvarsan (a.k.a. 606) was ready in 1910, and became available for general use after the first instance of large-scale medical testing, to prove the suitability of what was suspected to be a potentially toxic substance.[2]

Up to then, testing had been a long-term trial and error process which had eventually come up with adequate but not excessive dose rates which every student of pharmacy had to learn by rote. It was in part his or her job and liability to check the dose rate on those hurriedly scribbled prescriptions, a double check on errors which could prove fatal. Now, with new, never before heard of substances appearing on the market, the thousands of years of trial and error testing had to be circumscribed by laboratory assays with the use, unethical however well regulated, of millions of animals. Here also began the further demise of the use of herbal remedies: either one had to accept that long-term use and re-use gave old plant drugs scientific and legal acceptability, or they had to be tested all over again and eventually perhaps labelled with all their contents. If it was expensive to test a single new chemical, how about testing the simple, even in its eclectic form, let alone with all the botanical dross that went with it! To test a whole new plant drug, even if it had been used in Antiquity, would cost billions; indeed, if one had to list on the packet all the chemicals which give Garlic or Broccoli their distinctive taste, many of the flavourful components would be looked upon as poisons. Test them, nature's own food additives, would become the cry, and thank goodness for all those slaves and all those clay tablets. . . .

It was all very well to argue that with the plant simple you got not dross, but the whole tonic package, the active living principle of cytoplasm, sap and roughage; that the chemically produced drugs were of a single molecular type and so more readily caused allergy and engendered greater resistance in the target pathogen than the more diverse natural products; that the new drugs had not stood the test of time. These arguments and more were aired *ad nauseam*, but the fact of the matter was that once you had spent all the money on research and development, you could patent a chemical but you couldn't patent a plant.

Yet in the 1920s, right in the middle of the chemotherapeutic revolution, one of the biggest drug houses in America, Eli Lilley, began marketing a useful decongestant for asthma and a stimulant of the central nervous system: it was Ephedrine, active constituent of the Joint Pine, *Ephedra*, the pollen of which had laid so long in that grave in Shanidar. And in 1942 Harold Randall Griffith and G. Enid Johnson were opening up new vistas in heart surgery by the use of curare as a muscle relaxant – a major and exciting breakthrough, but curare extracted from the vines and lianas found growing in tropical rainforests had been used for millennia by Amerindian tribes as a fish and an arrow poison.[3]

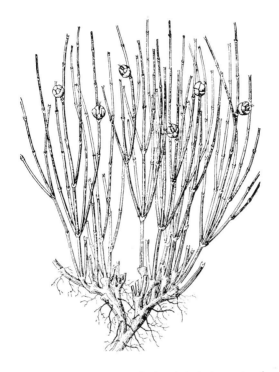

FIGURE 20.1 The Joint Pine (*Ephedra sinica*), the anti-asthmatic that spearheaded the resurgence of botanical pharmaceuticals in the 1920s.

At the same time, at the height of the Second World War, just as the Philippines were falling to the Japanese, Colonel Arthur F. Fisher, wracked with malaria, smuggled seeds of cultivated *Cinchona* out from Java to America, from whence their ancestors had come. One of the main enemies in that particular theatre of war was malaria, and at the time Java produced the world's best *Cinchona* bark, then the only prophylactic for that age-old scourge of people, white, yellow, black, brown or red. So began a true-life adventure acted out high in the Andes by a group of unsung heroes, botanists, naturalists, geographers, mining engineers and marines, who, with no time to start new plantations, explored, toiled and even gave their lives scouring the precipitous slopes of the High Andes for adequate supplies of Peruvian Bark, a plant product which had after its rediscovery by a Jesuit missionary in 1633 been

203

doing trojan service in the alleviation of malaria across Christendom, thanks to the high concentration of the alkaloid we now know as quinine.[4]

The story of the Fever Fighters must be amongst the most fantastic in the annals of economic botanical exploration. They were led by Dr William C. Steer, botanist with the American Board of Economic Warfare. Amongst some of the most awe-inspiring scenery in the world and immense physical hardship at altitudes which make even the fittest gasp for breath and where

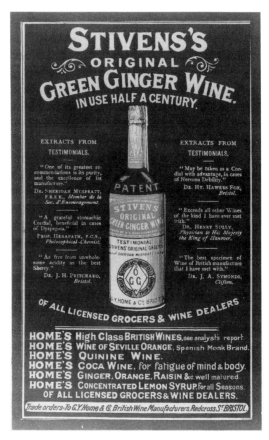

FIGURE 20.2 Quinine wine, coca wine . . . the two best-known Andean simples were well settled in usage as tonics long before they attained their modern importance.

equatorial hypothermia is a silent killer of the night, they found the precious *Cinchona* trees growing on precipitous cliffs. Locating, harvesting and transporting the wet bark was a nightmare which opened up the terrain to massive erosion and the workers to a plethora of diseases. They also found, like Culpeper and Withering before them, that biological variation was a problem, variation not only between the different species of *Cinchona* but also between different localities and even different stands when it came to the all-important yield of quinine, cinchodine, cinchonidine and quinidine. The latter was then in great demand for use in certain types of heart disease; the other three were used in the manufacture of Totaquine (still a successful antimalarial), a product which must contain at least 7 per cent quinine to be effective. (One of the earliest formulations we have for its use is thanks to Cardinal de Lugo: 'against quartan and tertian fevers accompanied by shivers, two drachms of the finely ground and sifted bark mixed in a glass of strong white wine three hours before the fever is due.'[5] These instructions were included in packets of Jesuit Bark which pilgrims took home with them from ague-wracked Rome to the ague-wracked rest of Europe.)

The fieldworkers of the Economic Warfare Board found that the best yields could be obtained from specific sites and specific localities between 8,000 and 10,000 feet above sea level, in areas in which there was adequate precipitation, which meant that it rained hard every day. In order to obtain sufficient supplies they employed the skills and knowledge of the locals and their mules, who could move with ease (but not without accident and disease) through the impossible terrain. They unfortunately had less success with the real 'locals' of the Oriente, the Jivaros, whose ancestors had pioneered the use of both curare and *Cinchona* perhaps 20,000 years before, when they had moved into the area while the world was still in the final grips of the last Ice Age and the rainforest was spreading back from montane and riverine refuges to reclothe what had been the savannahs of Amazonia. Above all, the scientists found, as the Incas had before them, that the only way to exploit the riches of the forest without harming the integrity of its resources was to set up small camps connected by simple walking trails which could then be supplied and serviced by the porters as they returned to collect the next crop of life-saving bark. If the tracks were opened up for traffic even to the hardy American Jeep, erosion soon brought the whole operation to a sticky end. So it was that the Allied armies were at least in part supplied with the bitter bark which helped them through to victory over Japan.[6] (It is also of interest to note that at the same time thousands of other unsung war heroes were busy tapping the latex of another rainforest tree, *Hevea brasilensis*, which cushioned the same war effort on rubber tyres.)

Despite such successes, the pleas of the then National Institute of Medical Herbalists and the British Herbal Union to be part of the British national health system, as we have already seen, fell on deaf ears. Those who legislate on these matters may have missed the point, but not so the pharmaceutical industry: plant products once more became all the rage, and very soon good pharmacognosists (scientists who knew their materia medica) were in short supply as age-old remedies were hauled out of the undergrowth into the light of modern research and media exposure.

The Green Hellebore, the plant which must never be taken with Mandrake, came under scrutiny once more and was shown to yield alkaloids effective against high blood pressure. The Swiss company Ciba-Geigy brought Reserpine onto the rising market in 1954. At first the product was extracted from the Indian Snakeroot, as it had been for centuries in the Caribbean where it was used as a sedative and a hypertensive. They soon learned to synthesize it – only to find that the natural product caused less patient problems and was cheaper to produce.[7]

Problems were looming on the horizon, for it may be easy to patent a pure synthetic chemical and so recoup the escalating costs of research, development and screening, but how can you patent a plant or the accumulated knowledge of 20,000 years? How could you, under mounting public concern (fanned by the superabundance of tablets and tabloids) over the new iatrogenic (drug- and doctor-induced) diseases which were beginning to fill more and more hospital beds in America and in Europe, ever screen all the myriad chemical components of a plant?

The trouble was that wherever the industry looked within the family of plants, they found a medicine chest overflowing with

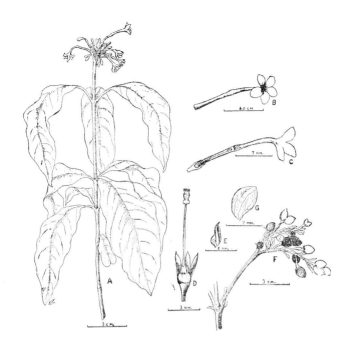

FIGURE 20.3 Indian Snakeroot (*Rauwolfia serpentina*), the Mahatma Gandhi's bedtime drink and highly effective against hypertension.

promise, giving scientific substance to herbal substances which had been in use across the centuries. Africa became a fount of hope. Another liana, this time from the rainforests of Nigeria (what little was left of them), produced the highly toxic Calabar Bean, *Physostigma venenosum*, which had been used in West Africa and in Madagascar (now down to its last 5 per cent of rainforest) as a trial-by-ordeal poison to determine guilt or innocence. This herbal ducking-stool is now a major tool of ophthalmology and is used in the treatment of glaucoma, as the physostigmine it contains produces protracted dilation of the pupil of the eye. From Madagascar too came the Rosy Periwinkle, *Catharanthus roseus*, now the species *célèbre* of herbal medicine. Researched in the depth it deserved, it was shown to contain vincristine and vinblastine, just two of what look like a whole family of drugs which are in their synthetic form already breathing longer life into 'terminal' cases of childhood leukaemia and Hodgkins' disease. *Strophanthus*, a number of species of which were used in arrow poisons, provides a source of ouabain, a stimulant used in cases of acute heart failure and cardiac oedema. African Snakeweed has now replaced its American counterpart as a source of reserpine, while in contrast the American May Apple, re-researched, is yielding a resin which may cure venereal warts and even come to the aid of people with AIDS. And – news to make all Thomsonians turn in their coffins – a species of *Lobelia*, Indian Tobacco, is now used to cure those addicted to the Virginian variety.[8]

Yet perhaps in all this the most significant discovery during this decade of the ascendancy of plants was that relating to human hormones. With the successful identification and isolation of insulin, the active principle of pancreatic tissue, back in 1923, the

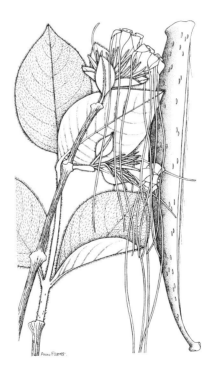

FIGURE 20.4 *Strophanthus kombe.*

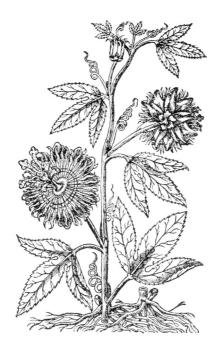

Figure 20.5 The May Apple (*Passiflora incarnata*).

search had begun for other useful products from slaughterhouse offal. Extraction proved very expensive and commercially almost impossible – for example, it took a tonne of bulls' testicles to provide a paltry 300mg of pure testosterone. Russell E. Marker, a brilliant biochemist, came to the amazing conclusion that it would be easier to obtain the chemical messengers which control so much of the bodily activity of humans from plants which contained their steroidal precursors. Investigation of hundreds of likely plants led him to the Mexican Yam (*Dioscorea* spp.), and to the fact that the diosgenin it contained could be chemically converted into the female hormone progesterone, which could itself be transformed into its male counterpart testosterone – the chauvinist's stone of biochemical alchemy at its best. Not only was the world of science, but also the company for which he worked, incredulous of his claims, so he left for Mexico, where he set up a company called

Syntex which produced the oral contraceptive pill. The rest is history – perhaps one of its most important chapters.[9]

No wonder that 1953 saw the founding in Germany of the Society for Research into Medical Plant Therapy and 1956 the launch of the American Society of Pharmacognosy. Each had its in-house journal, *Planta Medica* and *Lloydia*, to spread the good news of herbal renaissance. The public too were beginning to climb onto the bandwagon of environmental and personal concern: Rachel Carson had sown the very effective seeds of doubt about chemicals released into the food chain and pertinent questions began to be asked not only about pesticides and the likes of Agent Orange, but also about food additives and new and novel drugs like Thalidomide.[10]

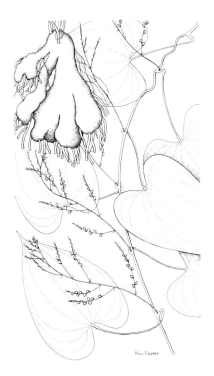

FIGURE 20.6 The Mexican Yam (*Dioscorea* spp.), possibly history's most important plant, which gave modern human society a measure of control over its own fertility.

Flower Power and Dr Bach's flower formulae were in the ascendancy as a young Zürich businessman tested the bullish market. Fred Pestalozzi had fallen ill with Menière's Disease and had been prescribed a terminal lifestyle. Hearing of a wonder herbal yeast tonic, and with nothing but debilitating time to lose, he tried it and was cured. Abandoning his previous life in the machine tool business, he set up Bio-Strath to make and market a whole range of herbal remedies to the world. A businessman at heart, he did his research and development with scientific precision and showed astonishingly good results and few side effects on all accounts. Because they were all tried and tested folk remedies (and perhaps because the ghost of Paracelsus still walked the herb-rich alpine pastures) he found no problems in marketing the full range of products, despite the maze of Swiss cantonal rules and regulations. However, as soon as he attempted to market them abroad, and especially in Britain and the USA, problems arose. The diehard chemotherapists there, perhaps overstimulated by the Thalidomide affair, and the nit-pickers of herbal rhetoric joined in to delay acceptance. Like the drugs they were marketing, or peddling depending from whose side you were looking, success bred the melancholy of contempt as it has done throughout this ptisane of herbal history. Vested interests, some for money, some for power and glory, and many for the impure mischief of jealousy fuelled by the fire of divergent opinion, shot their self-styled opponents in the back, and themselves and the whole movement of rational symbiotic medicine in the foot.[11]

The intricacies and inadequacies of the arguments for and against either side make pretty depressing reading, and rarely do we see anyone standing back and taking stock of the advances on both sides. Bad news has always made headlines, good news has always been relegated to the lower column inches. If this account has done anything we hope that it has provided an opportunity to look back, not in anger but in pity, and look forward, not in fear but in hope.

Today many humans in a cross-section of countries and societies are living longer and without the constant fear of painful remedies and painful death. Of course, there are still the ravages of congenital disease, accidents caused by new lifestyles and problems caused by new diseases, but there is no getting away from the fact that despite all those food additives more and more people survive to reproduce and to live on, fraught with the syndromes of old age, arthritis, rheumatism, Alzheimer's Disease, and of course cancer in all its manifestations. Unfortunately, or perhaps fortunately, none of the elixirs of long life which have been discovered to date keeps at bay the ageing process which attacks the muscles, joints, bones and brain. Little wonder therefore that today more and more of our hospital beds are being kept occupied by iatrogenic and geriatric diseases, which across an increasing spectrum must be regarded as one and the same thing. Survival of the unfit is now a growth industry on a First World scale.

Recycling of the gene stock at regular intervals has served the human species well over its few million years' existence. New bodies for old has been the way of natural selection, honing the fit towards the fitness of survival and the unfit along with all the pathogens to extinction. The only problem now is that with five billion plus recycling at an ever-increasing rate thanks to science, the pharmaceutical industry, medicine and, yes, the age-old and now reworked materia medica, the energy, the vital force which links all living things, is beginning to run out. The biosphere is dying, thanks to the devices, desires and aspirations of an exploding population, which are destroying the very hope we have for survival – let alone the healthful lifestyle, good food, not too much work, not too much play and airy spacious residences advocated in the Talmud twenty-three centuries ago.

The most terrible indictment of today's hi-tech multimedia society is that in every twenty-four-hour period 100,000 people, give or take a few, die of conditions relating to malnutrition and environmental pollution – in simple terms, due to starvation and dirty water. Or as put more eloquently by Robert McNamara, former president of the World Bank, when he reminded us that 25 per cent of the world's population live in 'A condition of life so characterised by malnutrition, illiteracy, disease, high infant mortality and low life expectancy as to be beneath any reasonable definition of human decency.'[12]

The amazing reality is that thanks to the resilience of the human genome, the advances of agricultural, medical and pharmaceutical science and the great band of traditional herbalists working away in the undergrowth from which they glean their wonder drugs, 250,000 do survive to swell the breakfast table of each new day: a quarter of a million new mouths to feed, new bodies to be clothed, housed and medically serviced, the vast majority thanks to herbal-based medicine. Little wonder that despite the smouldering antagonism of much of the medical profession the World Health Organization in 1974 announced that in order to reach the goal of adequate health care for everyone by the year 2000, part of their policy was to encourage all Third World countries to develop their own traditional systems of medicine. Four years later it recommended each country to begin a systematic study of their medicinal plants, the accent being on 'whole plant' drugs.[13]

In the years that have passed since then, years during which each minute has seen the premature death of at least 70 people and the destruction of some 60 hectares of natural vegetation (at least 40 hectares of which is moist tropical forest, which includes not only the richest diversity of plant and animal life but also the richest diversity of materia medica), less than 1 per cent of the plant species have been checked by modern science; and as the forest goes, so too does the knowledge of the local indigenous tribal people. Take note of the facts revealed by Brian M. Boom of the New York Botanical Garden. In a study of the Chacobo Indians of Bolivia, he refers to a study of a sample hectare containing 649 trees of 94 species with a diameter of 10cm or more (at breast height). He ascertained that the Indians were finding use for 75 species (82 per cent of the total), or 619 individual trees (95 per cent of the total). The species were grouped into five classes according to use: food, fuel, crafts and construction, medicinal and commercial. Some species, especially the palms, had uses in more than one category.

The problem was amply summarized in an advertisement placed in the *International Herald Tribune*, amongst other leading newspapers, in 1990. It reads:

THEY DIE, YOU DIE

Imagine your fate is entwined with that of a South American vine, or a fragile pink flower in far off Madagascar.

213

If these plants were threatened with extinction, you would spring to their defence.

What if we told you that many patients facing major surgery rely on a muscle relaxant extracted from an Amazonian vine, *Chondrodendron tomentosum*?

Or that four out of five children with leukaemia survive, thanks to the chemicals vincristine and vinblastine donated by the rosy periwinkle?

Would the fate of these plants still rouse your concern? If so, read on. It is essential that you be aroused beyond mere concern, to action.

Millions of people with heart ailments depend on foxgloves. These flowers provide the digitoxin which regulates their heartbeat.

Many sufferers of hypertension and high blood pressure owe a debt to the Indian Snakeroot shrub for its reserpine.

Extracts from an Amazonian oak tree coagulate proteins, immensely helping scientists in their search for an AIDS vaccine.

People sleep deeply and breathe easily during operations thanks to scopolamine derived from mandrake, henbane and thorn apples.

Cancer of the lung, kidney and testis responds to Etoposide, a drug synthesised from may apples. The Penobscot Indians of Maine have long found may apple useful against warts.

Women who take the contraceptive pill for granted would not be taking it at all were it not for the yam. This large tuber is the source of the Pill's active ingredient, diosgenin.

Peptic ulcers heal faster thanks to the pale blue petals and flat brown pods of the liquorice flower, origin of carbenoxalone.

Even the healthiest amongst us take compounds first discovered in fragrant meadowsweet and willow bark and now known as Aspirin.

Though these thirteen plants have healed and soothed millions of people, they're but the merest sample from nature's medicine chest. Over a quarter of all prescribed medicines are based on plants.

Yet, of the estimated 250,000 flowering plants believed to be in existence, tens of thousands remain undiscovered and only some 5,000 have been tested exhaustively for their pharmaceutical attributes. Now this vast store of known and potential medicines is under threat and we are all of us obliged to protect it.

You see, half of the earth's species thrive in the warmth and wetness of tropical rainforests. Just ten square kilometres of Amazonian jungle contain some 2,200 species of plant (numbers of lower plants like lichen and fungi are incalculable, as is their value: Cyclosporin, a product of two kinds of fungi, has helped revolutionise transplant surgery in the last decade).

Man is destroying these rainforests. 40 hectares a minute. An area the size of Austria every year.

Every day the bulldozing and polluting continues, countless lives are ruined, animal, bird, reptile, insect, not to mention human. Every day, in the midst of the carnage, five plants silently become extinct.

Chance alone kept alive those plants mentioned above long enough for them to help us.

Who knows what weapons against cancer, heart disease, AIDS or afflictions yet to come were lost forever in today's batch of five?

Join WWF – World Wide Fund For Nature and help reverse this process of destruction.

For almost 30 years WWF has lobbied governments and institutions, battling and educating in the name of conservation. What was once a worry about a few spectacular creatures is now a fight for man's survival.

Our latest battle plan covers 132 projects aimed at saving the earth's biological diversity, the intricate interdependence of ecosystems of which plants are the basis.

We need a further US$60 million to fund these projects through the next five years. (Already we are supporting 100 projects dedicated to conserving wetlands and 82 devoted to the management of national parks.)

Join our fight. Help save the plants and organisms which ease the pain and save the lives of humans. Help with your money, your work, your voice.

Start by writing to the WWF National Organization in your country or complete the form below and sent it to WWF International, CH–1196 Gland, Switzerland, *now*.

It's do or die.'[14]

Public reaction is also playing its part, for once again our retail outlets from grocery stores through drug stores to, yes, Boots the Chemists, are stocking and selling more and more homoeopathic and, excuse the word, alternative medicines. A list from the latter will suffice to show that many of the people's oldest plant friends, the simples, are hard at work once more, despite the fact that in some countries their virtues have to be tagged to a teabag thanks to drug legislation.

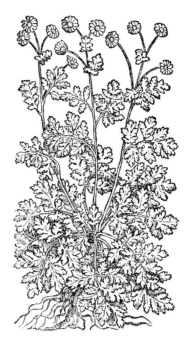

FIGURE 20.7 Feverfew (*Chrysanthemum parthenium*), another well-established source of salicylic acid.

Natural / homoeopathic / herbal / alternative products stocked in Boots the Chemists, UK

Boots Cod Liver Oil
Boots Almond Oil
Boots Clove Oil
Boots Castor Oil
Boots Cascara Tablets
Boots Coconut Oil
Boots Essence of Peppermint BPC
Boots Eucalyptus Oil
Boots Senna Laxative Tablets
Boots Senna Pods Tinnevelly
Boots Vegetable Laxative Tablets
Califig California Syrup of Figs
Braggs Medicinal Charcoal Tablets BPC

Fybogel Orange (Ispaghula Husk)
Herbal Feverfew Tablets
Heath & Heather: Catarrh Tablets; Feverfew Tablets; Indigestion and Flatulence Tablets; Inner Fresh Tablets; Quiet Night Tablets; Rheumatic Pain Tablets; Skin Tablets; Odourless Garlic Pearles
Hofels Garlic Pearles
Kamillosan Ointment (Chamomile extract)
Lustys Garlic Pearles
Mentholated Lozenges (Menthol)
Natracalm Tablets (Passiflora)
Nelsons Classical Series of Homoeopathic Medicines:
Arnica Cream; Calendula Cream; Evening Primrose Oil Cream; Graphites Cream; Haemorrhoid Cream; Hypercal Cream; Ointment for Burns; Ointment for Strains; Rheumatic Pain Cream;
Nelsons Specific Homoeopathic Remedies:
Diarrhoea/Food Poisoning Tablets; Flue-Cold Tablets; Hayfever Tablets; Noitura Tablets; Travel Sickness tablets; Teething Granules Tablets
New Era Homoeopathically Prepared Tissue Salts
Olbas Oil and Pastilles
Pierre's Monastery Herbs
Potter's Diuretabs
Catarrh Pastilles
Senokot Tablets, Syrup, Granules
Seven Seas Cod Liver Oil Capsules and Liquid
Seven Seas Natural Herb Remedies:
Backache Tablets; Catarrh Tablets; Feverfew Tablets; Laxative Tablets; Nerve Tablets; Restful Night Tablets; Rheumatic Tablets
Tiger Balm (Chinese Natural Medicine)
Stop Hemo Dressing (Sea Weed Calcium Alginate)
(Courtesy of The Boots Company PLC)

Ladies and gentlemen, this is our last chance. The world, our world, is dying from an iatrogenic disease caused by a pathogen called *Homo sapiens*, which is destroying the life support system of the Earth and the best-stocked pharmacy there has ever been. If the medical profession in all its guises can't see that its way ahead is through a new eclectic, the best of the old with the best of the new working in symbiosis to solve the real problems of this, the saddest of all centuries, the future hasn't a chance. We must use the greenprint of medicare handed down to the West over more than 30,000 years to reach a very attainable and respectable goal: every child a wanted child, growing up into an individual

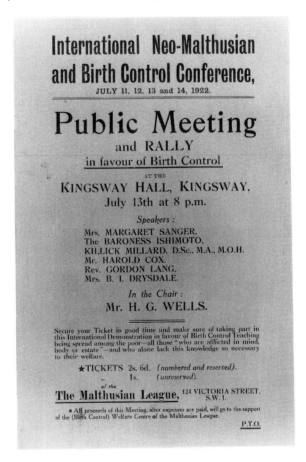

FIGURE 20.8 Thoughts about family planning may have begun with eugenic overtones, but now address a far more urgent problem: the overpopulation of a limited planet.

who can aspire to the dignity of a truly civilized world and an average active life of perhaps a little more than three score years and ten, leading on to an active old age, not sans eyes, sans teeth, sans everything, but sans the pain and the anguish of iatrogenic and geriatric syndromes.

Notes

1 *Encyclopedia Britannica*, 15th edn (Chicago: Encyclopedia Britannica Inc., 1985).
2 Ibid.
3 Ibid.; Ralph S. Solecki, 'Shanidar IV, a Neanderthal flower burial in northern Iraq', *Science*, 190 (28 Nov. 1975), p. 880; and Arlette Leroi-Gourhan, 'The flowers found with Shanidar IV, a Neanderthal burial in Iraq', *Science*, 190 (7 Nov. 1975), p. 562.
4 Froelich Rainey, 'Quinine hunters of Equador', *National Geographic Magazine*, 89.3 (1946), pp. 341–63.
5 Margaret Kreig, *Green Medicine* (London, 1965), p. 174.
6 Rainey, 'Quinine hunters of Equador'.
7 Barbara Griggs, *Green Pharmacy – A History of Herbal Medicine* (London: Robert Hale, 1981, 1987).
8 Ibid.
9 Farnsworth, 'The Plant Kingdom – suppliers of steroids', *Tile & Till*, 53 no.55 (Sept. 1967).
10 Griggs, *Green Pharmacy*.
11 Ibid.
12 Sir Edmund Hillary (ed.), *Ecology 2000 – The Changing Face of Earth* (New York: Beaufort Books, 1984), p. 197.
13 T. A. Lambo, 'Introduction – traditional medicine – a world survey on medicinal plants and herbs, *Journal of ethnopharmacology*, 2.1.
14 World Wide Fund for Nature (advertisement), *International Herald Tribune*, Wednesday, 13 June 1990.

How the Other Half Lives

21

SERENDIPITY –
THE AYURVEDIC LEGACY
OF SRI LANKA

Orthodox Modern Medicine, as now being practised throughout the 'western' world and those 'non-western' parts which have been influenced by it, has as we have seen grown up primarily in Europe, receiving and at times absorbing components from other climes and cultures as they gradually became available. There is of course a residuum, an underlayer of local medicine, which has been touched little if at all by the modern trends, and which crops up in practically any culture, whether in the shadow of palms or of skyscrapers. There are also other medical systems, however, which can boast at least as long a history as 'western' medicine, are based on highly sophisticated theoretical structures and, what is more, have a long and successful track record of relieving a sizeable proportion of mankind of an equally sizeable proportion of its ills and aches. The two which stand out amongst these are Traditional Chinese Medicine and modern Ayurveda. While the former is moderately well known in the West – if for no other reason than for its more exotic component, acupuncture – the latter is surprisingly unknown, despite the fact that it stems to a considerable extent from the same matrix as that of the West, and has had far more contacts with it than has its Chinese counterparts. Equally surprising, a considerable effort has been and is being made to integrate Traditional Chinese Medicine and Orthodox Modern Medicine into a coherent structure, both in China and in the West, while very little comparable can be said for Ayurveda.

One country which has given equal rights to different systems has been Sri Lanka, at other times known as Ceylon, Ceylan, Ceilao, Taprobane, Tambapanni, Lanka or Serendib, where a long tradition of Ayurveda medicine has coexisted with intense cultural contacts with the entire Indian Ocean basin and beyond.

At the time of the flowering of the study of anthropology at the end of the nineteenth century, the Veddahs, last remaining of the original Australid inhabitants of Sri Lanka, possibly descendants of mesolithic Balangoda man, still lived in caves and hunted and gathered the wealth of their forested lands around Bintenne. They are no more, their sustainable ways of life expunged by modern developments. Anthropological reports from the first half of the last century seem to indicate that they had no real concept of medicine apart from occult practices and exorcism, and that their knowledge of herbal lore stopped at the use of leaves and bark as purely physical bindings for injuries and wounds. It seems impossible to think that these were randomly selected, but that is unfortunately all the evidence we have. Excavations to date have revealed no more except caches of long pin-like copper rods called Kohl sticks. These were apparently used in the application of eye make-up, although their resemblance to certain instruments of acupuncture (or at least acupressure) cannot be overlooked.[1]

When the Indo-Aryans arrived in the island from North India sometime around the fifth century BC, they brought with them the Vedic medical skills already mentioned in chapter 5, which then appear to have undergone a similar development. This earliest form of healing is probably what lay at the root of the oldest system of medicine in Sri Lanka, referred to as Desiya Chikista, which in a tenuous form has survived to its present day. Handed down from generation to generation with the utmost secrecy, Desiya Chikista can be assumed to have been in part absorbed by later developments, and in part lost entirely due to breaks in the traditional chain of transmission.[2]

There also was, and never has ceased to be, a strong belief in the supernatural, both as the cause of illness and as its cure. Contemporary education and a high literacy rate have reduced its importance, but it is still there all right, and patients of all walks of life may be willing to make recourse to it, either in desperate cases or in unexplained ones. Similarly, in a culture as deeply permeated with religion as Sri Lanka's, it is not surprising that aspects of Buddhist ritual have assumed therapeutic roles. The sonorous chanting of *Pirith* (or *Paritta*), where extracts of the Buddhist Canon are recited by monks as a blessing and as a protection from danger, is one of these. Not only is it beneficial in terms of spiritually soothing and uplifting the patient, but it is also understood to banish any malign influence which might otherwise hinder the healing process.[3]

As in India, the medical system which eventually replaced the local folk remedies, sometimes absorbing them, was Ayurveda, with some minor adaptations to local conditions and to the by now mainly Buddhist ethos of the country. Indeed, the real history of Sri Lanka can be said to have started with the arrival of King Asoka's missionary envoys led by his son Mahinda sometime around 250 BC, which resulted in the island becoming one of the great centres of Buddhist civilization, actively involved in cultural exchanges and in missionary activities from China to the Red Sea, possibly to the Mediterranean. Initially in Pali (which remained the main religious language) and using the Brahmi script, later in Sanskrit, the new faith established itself as the cultural core of the Sinhala kingdoms, bringing with it, besides its philosophical work, a secular scholarship in which medicine played a major part.

Buddhism is not a religion, for Buddha is not a God to be worshipped or sought favours from. It is not a philosophy, for it provides no answers. Buddhism is a way of life in which people strive towards perfection while here on earth. Part of that process is for both the monks and the laity to perform good works, which include respect for all life and the relieving of the suffering and advancing of the welfare of all living things, plants, animals and people. The Lord Buddha himself said 'The Gain of Health is the Highest and the Best'. It is little wonder therefore that this way of life evolved hand in hand with the development of medicine, good works spearheaded by the Sinhalese royalty. We know much of this thanks to one of the most remarkable historical documents in existence.

The *Mahavamsa*, and its continuation the *Culavamsa*, was first written in classical Pali verse on *ola* leaves in the sixth century AD

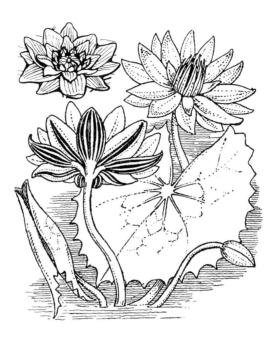

Figure 21.1 The Lotus (*Nymphaea lotus*), frequently taken as a symbol of Buddhism.

by a monk named Mahanama. It was continued by others up until the occupation by the British in 1815 and it details many of the kings' good works in the advancement of medicine. From it we learn that as early as the fourth century BC, King Pandukabaya (394–307 BC) set up a lying-in home and a hospital, and even something like a convalescent home in Anuradhapura, possibly history's first references to such institutions. The original centres of healing were the monasteries, where the presence of large communities of monks made some sort of medical facility a necessity. There is archaeological evidence that all monasteries had some sort of hospital attached to them, and most of them would have been open to the laity as well. Under such conditions, the financing and support of such establishments became one of the principal acts of charity in which a king could involve himself.[4]

While most Anuradhapura and Polonnaruwa monarchs left some medical legacy, it was Buddhadasa (AD 362–409) whose name is most firmly connected with the healing arts. An eminent physician himself, he is recorded as having built specific hospitals for the blind and the crippled, as well as having produced the Sanskrit compilation of all existing medical material, the *Sarasthasangrahaya*. His medical piety did not stop at man, for he is said to have been equally generous with veterinary institutions. By the ninth and tenth centuries AD the major hospitals, such as the ones at Mihintale, Medirigiriya and Anuradhapura, had become important official establishments, with regular staff, endowed lands for income, and at least in one case even legal extraterritoriality.[5]

What we learn from the *Mahavamsa* is backed up by the numerous inscriptions in Brahmi and in Sinhala which have been found in or around the medical centres. The earliest inscriptions date from the reign of Devampiyatissa (247–207 BC); they are in Brahmi script and are said to be contemporaneous with those of the reign in India of King Asoka, who himself showed a keen interest in matters of health, as we see from his inscriptions mentioning the establishment of a system of medical administration throughout his dominions as far as Tambaparni (Sri Lanka), in which medical treatment and medicines both for animals and for men are claimed to be provided by the state.[6]

Today no grand tour of Sri Lanka omits the highlight of a visit to at least one of these great hospital sites. There one can marvel not only at the size, the orderliness and the hygiene of these places of healing, but also at the strict rules of conduct of their physicians and helpers – rules which amongst other things record in stone that misappropriation of funds, goods and chattels has been the headache of every national health scheme since the dawn of history.

There one can also marvel at the stone medicine troughs designed on archimedean principles to minimize the amount of liquid required for full immersion therapy. It is these stone troughs and the querns used in the preparation of medicines which provide the most tangible proof of both the development of the medical methodology and the pharmacy of the time. A medicine based mainly on native plants was all part of the evolution of the Lankan civilization, a civilization dependent on the success of agriculture which was determined in part by the vagaries of the monsoon rains and to a great extent by the maintenance of a truly monumental system of irrigation, centred on a complex of earth dams built across streams and small rivers each empounding a 'tank' of water. The catchment of each tank was protected from erosion by a permanent cover of rainforest, which provided the local people with many things from fuel through food to most of their medicines. From the evidence to hand it would not seem wrong to conclude that for more than 2,000 years the 656 million hectares of land that is Sri Lanka supported the sustainable lifestyles and healthstyles of a population which may well have exceeded ten million people for much of that time – a phenomenal achievement both of tropical land use and of a system of public health engineering and medicare.

That the forested catchments of the tank systems were of great importance to all local physicians as their source of medicinal plants, there is no doubt; however, the existence of specific medicinal forests planted by the ancient kings has been called into doubt. A number of park-like forests identified as such due to their richness in trees of high medicinal value have been disqualified on the grounds that all the trees are fire-resistant: the argument goes that they are not plantations but are a by-product of slash-and-burn shifting agriculture; there is also no mention of such plantations in the *Mahavamsa* nor in any other contemporary literature or inscription. Then again, being fire-resistant, the trees in question – *Terminalia chebula*, *Terminalia belerica* and *Emblilica officinalis* (*aralu*, *bulu* and *nelli* in Sinhala respectively) – would be easily found in the vicinity of habitations, making their products readily available . . . [7]

If indeed there were no such special forests or plantations it must be concluded that the forested catchments, despite the problems of slash and burn, held adequate supplies of at least the majority of the commonly used medicinal plants. Others were definitely obtained from further afield. We know that 'precious ambrosial herbs' were among gifts sent by the Mauryan King Asoka on the inauguration of King Pandukabaya in Anuradhapura in 397 BC; that before the birth of Dutugemunu his mother gifted medicines to the Buddhist brotherhood in order that she would conceive, just as her son when reigning between 101 and 77 BC 'bestowed on preachers of the doctrine a handful of liquorice four inches long',[8] a well-known cure for sore throats and hoarseness. If this reference is to Spanish Liquorice (*Glycyrrhiza glabra*), which is a native of Persia, not Sri Lanka, then the import of medicinal plants must stretch from antiquity to the modern day: a conclusion backed up by the discovery of two blue glazed jars of Persian origin in the ruins of the Mihintale hospital, and by pieces of porcelain presenting Chinese characters revealed during excavations at Polonnaruwa.[9]

There is no doubt that both during the Golden Age of Sri Lanka, from about 200 BC to AD 1200, and in the more difficult centuries that followed up to the beginning of European penetration, the Ayurvedic system of health care came to full fruition. The Portuguese arrival in 1505 marked the beginning of the long period of European occupation, and the disruption it caused in local traditions. The decline of Ayurveda was limited at first, and mainly due to a general reduction of resources and patronage. The Portuguese, and the Dutch who replaced them by 1658, had relatively little influence on it; their numbers were moderate, they only occupied the coastal strip and anyway had little interest in the living conditions of the local inhabitants unless they resided in direct contact with them. Moreover, European medicine had less to offer at the time than might have been expected, and more than a little to learn. Nevertheless, the Europeans did introduce their own hospitals – and their own diseases. At the same time they often enough made use of local methods and medicines, either having run out of their own preparations or recognizing the native ones as superior under the circumstances. For example, the Portuguese viceroy's forces who captured the town of Jaffnapatam in 1560 were plagued by ill health and were short of food. Their Spanish physician, by the name of Dimas Bosque, having used all medicines carried by the fleet, turned to local remedies:

> Having nothing left with which to treat the sufferers from dysentery, whose sickness gave so much work to the army, I was forced to try experiments with these marmelos, of which I heard from the natives. I cured many cases with them, ordering plasters to be made for the belly and stomach. I also ordered a marmalade to be made which did

not taste bad, and had a pleasant acid flavour. I ordered the sick to eat it roasted, with sugar.[10]

The 'marmelo' in question was the fruit of *Aegle marmelos* (beli). In due time the skill of the local physicians and the efficacy of their remedies were fully recognized by the Portuguese, who eventually absorbed some of them into their own medical compendium. On his return to Portugal in 1680 João Ribero, soldier and historian, wrote:

> They are great herbalists, and in case of wounds, tumours, broken arms and legs they effect a cure in a few days with great ease. As for cancer, which is a loathsome and incurable disease among us, they can cure it in eight days, removing all viscosity from the scab without so much as leaving a mark anywhere to show that the disease had been there. I have seen a large number of soldiers and captains cured during my residence in the country, and the ease with

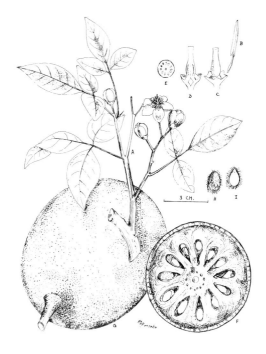

Figure 21.2 Dimas Bosque's local remedy for dysentery, beli (*Aegle marmelos*).

which this was done was marvellous. In truth the land is full of medicinal herbs and many antidotes to poison, which I have myself tried to learn as a remedy against snakebites.[11]

The Portuguese must be credited with the introduction not only of Western Medicine into Sri Lanka, but also of two diseases, as Pyrard de Laval tells us: 'Venereal disease is very prevalent but only where the Portuguese are. As for Pox it is no mark of shame there . . . they even make a boast of it. This malady prevails only among Christians.'[12] The other such disease was yaws or parangi, a disease caused, like syphilis, by *Treponema* spp., which, however, was introduced through Negro slaves from Mozambique, and was to cause untold misery to thousands of rural people for several centuries. We may add a third, Tobacco, which was initially introduced as a medicinal plant but, as elsewhere, just stayed on. At the same time, Portuguese records frequently mention epidemics attacking both Europeans and locals, whose description could fit equally well cholera, beriberi, dysentery or plague – smallpox, on the other hand, was readily recognized. For these and other ailments the Portuguese made use of a number of oriental products, partly imported via their main base at Goa, partly obtained locally. The Portuguese physician García da Orta, in his important work *Colloquies on the Simples and Drugs of India* (1563) mentions amongst others the Coconut (*Cocos nucifera*), Cinnamon (*Cinnamomum zeylanicum*), Cardamom (*Elettaria cardamomum*), Nutmeg (*Myristica fragrans*), Cloves (*Syzygium aromaticum*), Tamarind (*Tamarindus indica*), Betel (*Areca catechu*), Opium (*Papaver somniferum*) and Cannabis (*Cannabis sativa*), as well as other less orthodox substances such as gems, pearls and ivory.[13]

When the Dutch replaced the Portuguese in 1656, there was little change in things medical, apart from the fact that there were more hospitals (for the Dutch) and that they were run more professionally, as part of the Vereenighte Oostindische Companie medical structure. The surgeons and physicians attached to these hospitals, of which Colombo was by far the most important, had ample opportunities to study the local materia medica. Probably the most famous of them was Paul Hermann, who regardless of his unpopularity as a medical practitioner is remembered as the

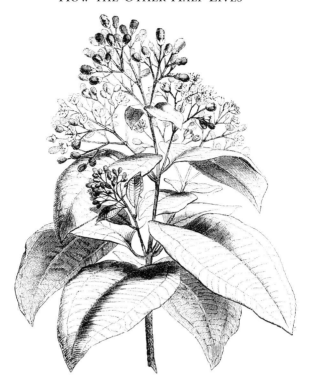

Figure 21.3 Cinnamon (*Cinnamomum zeylanicum*), Sri Lanka's spice *par excellence*.

Father of Sri Lankan Botany for his studies between 1672 and 1680 when he obtained the chair of Botany at Leyden, where he brought his extensive herbarium. His main interest, evidently to the detriment of his healing work, was the local flora, and of the plants he saw in Sri Lanka all except three were new to him.

Other physicians with a botanical bent left their mark as well. The Flemish doctor Aegidius Daalmann was sent to Sri Lanka especially 'to look for new herbs and roots that grew there wild'. He succeeded and presented his *Pharmacopoeia of Ceylon* to Governor Pyl. This included both external and internal remedies and a statement that 'no more, not a single one, need be sent out from the Fatherland'. One of the drugs recommended by Daalmann was *Coscinium fenestratum*, False Columbo Root, an import into India from South America by seventeenth-century missionaries. He prescribed it for inflammation of the throat, and it is still used nowadays as a prophylactic against tetanus. In a similar vein, Charles Peter Thunberg, a professor from Uppsala University in Sweden, made a study of medicinal plants during his visit to Sri Lanka in 1777. He describes, for example, how 'shingles are cured with the capsules of *Hibiscus tiliaceus* by rubbing the juice of them over the eruption.'[14]

Just as the Sinhalese learnt to respect certain aspects of Western medicine, which however always remained a luxury, the Dutch reciprocated, and towards the end of their rule, they showed their appreciation of the knowledge and skill of local Ayurvedic doctors by appointing one 'native physician' to each of their hospitals. His duty was to assist the chief surgeon in his daily visits to the sick, so that his knowledge could best be put to use.[15]

Conquest by Britain, begun in 1796 and completed in 1815, was to bring the most far-reaching changes both in medicine and in Sri Lanka's sustainable society. The British occupied the entire island, and their intrusion went far deeper into Sinhalese culture than the Portuguese and Dutch ever had, as they saw the country as a colony to be administered rather than as a conquered resource which, as long as it produced, could by and large be left to take care of itself. Also, times had changed, and the Europeans saw themselves very much in a 'civilizing' role. An organized medical establishment was set up, initially on the lines of the Army Medical Service and intended for the care of the Europeans, but it was soon joined by a Native Medical Establishment, under whose care came the local workers on whom the Europeans were dependent.

And not only local: the massive influx of workers from South India to service first the coffee, then the tea and rubber plantations, brought with them epidemics on a hereto unknown scale, diseases like smallpox and cholera which though extant previously were not endemic, and had not presented such a problem. Also, the new plantations replaced much of the forest which had protected the catchments from erosion and had been the traditional source not only of tank-based irrigation but also of native medicines, fuel and food. The age-old sustainable ways of village life based on clean water, good sanitation, healthy eating and Ayurvedic Medicine went into rapid decline. So much so that in the face of onslaught after onslaught by smallpox in 1802, the British set about the awesome task of inoculating the whole population. To this end Sir Alexander Johnston, later to become Chief Justice, appointed a Muslim physician as the native superintendent of the medical department.

> The chief of this (Mohammedan) family was appointed by me, in 1806, native superintendent of the medical department, under the control of the Supreme Court. He was considered by the natives of the country as one of the best informed of the native physicians on the island, and possessed one of the best collections of native medical books, most of which had been in his family between seven and eight hundred years, during the whole of which period it had been customary for one member of his family at least to follow the medical profession. This same person made me a very detailed report of all the plants in Ceylon which have been used from time immemorial for medical purposes by Mohammedan native physicians on that island. The cultivation and improvement of these plants, as well as of all other plants and vegetables on the island which might be used either for food or commercial purposes was one of the great objects for which His Majesty's Government, at my suggestion, in 1810, established a Royal Botanical Garden in Ceylon.[16]

So the links with past practices were maintained, but four centuries of foreign rule, of wars and rumours of wars, had replaced and sapped the strength of traditional culture, including that of native medicine. This was sadly true especially under British rule, during which time Western Medicine not only replaced Ayurveda over large area, but also sought to ridicule it wherever possible. That it survived at all was due more than anything else to the half-heartedness of the authorities' efforts, for indeed there was a policy to replace traditional medicine, seen by and large as uncivilized quackery, across the board with Western practices.[17]

From the second decade of the twentieth century onwards, however, there has been a strong revival of national identity and traditional culture, and Ayurveda has played a significant part in it. Having gained the active support of some national leaders in

1925, it has never looked back, except to its roots deep in the culture and the soils of the country. The setting up of the Ayurvedic College and Hospital at Borella in 1929 was an important foundation-stone of this revival, and the enactment of the Ayurveda Act No. 31 of 1961 provided, amongst other things, the establishment of the Department of Ayurveda and three statutory bodies: the Ayurvedic Medical Council, the Ayurveda Educational and Hospital Board and the Ayurvedic Research Committee. It also envisaged the establishment of a Ministry of Indigenous Medicine, a body which was finally appointed in 1980, another first in modern medical history. Since then, Ayurveda has been considered as official a medical system as Orthodox Modern Medicine, and given equivalent priority in the country's health scheme.[18]

Ayurvedic Medicine in Sri Lanka today is a composite of Traditional Indian Medicine (Ayurveda), Traditional Tamil Medicine (Siddha), Traditional Sinhalese Medicine (Desiya Chikitsa) and medicine derived from the Moorish tradition and therefore of Arabic origin (Unani). On the whole, the basic concepts of Sinhalese Ayurveda do not deviate significantly from those of Indian Ayurveda, apart from where differences arise because of floral variations. Of the others, Siddha is popular among the Tamil-speaking population, being almost identical to Ayurveda except for the language of its ancient works, Tamil instead of Sanskrit, and its greater use of metals and minerals in its formulations. Unani, on the other hand, is a fairly straightforward derivative of Persian, in other words Arabo-Hippocratic, Medicine. It is practised almost exclusively by the Muslim community, uses Avicenna's *Canon* as its basic text, and stands out for its abundant use of syrups and electuaries.[19]

Today there are five well-known Ayurvedic educational institutes, the diplomas of two of which are recognized by the government. The graduates from these are backed up by 10,000 registered Ayurvedic practitioners, 7,500 of which are traditional physicians in the mould of those described by the Reverend Phillipus Baldeus, a Dutch clergyman, in 1672:

There is no lack of artzen or doctors, though ignorant of anatomy . . . All their cures consist of pure empirics and experience. They possess great written folios which have passed to them from their forefathers to which they have added the results of their own researches.[20]

Like them, their modern counterparts have no formal institutional training, but acquire proficiency by serving a long period of apprenticeship under a teacher. The emphasis is on the practical aspects of medical care, and the pupil acquires a sound knowledge of the preparation of herbal medicine through long association with the teacher and by assisting him in his work, where he learns clinical methods by observation of patients. Since 1979 this apprenticeship scheme has been advanced and developed by the institution of seminars and of a new scholarship scheme. Together this dedicated body of men and women in 1982 alone serviced sixteen medical institutions and 233 free dispensaries maintained by local authorities.[21]

One good example of such centres is the 'Ayurvedic Village' of Wedagama. This is an admittedly somewhat artificial concentration of Ayurvedic practitioners housed in traditional homes-cum-practices, where they treat their patients for a token sum wrapped in the traditional Betel leaf. The intent is that of creating a Centre of Excellence for Ayurveda, and to offer students the possibility of learning from a wide selection of traditional healers; as these frequently owe their fame to 'secret' methods and formulations, this increases the chance that such 'secrets' will be passed on and hopefully in some future time come into the public domain. The village also houses an Ayurvedic school, where along with the traditional knowledge students receive the standardized 'scholastic' Ayurvedic curriculum. In addition, the entire village area has been planted with medicinal plants for local use, as every practitioner is also his own pharmacist. Such teaching may lack many of the refinements which Western medicine has made us accustomed to, but then we are talking of two approaches differing in more than just medical terms. Comparing Orthodox Modern Medicine to Ayurveda means comparing a high-tech, high-cost, high-profit profession within a hierarchical structure to a low-cost, low-profit activity best carried out individually at the village level; the two are unlikely to attract the same sort of practitioners. This may also be one of the reasons for the fact that Ayurveda is practically unknown outside the Indian subcontinent and its cultural outliers.[22]

Equally important has been the establishment of a research institute for the purpose of investigating Ayurveda in the light of modern science. The Bandaranaike Memorial Ayurvedic Research Institute (BMARI) in Nawinna, Maharagama, operates as an Ayurvedic hospital in which selected patients undergo Ayurvedic treatment under Western-style clinical monitoring for research purposes. Also, the Institute is involved in reproducing, cataloguing and as far as possible translating the ancient medical texts, and its gardens act as a reservoir of type specimens of medical plants used for propagation.[23]

The Department of Ayurveda's brief also covers the production and supply of Ayurvedic drugs used by the public hospitals and

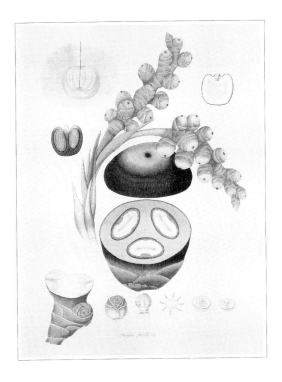

FIGURE 21.4 The Toddy Palm (*Arenga saccharifera*), source of Sri Lanka's jaggery sugar, which puts more than alcohol into their toddy and arak.

237

dispensaries. Beyond this, a number of firms are now engaged in the manufacture of the traditional medicines both at home and abroad. In fact, Ayurveda has even penetrated the fortress of so many of the Western pharmaceutical giants: Ayurveda Natura Medicin, based in Switzerland, now serves the international market, in part thanks to the World Health Organization's increasing recognition of the efficacy of traditional medicine and the fact that it can cost less and cause fewer side effects.[24]

One of the main problems holding up further development of Ayurveda in Sri Lanka is the almost complete destruction of the native forests by plantations, slash and burn cultivation and, more recently, by plantations of Pine and Eucalyptus. This has led to an alarming decrease in the supply of herbs and has necessitated their import from India and other sources, itself causing a large increase in their price to consumers. It has also fortunately led to concern for the training of taxonomic botanists, for the setting up of at least rural-plot-sized medical gardens and plantations and to the conservation of those forest areas still left in a semi-natural state. The importance of the latter cannot be overestimated, for it is from the diversity of the natural populations of those plants which have provided the Ayurvedic materia medica for more than two millennia that any future hope for sustainability now lies.

Notes

1 C. G. Uragoda, *A History of Medicine in Sri Lanka* (Colombo: Sri Lanka Medical Association, 1987).

2 Ibid.; and *Encyclopedia Britannica*, 15th edn (Chicago: Encyclopedia Britannica Inc., 1985).

3 Uragoda, *A History of Medicine in Sri Lanka.*

4 Ibid.; P. B. Wanninayaka, *Ayurveda in Sri Lanka* (Sri Lanka: Ministry of Health, 1982); and A. Lyanagamage, personal communication (1989).

5 Uragoda, *A History of Medicine in Sri Lanka*; and Rohan Gunaratna, *Sino-Lankan Connection: 2000 Years of Cultural Relations* (Colombo: Department of Information, Ministry of State, 1987).

6 Uragoda, *A History of Medicine in Sri Lanka.*

7 Ibid.; and Wanninayaka, *Ayurveda in Sri Lanka.*

8 Uragoda, *A History of Medicine in Sri Lanka*, p. 38.
9 Uragoda, *A History of Medicine in Sri Lanka*; and Gunaratna, *Sino-Lankan Connection*.
10 Uragoda, *A History of Medicine in Sri Lanka*, p. 46.
11 Ibid., pp. 46–7.
12 Ibid., p. 55.
13 Uragoda, *A History of Medicine in Sri Lanka*; and V. H. Heywood (ed.), *Flowering Plants of the World* (Oxford: Oxford University Press, 1978).
14 Uragoda, *A History of Medicine in Sri Lanka*, pp. 68–9.
15 Uragoda, *A History of Medicine in Sri Lanka*.
16 Ibid., p. 82.
17 Uragoda, *A History of Medicine in Sri Lanka*; and Wanninayaka, *Ayurveda in Sri Lanka*.
18 Wanninayaka, *Ayurveda in Sri Lanka*.
19 Ibid.; and Upali Pilapittiya, personal communication (1989).
20 Wanninayaka, *Ayurveda in Sri Lanka*, p. 32.
21 Wanninayaka, *Ayurveda in Sri Lanka*.
22 Anuradha Sirisena, personal communication (1989).
23 Upali Pilapittiya, personal communication (1989).
24 Wanninayaka, *Ayurveda in Sri Lanka*.

General information

Gananath Obeyesekere, 'The Theory and Practice of Psychological Medicine in the Ayurvedic Tradition', *Culture, Medicine and Psychiatry*, 1 (1977), pp. 155–81.

Dharamit Singh, 'The traditional medicine in India', *Impact of Science on Society*, 26.4.

Vernon L. B. Mendis, *Foreign Relations of Sri Lanka from Earliest Times to 1965*, *Ceylon Historical Journal* Monograph Series, vol. 2, *Dehiwela* (Sri Lanka: Tisara Prakasakayo, 1983).

J. B. Disanayaka, *Mihintale – Cradle of Sinhala Buddhist Civilization* (Colombo: Lake House Investments, 1987).

H. V. Savnur, *Ayurvedic Materia Medica* (1950; Delhi: Sri Satuguru Publications, 1988).

22

CHINA SYNDROME
– TO RECAPITULATE THE ESSENCE
OF THIS PTISANE AND TO PROVE
THAT AT LEAST IN PART
THE PROBLEMS CAN BE SOLVED

China seems to have gone its own way in medicine as in so many other fields. Size, relative stability, and remoteness have all played a historical part in keeping Chinese culture relatively isolated from the rest of the world. Its medical system developed on its own individual path, in keeping with the synthetic nature of its philosophical schools. On the other hand, apart from China, this system and its derivatives have served – and frequently well served – Japan, Korea, most of Southeast Asia, the very large community of Overseas Chinese, and a growing number of Western patients. It can therefore be said that around one-third of humanity has relied on it to some extent – far from a minority interest indeed![1]

The history of Chinese Medicine can be defined in three stages: Chinese Folk Medicine, Min-chien i-hsueh, which is based on the plant lore and magico-religious healing techniques which have their roots in the early neolithic and was probably still dominant until around 1000 BC; Traditional Chinese Medicine, Chung-i, which arose out of Chinese Folk Medicine round about the Shang-Yin dynasty (1500–1027 BC) and lasted more or less until the beginning of the twentieth century AD; and the New Chinese

Medicine (Chung-kuo i-hsueh), which is the current attempt at creating a twentieth-century amalgam of Eastern and Western systems of medicine.[2]

The fundamental concepts of Chinese Medicine are homoeostasis, balance and integration, making it synthetic rather than analytic. In general terms, the Western scientific approach has always tended towards an increasing objectivity and a strict division between subject and object – as can be seen by the 'wrongness' which so many Westerners still feel when faced with a concept which seems to blur this division, such as the theory of relativity. Applied to medicine, this attitude means that disease is seen as an independent entity impinging onto an equally independent body. To the Eastern scholar, trained in a naturalistic and synthetic outlook, disease is seen as the visible aspect of a dysfunction of the body itself, both in its material and immaterial aspects, a dysfunction for which the patient is himself partly responsible. The healer's purpose is not to cure a disease, but to restore the natural balance; the cure will follow of its own accord. As Frederick K. Kao puts it: 'The overall Western Ethos has led to the concept of hardware, whilst that of the East has led to the concept of software.'[3]

Some of the earliest archaeological evidence of recorded history in China seems to point towards a medical theme, with the finds in Anyang, dating around 1700 BC, including objects which might have been stone 'acupuncture needles' of some sort. Appropriately, the origin of medical theory is intermingled with the myths concerning early Chinese civilization, generally concentrated in the figures of Fu Hsi, Sheng Nung and Huang Ti.[4]

Fu Hsi (supposedly around 4000 BC) is the mythical inventor of the basic elements of civilization: agriculture, family structure, record-keeping and the calendar. Sheng Nung (c.3000 BC), the 'Divine Peasant', is accredited with the introduction of rice and grain culture and with the invention of herbal medicine through the attributed authorship of the *Pen Ts'ao*, or *Great Herbal*, as well as of other texts in dealing with longevity and dietetics. Huang Ti, or the 'Yellow Emperor', is claimed to have lived around 2700 BC, and is deemed the founder of the Chinese state, the inventor of writing, and the inspiration behind the *Huang Ti*

Nei Ching, or *Yellow Emperor's Canon of Internal Medicine*, the first major Chinese medical compendium.[5]

Sheng Nung's *Pen Ts'ao* – a term which means approximately 'pharmaceutics whose basis is herbs' – can be safely taken to be an evolving collection of herbals and lists of materia medica which were turned into a usable manual of drugs usage with T'ao Hung Ching's (AD 452–536) commentary, *Sheng Nung Pen Ts'ao Ching*, and were eventually to find their way into Li Shi Chen's *Great Herbal*, a definitive compilation published under the emperor Shen Tsung in AD 1596. The *Huang Ti Nei Ching*, on the other hand, can probably be dated to the Chou Dynasty (1066 to 221 BC), around the middle of which so many of the Chinese civilization's philosophical and religious foundations were laid.[6]

The *Huang Ti Nei Ching* can be compared to the Western Hippocratic corpus, systematizing existing knowledge and fitting it into the current philosophical and religious structure, though separating it clearly from the earlier magical interpretations. Amongst other things, acupuncture is already here dealt with in depth, and is clearly considered one of the principal medical techniques.[7]

The philosophical developments of the time played a significant part in the development of medicine, both directly and indirectly. Kung Fu-tse (551–479 BC), known in the West as Confucius, had and still has a monumental influence on Chinese thought and, by developing a philosophy based entirely on human and social structures and therefore defining non-human phenomena as elements of minor importance, was probably responsible for the long stability and immobility of Chinese culture. Lao Tse (*c.*600 BC), on the other hand, syncretized Taoism out of what must have been a vast base of pre-existing mythical and religious concepts. Mystical and poetic, the Tao was at the same time open to nature, experience and ethically neutral experiment, and therefore opened the way to proto-science, in particular through Chinese alchemy. It was a Taoist philosopher, Chuang Tze (369–286 BC), who first formulated the concept of the cycle of life out of which Chinese Medicine's principal tenet, the concept of Ch'i, arose. The fortunes of the two schools of thought alternated, but between them they could create a medical discipline capable both of accumulating empirical knowledge and of applying it 'to the benefit of society' – and beyond, as the story of Mah Shih Huang tells us. This worthy veterinary doctor is remembered for successfully applying acupuncture to an ailing dragon which had visited him with drooping ears and gaping mouth. Just how much of the early stories can be considered historical fact is difficult to say, but they do speak of a fairly advanced knowledge of surgical technique and anaesthesia, apart from elements of hygiene, herbal treatment and diagnostics which are still valid in today's practice.

The point of origin of Chinese medical thought – as for any science – was magic and religion, continuously modified and revised in the attempt to gradually exclude supernatural interpretations wherever natural ones become available. Throughout this process, what has lasted longest is the basic Chinese cosmological scheme, derived from the concept of the Wu-chi, the Great Void, giving rise to the T'ai Chi, or Great Absolute, which in turn differentiates itself into the two mutually interdependent opposites, the Yang and the Yin, which finally combine to form every other existing entity – the Wan-wu, or Myriad of Things. It is worth mentioning that this concept is seen to parallel, as a philosophically satisfactory metaphor, both in the East and in the West, some of the theories of cosmogony put forth by modern physics. Next to the Yin-Yang doctrine is the doctrine of Wu-hsing or Five Elements, in which entities material and immaterial are seen to be the result of the interaction of the five 'Elements' – Water, Fire, Metal, Wood and Earth are the terms most often used, but their exact meaning is exceedingly vague, varied and open to interpretation; though having been of considerable importance in the past and offering interesting similarities with Indian and Western concepts such as Elements, Humours and the *Panchamahabhuta*, the Five Elements doctrine does not seem to have found a place in the more modern interpretations of Chinese medicine, apart from the fivefold classification of flavours/tastes, Wu-wei (*hsien* or 'salty', *k'u* or 'bitter', *suan* or 'sour', *hsin* or 'acrid' and *kan* or 'sweet'), which is still significant in the description of herbal remedies.[8]

Out of this background two fundamental concepts have been derived. The first concerns the roles of the different organs in the

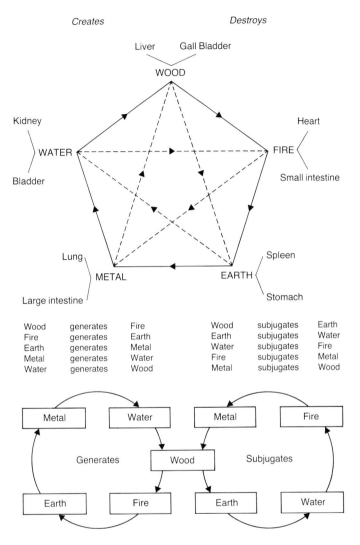

FIGURE 22.1 The relationships of the Five Elements in Traditional Chinese Medicine.

body, roles which have been assigned through a macrocosm-microcosm scheme resembling that of alchemy, with the marked difference that while alchemy searched for correlations between man and the cosmos, Chinese Medicine is more likely to see

244

parallels between the body and the social macrocosm and interpret it in terms of function, as described by Ko Hung in the *Pao Pu Tse* in AD 400:

> Thus, the body of a man is the image of a State. The thorax and abdomen correspond to the palaces and offices. The four limbs correspond to the frontiers and boundaries. The divisions of the bones and sinews correspond to the functional distinctions of the hundred officials. The pores of the flesh correspond to the ministers, and the Ch'i to the people. Thus we see that he who can govern his body can control a kingdom. Loving his people, he will bring peace to the country; nourishing his Ch'i, he will preserve his body. If the people are alienated, the country is lost; if the Ch'i is exhausted, the body dies.[9]

The Ch'i Ko Hung mentions is the second of these concepts, and the thread joining Traditional Chinese medical theory with its practical applications. Meaning literally 'air', and written with radicals of 'rice' (or 'food') and of 'gas', the term covers a gamut of meanings ranging from breath or breathing through to vital energy, and can be seen as a kindred concept to the *pneuma* of Classical Medicine and the *prana* of Ayurveda. Most of Traditional Chinese Medicine is somehow involved in measuring, preserving, encouraging, balancing, redirecting or cultivating the Ch'i.

This Ch'i is the essence of the body's life functions, flowing in a spatial and periodic pattern through organs and tissues. Any disturbance of this flow involving either deficiency or excess is a cause of disease, and the treatment involves either removing the disturbance or restoring the flow around it. While drugs or surgery may on occasion be more appropriate, by far the most important mechanism used is acupuncture and its related systems such as acupressure and moxibustion (the application of heat through slow-burning Moxa leaves), by which the flow of Ch'i is affected by stimulating specific loci along its flow pattern, either through tonification or through sedation. Thus the Ch'i and the meridians through which it flows, the Ching Lo, can be interpreted as a concept of circulation embracing the circulatory, nervous and endocrine systems, and encompassing all of the body's regulatory functions.[10]

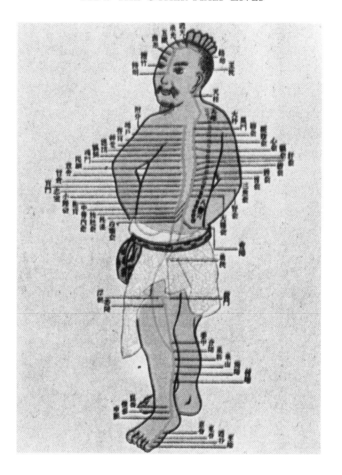

FIGURE 22.2 The Ch'i channels, along which its flow can be influenced by acupuncture and kindred techniques.

The next burst of Chinese medical discoveries took place in the early centuries of our era, possibly aided by an increase in anatomical knowledge gleaned from warfare – the story is told that circulation was discovered by the physicians who were ordered to dissect the exhumed and desecrated bodies of Han princes by the usurper Wang Mang in the year 7 AD. Whatever the cause, from then on Chinese Medicine developed fairly rapidly. Pulse reading was developed to a fine art, and major advances in materia medica become apparent: amongst others, Ma Huang (*Ephedra vulgaris*) was already being used to treat fever and asthma.

At this time, three figures seem to dominate the medical scene. The first, Chun Yu I (*c*.AD 216), began what can be called clinical medicine by keeping medical records – which incidentally seem to show that alcoholism and venery were the main causes of disease at the time, or at least the main causes for which a member of the aristocracy would seek a cure – and promoted the use of herbal drugs. The second, Chang Chung Ching, was born at the end of the century and thus was a contemporary of Galen; a prolific writer, he classified diseases according to their symptoms and compiled the *Shan Han Lun*, or *Treatise of Fevers*, in which 170 drugs in various formulations are described. He is also accredited with the recognition of the concept of public health, by regulating the quality of food on public sale. The third, Hua T'o (AD 110–207), is considered the father of Chinese surgery, and to him are ascribed major advances in surgery and anaesthetics.[11]

Throughout the Sui and Tang periods, China enjoyed an unprecedented degree of foreign contact, in particular through the introduction of Buddhism from India. Its main effects on medicine were the continuous and at times acrimonious struggle between Taoism and Buddhism, in which medical schools and doctrines were frequently involved, and the contact with Indian medicine (Ayurveda). Together with the invention of printing in about AD 800, these induced a period of reform which culminated in the setting up of a Grand Medical College in AD 1300. The peak of Traditional Chinese Medicine was reached in the sixteenth and seventeenth centuries with the *Materia medica* of Li Shih Chen (1518–1593) and Wou Yu Ke's work on infectious diseases published in 1642. The latter recognized the concept of infection and postulated the existence of external pathogens – a radical departure from traditional concepts. Unfortunately, the cultural ground (and the absence of experimental tools such as the microscope) was not receptive to such major changes, and in the following centuries Traditional Chinese Medicine found itself first stagnating, and then being ousted by Western medicine. In 1822 the Grand Medical College suspended the use of acupuncture on

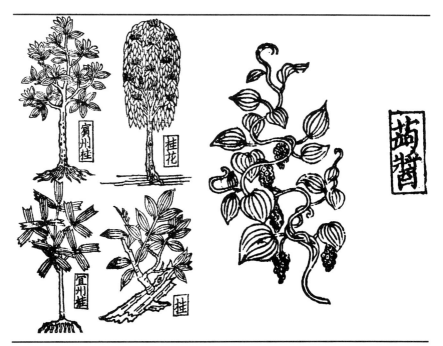

Figure 22.3 *Kuei* (*Cinnamomum cassia*, Cassia) and *Chu-chiang* (*Piper nigrum*, Black Pepper), shown in an early flora of Southeast Asia – proof both of fourth-century medico-botanical and ethnomedical knowledge.

internal ideological grounds and concentrated on herbal medicine – though acupuncture thrived further without the need for official sanction – and in 1929 Traditional Chinese Medicine was in theory officially abolished. Ironically, it was during this period of decline that Traditional Chinese Medicine found its way to the West.[12]

Some contact with foreign cultures had taken place already. The communications with India did not go only one way. Japanese medicine developed in the seventh and eighth centuries AD as a direct derivative of the Chinese, and in the eighth and ninth centuries Chinese influence (and naval presence) throughout the Indian Ocean brought some elements of Traditional Chinese Medicine into contact with the Arabic world. Nevertheless, it was the writings of seventeenth-century travellers and Jesuit missionaries which brought the first detailed descriptions of Traditional

Chinese Medicine to the West. The first treatise on acupuncture to reach Europe was the Reverend Father Harview's *Les Secrets de la Médicine des Chinois consistant en la Parfaite Connaissance du Pouls, envoyés de la Chine par un Français, Homme de Grande Merite* (1671). Such books and reports multiplied, and eventually it was Georges Soulie de Morant (1878–1955) who, after twenty years in China, introduced acupuncture in Europe as a formally taught discipline. The Western interest in Chinese Medicine is welcome to its present practitioners, but it must be remembered that for the most part it is concentrated on Traditional Chinese Medicine, which is rather like describing Western Medicine on the basis of the Hippocratic Corpus.[13]

In China in the meantime, the general attempt at westernization throughout the first half of the twentieth century involved medicine as it did other aspects of material life. The establishment of Western-style medical schools and the training of Western-oriented physicians proceeded apace, while the majority of the population continued to resort to traditional methods where Western medical care was unavailable. During the Second World War and the subsequent Communist revolution, the realities facing the new government meant that medical care was needed regardless of its form, and the resources for introducing widespread Western medical care were simply not there. In 1950 a major policy was therefore formulated, to the effect that all the resources, Western and Traditional, were to be mobilized, and that future medical education should aim to integrate the two. Since then, the slow fusion between the two systems has brought about first of all considerable benefits to the population, which has had access to medical care to an unprecedented extent, and secondly the gradual exposure of Traditional Chinese Medicine to formal scientific enquiry in the hope of abstracting from it those elements which appear to offer valid alternatives to Western practice or useful integration with it. For example, there is growing experience in the non-surgical treatment of acute diseases through herbal remedies and in the use of acupuncture as an analgesic and anaesthetic, even though some of the claims which arose during the Cultural Revolution were somewhat over-enthusiastic. In the same way, traditional remedies are finding new or extended applications, such as with *Artemisia annua*, long used as an antipyretic, which has now been recognized as a useful antimalaric. It is this synthesis which forms the New Chinese Medicine, Chung-kuo i-hsueh. The same twin approach, Western and Chinese, underlies the training of the 'Barefoot Doctors', medical auxiliaries who are now more often than not the first line of contact between the patient and the available medical care.[14]

While Chinese Folk Medicine has left its mark and in some way survives in the 'temple medicine' still practised to some extent both in Taiwan and amongst Overseas Chinese communities, and most probably in the People's Republic as well, and the New Chinese Medicine offers considerable hopes for the future, it is Chung-i, the Traditional Chinese Medicine, which is the most important both from the historical perspective and in the history of Chinese herbalism, if for no other reason than for its extremely long persistence and massive corpus of literature: a bibliography published in 1936 (Tamba Mototane's *Chung-kuo i-chi k'ao*) mentions 2,605 titles – of which, however, only a relatively small portion actually refers to pharmaceutics.[15]

Here one can follow the gradual development of an *a priori* formalized structure in which remedies and their effects were classified, a structure which was initially meant to mirror the hierarchies both of the heaven/man/earth macrocosm and that of the Imperial state. Considering the timescale over which the system evolved, one can envisage three conceptual steps: first, the empirical discovery ('Has this medicine any effect on the patient?'); second, its classification ('Where can it be fitted in the Heavenly Scheme?'); and third, usually much later, the gradual evolution of the classification through commentaries and glosses, which more often than not claim to point out an older and more original interpretation so as to maintain the claim of antiquity ('How should this scheme be interpreted so that it makes more sense?'). The principle of these structures is that of dividing drugs into Yin and Yang (and their related properties, 'heat' and 'cold' – which have no thermal implications in the Western sense), therefore giving them the property of replenishing an insufficiency of either of the two opposing components, or, conversely, balancing out an excess. The next to stand out is categorizing drugs as belonging either to the upper-class 'rulers', *chung*, middle-class 'ministers', *ch'en*, and lower-class 'assistants', *tso*, and 'aides', *shih*. The first are those drugs involved in the maintenance of health, such as tonics, rather than its restoration; as such, they have only limited medicinal effect, act slowly, and can be taken over long periods of time. The last two are curative, with strong medicinal effects, and only to be used for short applications. The *ch'en* class involves both kinds and is somewhat indefinite in nature, and it could be that it exists more to satisfy the macrocosmic image than because of any real practical differentiation. Through the various commentaries on the classics these terms evolve in their meaning, and *chung* is now applied to the principal active ingredient, be it a tonic or a curative. In either case, the remedy was and is almost invariably composed of a number of different drugs, the specific 'ruler' being supported in its action by a number of 'ministers', 'assistants' and 'aides' which modify its action or diminish its side effects. The role of 'rulers' given to those drugs involved in the maintenance of life – and therefore helping towards longevity – is a direct influence of the early Tao aspirations to immortality, and a similar religious basis can be seen in the fact that the early *Pen Ts'ao* describes exactly 365 drugs.

In practical use, the properties of the individual drugs are not only modified by admixture, but also by the preparation, both of the single components and of the remedy itself; for example, Aconite root is used as a cardiac tonic after boiling, which converts aconitin to benzylaconin with a massive lowering in toxicity.[16] Such changes are only now being described in scientific terms, but were nevertheless well known in the past and explained within the existing schemes. To quote Liu Chang-Xiao:

> *Amomum xanthoides* . . . can promote circulation of the vital energy, activiate the function of the spleen and improve appetite. After being broiled in salt, it is endowed with the action of conducting vital energy to the kidney and then it warms that organ and eliminates dampness, so it is clinically indicated for polyuria.[17]

An obvious offshoot of herbal practice has been the preparation of patent medicines. Pills, syrups and whatever other formulation might strike a pharmacist's fancy have been and are currently being produced and consumed in Asia and to a lesser extent in the West. These contain proprietary formulations of the traditional drugs, animal, vegetal and mineral; though the plant component is preponderant, a fairly wide selection of sometimes exotic animal components, such as 'Fossilized Bones of Dinosaur' ('Dragon's Bones'), 'Scales of Anteater', 'Genitalia of Male Sea Lion' and 'Clear Urine of Healthy Boys Under 12 Years of Age', have been used in the past and are in part still used. In practice, most of the animal and mineral components tend to fall out of the formulation of those remedies which have undergone some sort of clinical testing or whose manufacture has been re-established recently under modern production conditions, as for example those Chinese patent medicines being produced in the USA so as to circumvent the FDA's controls on imported 'medicines'. In a similar vein, a considerable effort has been put into developing the cultivation of medicinal plants on a sound agricultural basis, with selection both for higher production and for enhanced activity.

Proof of the success of Chinese Medicine in biological terms came when it was decided in 1979 that every non-minority-group family in the People's Republic should have only a single child. If only the decision had been taken forty years earlier, the figure could have been two.

Notes

1 Joseph P. Hou, 'The development of Chinese herbal medicine and the Pen-ts'ao', *Comparative Medicine East and West*, 5.2 (1977), pp. 117–22.

2 Frederick K. Kao, 'China, Chinese Medicine, and the Chinese medical system', *American Journal of Chinese Medicine*, 1.1 (1973), pp. 1–59; and John W. Schiffler, 'An essay on some of the fundamental philosophical tenets found in Traditional Chinese Medicine', *American Journal of Chinese Medicine*, 7.3 (1979), pp. 285–94.

3 Kao, 'China, Chinese Medicine, and the Chinese medical system'.

4 Ibid.

5 Ibid.; and Paul U. Unschuld, 'The development of medical-pharma-

ceutical thought in China', *Comparative Medicine East and West*, 5.2 (1977), pp. 109–15 (Part I), and 5.3–4, pp. 211–321 (Part II).

6 Ibid.
7 Kao, 'China, Chinese Medicine, and the Chinese medical system'.
8 Ibid.; and Schiffler 'An essay on some of the fundamental philosophical tenets found in Traditional Chinese Medicine'.
9 Kao, 'China, Chinese Medicine, and the Chinese medical system'.
10 Ibid.
11 Ibid.
12 Ibid.
13 Ibid.
14 Ji Zhongpu, 'Review and prospect of integration of Traditional Chinese and Western Medicine in past 30 years' *Chinese Journal of Integrated Medicine*, 8 (1988), pp. 88–9 (Special Issue 2).
15 Unschuld, 'The development of medical-pharmaceutical thought in China.
16 Hong-Yen Hsu and William G. Peacher, *Chinese Herb Medicine and Therapy* (Hawaiian Garden, CA: Oriental Healing Arts Institute of the USA, 1976).
17 Liu Chang-Xiao, 'Development of Chinese Medicine based on pharmacology and therapeutics', *Journal of Ethnopharmacology*, 19 (1987), pp. 119–23.

General information

Jiang Tingliang, 'Research on Chinese materia medica with Traditional Chinese and Western Medicine', *Chinese Journal of Integrated Medicine*, 8 (1988), pp. 193–6 (Special Issue 2).

Paul U. Unschuld, *Medicine in China – A History of Ideas* (Berkeley, CA: University of California Press, 1985).

Frank Liu and Liu Yan Mau, *Chinese Medical Terminology* (Hong Kong: The Commercial Press, 1980).

Shi Jizong and Chu Feng Zhu, trans. Shi Jiaxin, *The ABC of Traditional Chinese Medicine* (Hong Kong: Hai Feng Publishing Co., 1985).

Ron Teeguarden and Caroline Davies, *Chinese Tonic Herbs* (Tokyo: Japan Publications Inc., 1984).

Daniel P. Reid, *Chinese Medicine* (Wellingborough, Northants: CWF Publications/Thorsons, 1987).

Postscript

23

Hello, *Homo Sapiens*! This Is Your Largest Endocrine Gland Calling

Louis Pasteur's early work on the diseases of silkworms made him very aware of the fact that the organism's resistance plays as large a part as the pathogen in defining mortality. He was also aware of the fact that his Germ Theory relegated this resistance to a lesser role than it deserved, as was maintained by his contemporary, Paul Bernard. This fact is now being thrown in the face of society again and again as AIDS takes away the inbuilt resistance of the immunological system of its victims.

It was at the turn of the century that the well-known physician Oliver Wendell Holmes claimed that if all the drugs available were tossed into the ocean, it would be all the better for mankind and all the worse for the fishes. Nevertheless, with all the dubious treatments both herbal and chemical which medicine has offered through the ages, be they useless, dangerous, painful, or indeed damaging, the patients (and never was a word better applied) felt better for them and, at least often enough to notice, got better. Had they failed to do so, the institution of medicine would not have survived. That healers, from neolithic shamans to late-twentieth-century consultants, continue to live, practise and thrive, and are moreover given a major status in society regardless of the uncertainty of their tools, means that the most important component of the healing process is, and always has been, something resident within the patients themselves. Could it be that the majority of medicines used throughout history had no physical effect, but only served to focus the mind and the body's capacity for self-healing?[1]

We all know by now about the placebo effect, and how the expectation of cure can itself work wonders. Less well known is just how far this effect can go: there have been instances where mock heart surgery – in which the anaesthetized patient was opened and closed again, with all the trappings of surgery and convalescence but without the deep intervention – has proved as effective as the full operation. Nor is it a one-way road, either, as there have been recorded occasions where it was the doctor's expectations rather than the patient's which made the difference – and here really the only way the patient's health could have been affected would have been through his perception of the doctor's behaviour, in other words through the mind. The same can be said for the observation that the meaning of an injury for the patient can influence his response: for example, a soldier suffering a serious wound that implies a ticket home is likely to require less painkillers than one suffering from a minor injury which is likely to see him back in action after recovery. The brain and the mind it cannot contain may well be not only part of the healing process but also a very large part of our resistance to disease.[2]

How many of us have not read one of those fascinating *Reader's Digest*-type medico-anatomical articles and then sat worrying about the described symptoms which may or may not have been there already, but certainly have erupted like a mote in your mind's eye? The reason that we can indulge in such fantasies is that we have a large and highly sophisticated brain. That we seldom consider its full implications is perhaps the fault of the Descartian principle which separates mind and body, and which has steered our way of thinking to a greater or lesser extent over the past four centuries. As a result, both medicine and psychology have always undervalued the fact that the brain is not only the seat of thought and the centre of behaviour, but also the body's largest endocrine gland. In survival terms the brain's primary responsibility is to help its individual avoid trouble. Ill-health is a major source of trouble and probably has been throughout evolution, and certainly there are enough behavioural traits in man as well as in other animals aimed at the maintenance of health. It would seem unlikely therefore that the endocrine aspect of the brain would lack an important function in this sphere as well.[3]

The growing evidence of biochemical links between the hypothalamus, the oldest and 'deepest' part of the brain, and the immune system might perhaps be the breakthrough in the understanding of the mind–body interaction which physicians and psychologists have been waiting for, consciously or not. These links, moreover, would appear to be mediated both by the body's normal messengers, the hormones, and by endorphins, the brain's own 'internal' messengers known to underlie amongst others the feelings of pleasure and pain, and whose structure the plant-derived opiates so closely resemble as to imitate their action when taken by a not surprisingly addicted user.

There is, however, another aspect of the brain–body relationship which Descartes never envisaged, and that relates to the fact that the success of people has gone hand in hand with the survival requirements of a social primate with a menstrual cycle and a prolonged infancy. So it is little wonder that the social environment, in other words the amount of support and interaction one can count upon, has a significant effect on health, both in terms of avoiding disease and in easing recovery from it. Such interactions may be as close and emotionally demanding as those involving the immediate family, or may be as generic as those with work colleagues, neighbours or pets.

The fact that I as a child was taken to the doctor in my best clothes and I and the family firmly believed that he could make me better is part of that social package, naive as it may seem. In a similar vein, Albert Schweizer wrote: 'The witch doctor succeeds for the same reason all the rest of us succeed. Each patient carries his own doctor inside him. They come to us not knowing that cure. We are at our best when we give the doctor who resides within each patient a chance to go to work.'[4]

The brain may well be an all-important part of our internal health system and work in symbiosis with whatever medicare is on offer. There is, however, to date no proof that it can help us to make rational decisions either about our health or about our future.

The simple facts presented in this ptisane of history tell us unequivocally that better health and longer life expectancy in the nineteenth and twentieth centuries have for the most part not been the result of improved medical practice. The decrease of death by infective diseases was brought about by better social and hygienic conditions before the advent of modern pharmaceutical and medical developments. As an example, by the time streptomycin was introduced as a cure for tuberculosis in 1945, the number of deaths by tuberculosis had already shrunk by 97 per cent compared to what it had been in 1840; modern pharmaceutical and medical techniques can only account for the defeat of the residual 3 per cent. Similar curves can be drawn for a number of other infectious diseases, with the notable exception of poliomyelitis. Modern medical practices have allowed a large number of people to overcome illness, but the real cause of the health improvement over the last two centuries is that, at least in the developed world, fewer people tend to become seriously ill in the first place.[5]

As more and more medical effort is made to treat the residual cases of ill-health, society faces both a serious problem of diminishing returns, and a rapidly growing proportion of iatrogenic diseases. Also, lifetime factors, once absorbed in a generally high level of morbidity, stand out now as one of the main discriminating factors between the ill and the healthy. 'Health' is more and more being confused with 'Disease Being Cared For' – and the two things are not synonyms, and indeed never have been. One is therefore forced to ask, for example, does Britain have a National Health Service, or a National Diseases Being Cared For Service?[6]

Of course, we have both: our sewage systems, our waterworks, our pre- and post-natal clinics, weight watchers' clubs, geriatric counselling, aerobic and Tai Ch'i classes etc, etc., the requirements for the vast majority of which were already spelled out in the Talmud and in the Chinese Classics, are certainly the former. The increasing plethora of diagnostic equipment, from the colour-coded LCD thermometers at last banishing mercury from the sickroom to the great and unbelievably expensive body scanners, must be considered as part of an intermediate stage screening the *Reader's Digest* symptoms out from the real thing, while the rest of medical and health care comes into the latter category. If we omit the works of civil engineering – many of which, though in need of urgent repair, are still a legacy from our Victorian era – and omit the vast amount of money raised by charity to fund diagnostic and even what is now regarded as routine treatment equipment, the cost to the UK – 4.8 per cent of GNP in the early 1980s – was almost exactly the same as the amount spent on military defence, and less by 0.2 per cent than that spent on education.

An analogy with military defence is perhaps worth pursuing a little further. Each year we spend all these billions on maintaining the health of the corporate body called The Nation, protecting it and readying it against possible attack and in effect making it immune and diagnosing from whence attack may come. If attacked, the cost of warding off the predator and defeating it will escalate manyfold: a cost which very few, at least on the winning side, would consider out of proportion. The same is true of the health bill: we must spend money in maintaining our drains and water supplies and any expenditure is surely worth while to alleviate the symptoms and effect a cure, especially when viewed from the sickbed or from the visitors' chairs round it. But how is it all to be paid for? And how do you make rational decisions about iatrogenic and geriatric conditions? Where does ethics stop and euthanasia start, and certainly where does rationality get a look in? Nuclear missiles, which may well have been the most effective part of our enormously expensive national 'immune' system, can travel from Western Europe to Moscow in six minutes, yet everyday tens of millions of rural women and children spend long hours carrying water, leaving little time or energy to tend their crops or their education. What is more, for more than half of the world's poorest people, the water they carry is not safe to drink.

Earthwatch warns us that at any one time there may be:

500 million people with trachoma
250 million people with elephantiasis
200 million people urinating blood thanks to schistosomiasis
160 million people incapacitated with malaria
100 million people aching with constant diarrhoea and unable to work
30 million people already blind or succumbing to river blindness

Several million people have a combination of these sicknesses, to which may be added the waterborne diseases such as typhoid, cholera, dysentery, gastroenteritis and hepatitis, and those diseases aggravated by the lack of sufficient water for washing, such as scabies, yaws, leprosy and conjunctivitis. Over ten million people die each year – and that is 30,000 a day – from diseases caused or aggravated by impure water.

All this could be stopped by the expenditure of an amount that is peanuts in global warfare terms. A rational decision, yes; but think of the other 70,000 a day that die from conditions relating to malnutrition. The early 1960s saw rational jubilation as the new high-yielding crop varieties helped the world produce more food than ever before. The US Council for Environmental Quality estimates that in the year 2000 food production will be 90 per cent higher than it was in 1970. The other side of the coin is that in 36 years world consumption of fertilizers has already risen tenfold and the annual consumption of tractors quadrupled, increases which can in no way be maintained on a global scale. And so the World Bank estimates that the number of malnourished could rise from some 400 million in the mid-1970s to 1.3 billion by the turn of the century. Our brains must remind us of the fact that malnutrition and poor living conditions are key factors increasing the incidence of disease and premature death.

It is for this reason that there should be no doubt that the greatest landmark in the history of modern medicine, both herbal and regular, was that tropical Yam planted by Russell E. Marker, providing hope for a future both ethical and rational.

For anyone who might find fault with this conclusion welling up in their largest endocrine gland, please think about the following statistics:

Chance of death in a year:

1 in 5	Being a child under 12 months of age in Sierra Leone
1 in 10	Being a child under 12 months of age in Egypt
1 in 20	Being a child under 12 months of age in São Tomé & Principe
1 in 50	Motorcycling
1 in 75	Being a child under 12 months of age in Hong Kong

1 in 200	Smoking (20 cigarettes a day)
1 in 3,000	Preventing pregnancy by illegal abortion
1 in 6,000	Driving a car
1 in 7,500	Rock climbing
1 in 10,000	Preventing pregnancy by legal abortion (after 16 weeks)
1 in 10,000	Tubal ligation*
1 in 16,000	Preventing pregnancy by oral contraception: smoker*
1 in 25,000	Playing football
1 in 25,000	Preventing pregnancy by legal abortion (13–16 weeks)
1 in 63,000	Preventing pregnancy by oral contraception: non-smoker*
1 in 100,000	Preventing pregnancy by legal abortion (9–12 weeks)
1 in 100,000	Preventing pregnancy by intra-uterine contraceptive device*
1 in 400,000	Preventing pregnancy by legal abortion (9 weeks)
None	Barrier methods of contraception*
None	Natural methods of contraception*
None	Vasectomy*

* The failure of these methods could lead to death in pregnancy, but the likelihood of failure is very much greater for some methods than for others.[7]

Notes

1 R. Ornstein and Daved Sobel *The Healing Brain* (London: Macmillan, 1988).
2 Ibid.
3 Ibid.
4 Ibid., p. 258.
5 Ornstein and Sobel, *The Healing Brain*.
6 Ibid.
7 Eric McGraw, *Population: The Human Race* (London: Bishopsgate Press, 1990).

The Green Family Doctor
– or, The Families of
Healing Plants

INTRODUCTION

There is no complete list of the Planet Earth's materia medica. Each culture and sub-culture throughout history has dipped into the patrimony of plants at his disposal for better or for worse, a patrimony which has varied between the strictly local and the global. Knowledge was accumulated, knowledge was lost, and in some areas is at present being lost at an ever-increasing rate. What information is available is recorded in a bewildering variety of contexts, languages and media, and its reorganization in a usable form is perhaps one of the major tasks facing ethnobotanists, on a par with that of preventing the loss of otherwise unrecorded oral knowledge. It is a wide field, where brief examples risk being trivial, and thorough examples are in danger of becoming overbearing; what follows falls unavoidably in the second category.

The following list (Table 1) centres on all the families of flowering plants, dealt with in evolutionary order according to Heywood's arrangement.[1] Relevant families in the other plant groups are included wherever important materia medica is found in them. All the families of flowering plants are included for, as ethnobotanical research continues, we are sure that most if not all of them will be found to have been used, at least in the past if not in the present, and are therefore worthy of further investigation. Under each brief family description we append some of its alimentary or otherwise non-medicinal uses, with a few examples if appropriate. When the word 'some' is used in reference to species, it means that its taxonomic study is incomplete; when it is used in reference to genus, it should be carried over to species as well.

For each family, we have summarized the relevant entries from several different sources, so as to give an idea both of the spread of medicinal properties throughout the plant kingdom (plus some), and the varying importance which they have had in Western medicine. The sources are the 1988 edition of the *British Pharmacopoeia*,[2] the 1979 and 1907 editions of the *British Pharmaceutical Codex*,[3] and a 1966 edition of the first Book of Avicenna's *Canon* as used in Unani Medicine,[4] chosen for its 'nearness' to the roots of Western Medicine regardless of its contemporaneity.

In the numerical 'Summary of the simples' that follows the list of plant families (Table 2), the relative frequencies of medicinal plants occurring in families has been noted. In addition, the last two columns show the number of species within the family which are referred to in two major catalogues of materia medica referring to the two other principal medical systems, Chinese Traditional Medicine, represented by the medical flora of Hong Kong,[5] and Ayurveda, based on the medicinal flora of Sri Lanka.[6]

Our sources of taxonomic and economic information have been multifarious, but the main authority on Angiosperms has been Heywood,[7] with several other sources, both generic and specific, to other divisions and kingdoms.[8]

The codings are as follows:

1988 refers to *The British Pharmacopoeia* (1988)
1979 refers to *The (British) Pharmaceutical Codex* (1979)
1907 refers to the *British Pharmaceutical Codex* (1907)
In these three cases the reference and the uses quoted are given.
Canon refers to Book I of Avicenna's *Canon*, for which the reference is given both in English and in Urdu, together with the part used and its Temperament, according to Avicenna's Humoral system.

Notes

1 V. H. Heywood (ed.), *Flowering Plants of the World* (Oxford: Oxford University Press, 1978).

2 The British Pharmacopoeia Commission, *The British Pharmacopoeia* (London: HMSO, 1988).

3 The Pharmaceutical Society, *The Pharmaceutical Codex*, 11th edn (London: The Pharmaceutical Society, *The British Pharmaceutical Codex* (London: The Pharmaceutical Society, 1907).

4 Mazar H. Shah (ed.), Avicenna, *The General Principles of Avicenna's Canon of Medicine* (Karachi: Naveed Clinic, 1966).

5 Cheung Siu-cheong and Li Ning-hon (eds), *Chinese Medical Herbs of Hong Kong*, vols 1–5 (Hong Kong, 1978).

6 D. M. A. Jayaweera, *Medicinal Plants (Indigenous and Exotic) Used in Ceylon* 5 vols (Colombo: The National Science Council of Sri Lanka, 1981).

7 Heywood, *Flowering Plants of the World*.

8 Peter H. Raven and George B. Johnson, *Biology* (St Louis, MO: Times Mirror/Mosby College Publishing, 1986); Lilian E. Hawker, *Fungi, an Introduction* (London: Hutchinson University Library, 1966); Mirko Svreck, *The Hamlyn Book of Mushrooms and Fungi* (London: Hamlyn, 1983); A. J. E. Smith, *The Moss Flora of Britain and Ireland* (Cambridge: Cambridge University Press, 1978); K. R. Sporne, *The Morphology of Pteridophytes* (London: Hutchinson University Library, 1962, 4th edn); and K. R. Sporne, *The Morphology of Gymnosperms* (London: Hutchinson University Library, 1965, 2nd edn).

Table 1
The Families of
Healing Plants

KINGDOM: PROTISTA

BROWN ALGAE – PHYLUM PHAEOPHYTA

Worldwide, mainly marine (brown seaweeds), some 1500 species.

Wrack family – Fucaceae

> *Fucus vesiculosus*   Origin: Europe
> 1907:   Fucus, Bladder-wrack
> Uses: Has been used to reduce glandular swellings; is the basis for most current 'anti-fat' nostrums.

Kelp family – Laminariaceae

> *Laminaria* spp.: sections of its stipes are used for plugging open wounds.

RED ALGAE – PHYLUM RHODOPHYTA

Worldwide, mostly marine (red seaweeds), some 4000 species.

Gelidium family – Gelidiaceae

> *Gelidium* spp.   Origin: Asia
> 1988:   Agar
> Uses: Pharmaceutical aid.
> 1907:   Agar-Agar
> Uses: Culture media, gelatin.

Gigartina family – Gigartinaceae

Chondrus crispus   Origin: Europe
1907:   Chondrus, Carragheen, Irish Moss
Uses: Demulcent and emulsifying agent.

KINGDOM: FUNGI

Microscopic, filamentous, multinucleate true cells, with cell walls rich in chitin, saprophytes living on decaying organic material, some parasites. Worldwide from the sea to the mountain tops, some 100,000 named species.

DIVISION EUMYCOPHYTA

Sac Fungi – Class Ascomycetes

Sac fungi, yeasts and moulds; many parasitic plant pathogens, some 30,000 named species.

SUB-CLASS EUASCOMYCETIDEAE

Series Plectomycetes

ORDER PLECTASCALES

Family – Aspergillaceae

Penicillium spp., the source of penicillin and all that followed.

Series Hymenoascomycetes

Sub-series Pyrenomycetes

ERGOTS – ORDER CLAVICIPITALES

Ergot family – Clavicipetaceae

Claviceps purpurea   Origin: Europe
1907:   Ergota, Ergot, Ergot of Rye
Uses: Contains ergotoxine and ergotinine. Plain muscle stimulant, vasoconstrictor.

Mushrooms – Class Basidiomycetes

Mushrooms, toadstools, brackets, rusts and smuts, worldwide some 25,000 species.

SUB-CLASS HOMOBASIDIOMYCETIDEAE

Series Hymenomycetes

ORDER AGARICALES

Family – Agaricaceae

Agaricum officinale　　　　　　　　　　Origin: North Temperate
Canon: Agaric (Urdu: Gharoqoon)
Parts used: Fruiting body.
Temperament: Hot and Dry in the First Degree.

LICHENS – DIVISION LICHENES

Symbiotic associations between green algae, cyanobacteria and fungi, the latter mostly ascomycetes though some basidiomycetes; worldwide, some 25,000 species.

Cetraria islandica　　　　　　　　　　Origin: Europe
1907:　　Cetraria, Iceland Moss
Uses:　　Decoction forms a nutritious and demulcent drink.

Roccella spp.　　　　　　　　　　　　Origin: Africa
1907:　　Persio, Cudbear
Uses:　　Purple-red colouring agent, litmus indicator.

KINGDOM: PLANTAE

MOSSES AND LIVERWORTS – DIVISION BRYOPHYTA

Worldwide, some 10,600 species

Class Sphagnopsida

ORDER SPHAGNALES

Bog Moss family – Sphagnaceae

Cosmopolitan but favouring temperate and cold regions and mountains. Many species of Bog Mosses have been used as absorbents, both as babies' diapers and in wound dressings. Some claim to a factor speeding the healing process. Peat, mainly derived from the Bog Mosses, is highly prized in balneotherapy in central Europe and in Poland claims have been made in the use of peat extracts against skin cancer.

CLUB MOSSES – DIVISION LYCOPHYTA

Worldwide, 5 genera with some 1000 species.

ORDER LYCOPODIALES

Club Moss family – Lycopodiaceae

2 genera with some 200 species, cosmopolitan, from creeping bog plants to pendulous epiphytes.

Lycopodium clavatum   Origin: Europe *et al.*
1907:   Lycopodium
Uses: Covering for pills; dusting powder; insufflation diluent, basis for snuffs. Tincture has been prescribed for bladder disorders.

FERNS – DIVISION PTEROPHYTA

Cosmopolitan, found across the complete range of climates and habitats from brackish to freshwater to mountain tops, some 12,000 species.

Class Leptosporangiata

ORDER FILICALES

Male Fern family – Dennstaedtiaceae

Dryopteris filix-mas   Origin: Europe
1979:   Male Fern, Filix Mas
Uses: Violent anthelmintic.
1907:   *Aspidium filix-mas*, Filix Mas, Male Fern, Aspidium
Uses: Astringent, occasionally used as powder. Liquid extract is used to expel tapeworm, to all varieties of which it is an acute poison.

Maidenhair Fern family – Adiantaceae
Adiantum capillus-veneris
Canon: Maidenhair Fern (Urdu: Hansraj)
Parts used: Plant.
Temperament: Hot and Dry.

Polypod family – Polypodiaceae

Polypodium vulgaris
Canon: Polypody (Urdu: Bisfaij)
Parts used: Root.
Temperament: Hot in the Second and Dry in the Third Degree.

CONE-BEARING PLANTS – DIVISION CONIFEROPHYTA

Worldwide, some 50 genera with 550 species.

ORDER CONIFERALES

Pine family – Pinaceae

Abies balsamica   Origin: North America
1907:   Terebinthina Canadensis, Canada Balsam
Uses: Pill exipient, flexible colloidon source; microscopy medium.

Picea excelsa   Origin: Europe
1907:   Pix Burgundica, Burgundy Pitch
Uses: Mild counter-irritant, used in the preparation of plasters.

Pinus spp.   Origin: southern Europe
1988:   Turpentine Oil
Uses: Rubefacient.
1979:   Colophony Resin, Turpentine Oil
Uses: Ingredient in plaster masses and colloidons. Turpentine Oil is
        a counter-irritant and rubefacient.
1907:   Oleum Terebinthineae, Turpentine Oil
Uses: Antiseptic, germicidal in high concentration. External irritant
        and rubefacient. Inhaled, arrests profuse secretion and relieves
        bronchioles; salivatory, expectorant, diuretic and urinary
        stimulant.

Pinus mugo var. *pumilo*   Origin: Austria
1979:   Pumilo Pine Oil
Uses: Aromatic, used for inhalations to relieve cough.
1907:   Oleum Pini, Oil of Pine
Uses: Antiseptic, germicidal in high concentration. External irritant
        and rubefacient. Inhaled, arrests profuse secretion and relieves
        bronchioles; salivatory, expectorant, diuretic and urinary
        stimulant.

Pinus palustris   Origin: North America
1907:   Thus Americanum, American Frankincense, Gum Thus
Uses: Oleoresin used in the preparation of plasters.

Pinus gerardiana
Canon: Pinenuts (Urdu: Chilghoza)
Parts used: Nuts.
Temperament: Hot in the Third Degree and Dry in the First.

Tsuga canadensis   Origin: North America
1907:   Pini Canadensis Cortex, Hemlock Spruce Bark
Uses: Astringent in catarrhal diseases.

Cypress family – Cupressaceae

Callitris quadrivalvis   Origin: North-west Africa
1907:   Sandaraca, Sandarac, Gum Juniper
Uses: Gum used as pill-coating and as temporary stopping for teeth.

Cupressus sempervirens
Canon: Cypress (Urdu: Saroo)
Parts used: Leaves.
Temperament: Cool and Dry.

Juniper communis   Origin: Europe
1907:   Oleum Juniperi, Oil of Juniper
Uses: Employed chiefly as a stimulating diuretic in cardiac and
         hepatic dropsy.
Canon: Juniper (Urdu: Shamshad ka phal)
Parts used: Berries.
Temperament: Hot and Dry in the Third Degree.

Juniperus oxicedrus   Origin: Mediterranean
1979:   Cade Oil, Juniper Tar Oil
Uses: Local application for the treatment of psoriasis.
1907:   Oleum Cadium, Oil of Cade, Juniper Tar Oil
Uses: Stimulant antiseptic in chronic skin diseases.

Juniperus virginiana   Origin: North America
1907:   Oleum Cedri, Cedar Wood Oil
Uses: Has been recommended for use in place of oil of sandalwood
         in gonorrhoea. Useful as perfuming agent, and in microscopy.

Juniperus sabina   Origin: southern Europe
1907:   Oleum Sabinae, Oil of Savin
Uses: Powerful irritant, both externally and internally. Employed in
         amenorrhoea with other emmenagogues, with caution.

JOINT PINES – DIVISION GNETOPHYTA

ORDER GNETALES

Joint Pine family – Ephedraceae

Distributed disjunctly worldwide, 3 genera with some 70 species.

Ephedra spp.   Origin: China, India
1979:   *E. sinica, E. equistina, E. gerardiana*
Uses: Source of ephedrine. Sympathomimetic amine. Resembles
         adrenaline and amphetamine in its effects.

FLOWERING PLANTS – DIVISION ANTHOPHYTA

Worldwide, some 235,000 species.

Class Angiospermae

SUB-CLASS DICOTYLEDONEAE

Superorder Magnoliidae

ORDER MAGNOLIALES

Magnolia family – Magnoliaceae

Trees and shrubs, about 220 species. Native in Asia and America,
produces many horticultural shrubs and trees and some timber.
Magnolia officinalis, bark and flower buds yield an essential oil and
ho-curare, a valuable drug being exported from China.

Winter's Bark family – Winteraceae

7 or 8 genera with up to 12 families found in montane and temperate
forests bordering the Pacific, with an outlier on the southern Brazil
coast. They lack vessels, and are possibly the most primitive of
flowering plants. The leaves and bark of some species are used as
medicinals.
Drymis winteri was used as an antiscorbutic.

Galbulimima family – Himantandraceae

A monogeneric family with only 3 species, all occurring in the tropical forests of north-eastern Australia and the adjacent islands, New Guinea and the Moluccas. A botanical relict of the early development of the flowering plants.

White Cinnamon family – Canellaceae

A small family of some 17 species of aromatic trees, restricted to the tropics but in Madagascar, East Africa, the West Indies and Central America.

Canella alba   Origin: Caribbean
1907:   Canellae Cortex, Wild Cinnamon Bark
Uses: Aromatic bitter.

Soursop family – Annonaceae

Some 2000 species of trees and shrubs, widely distributed throughout the forested tropics. The family has given the world the Soursops and Sweetsops which are now being commercially grown.
Monodora myristica fruits are used as a nutmeg substitute; *Xylopia aethiopica* fruits provide the so-called 'Negro Pepper'.

Nutmeg family – Myristicaceae

Some 380 trees, mainly found in lowland rainforest throughout the tropical belt.

Myristica fragrans   Origin: Moluccas
1988:   Nutmeg Oil
Uses: Flavouring.
1979:   Nutmeg, Myristica, Nutmeg Oil
Uses: Carminative and flavouring agent.
1907:   Myristica, Nutmeg
Uses: Aromatic and carminative. The oil has some stimulant action on the cerebral cortex.

Degeneria family – Degeneriaceae

Monogeneric family with a single species of tree found in Fiji, *Degeneria vitiensis*.

ORDER ILLICIALES

Star Anise family – Illiciaceae

A single genus of about 40 species of small trees and shrubs, from south-eastern USA, West Indies, Japan, China and Southeast Asia.

Illicium verum   Origin: China
1988:   Anise, Aniseed
Uses   Carminative, flavouring.
1979:   Star Anise
Uses: Carminative, expectorant.
1907:   Star Anise
Uses: Same use and active principles as Anise (*Pimpinella anisium*).
        Aromatic carminative, to decrease flatulence.

Schisandra family – Schisandraceae

2 genera of perhaps 50 species of trailing and twining shrubs, found in tropical and subtropical India, Southeast and East Asia and south-eastern USA.

ORDER LAURALES

Austrobaileya family – Austrobaileyaceae

A single genus with 2 species of liana-like climbing shrubs from the rainforest of north Queensland.

Eupomatia family – Eupomatiaceae

1 genus, 2 species of shrubs and small trees from the rainforests of eastern Australia and New Guinea.

Gormotega family – Gormotegaceae

A single evergreen tree species found in the forests of south central Chile, perhaps related to the Laurels.

Boldo family – Monimiaceae

Some 30 genera many with only 1 species distributed throughout the tropics with the exception of India.

278

Peumus boldus   Origin: Chile

1907: Boldo Folia, Boldo Leaves
Uses: Used in South America in chronic hepatic congestion and as an aromatic tonic and diuretic in genito-urinary disorders. Also a hypnotic.

Carolina Allspice family – Calycanthaceae

8 species of hardy deciduous and evergreen shrubs, from North America, East Asia and north-east Australia. *Iodospermum australiense* has been recently found again in the Queensland rainforest after it was believed to be extinct.
Calycanthus floridus bark was used as a spice by the American Indians; *Calycanthus fertilis* bark, leaves and roots are used in medicine.

Chloranthus family – Chloranthaceae

5 genera and 65 species of herbs, shrubs, and small trees. Found in the humid tropics and south temperate region except Africa and Australia. *Chloranthus inconspicuus* leaves are used to flavour tea, and in an infusion to treat coughs in eastern Asia; *Hepyosmum brasilense* extracts of leaves are used as a tonic, diuretic, aphrodisiac, to induce sweating and for stomach disorders.

Laurel family – Lauraceae

A medium-sized family of 32 genera and some 2500 species of shrubs, trees and a few parasitic climbers widely distributed throughout the tropics and subtropics. The family has given the world Avocados, Cinnamon, Bay Leaves, Camphor and Sassafras Oil.

Cinnamomum camphora   Origin: southern China
1988: Camphor
Uses: Counter-irritant.
1907: Camphor
Uses: Carminative, antiseptic for the alimentary canal, mild vaso-dilatant, directly excites the cerebrum. Taken as relief for colds. The oil is rubefacient and a mild counter-irritant.
Canon: Camphor (Urdu: Kafoor)
Parts used: Resin.
Temperament: Cool and Dry in the Third Degree.

Cinnamomum cassia   Origin: Southeast Asia
1907:   Cassiae Cortex, Cassia, Chinese Cinnamon
Uses: Mildly astringent, carminative, antiseptic. The oil is carminative
        to the gastro-intestinal tract and antiseptic; taken internally
        against influenzal colds, and inhaled for phtisis.
Canon: Cassia Bark (Urdu: Taj)
Parts used: Bark.
Temperament: Hot and Dry in the Third Degree.

Cinnamomum olivieri   Origin: Australia
1907:   Oliveri Cortex, Oliver Bark, Black Sassafras
Uses: Australian substitute for cinnamon: Carminative, antiseptic,
        flavouring. Oil is carminative to the gastro-intestinal tract and
        antiseptic. Taken internally against influenzal colds, and
        inhaled for phthisis.

Cinnamomum zeylanicum   Origin: Sri Lanka
1988:   Cinnamon
Uses: Carminative, flavouring.
1979:   Cinnamon
Uses: Carminative, slightly astringent.
1907:   Cinnamomi Cortex
Uses: Carminative, antiseptic, flavouring. The oil is carminative to
        the gastro-intestinal tract and antiseptic; taken internally
        against influenzal colds, and inhaled for phthisis.
Canon: Cinnamon (Urdu: Darcheeni)
Parts used: Bark.
Temperament: Hot and Dry in the Third Degree.

Cryptocarya spp.   Origin: Bolivia
1907:   The probable source of Coto Bark
Uses: Said to increase the appetite by gastric vasodilatation. Used in
        the treatment of diarrhoea, marasmus, and intestinal catarrh.

Laurus nobilis   Origin: Europe
1907:   Lauri Fructus, Laurel Berries
Uses: Volatile oil used on account of its pleasant odour; the fixed oil
        has been used for rubbings, in rheumatism.

Nectandra rodiaei   Origin: Guyana
1907:   Bebeeru Cortex
Uses: Source of berberine and siperine. Aromatic bitter tonic, used
        as substitute for quinine.

Sassafras officinale   Origin: North America
1907:   Oleum Sassafras, Oil of Sassafras
Uses: Perfuming and flavouring agent; rubefacient and anodyne
        liniment in chronic rheumatism. Pith of plant is demulcent.

Hernandia family – Hernandiaceae

A pantropical family of 76 species and 4 genera of trees, shrubs and
some lianas which like to grow near the coast.

ORDER PIPERALES

Pepper family – Piperaceae

A pantropical family of some 5 genera and some 2000 species of trees,
shrubs and woody climbers growing mainly in rainforests.

Piper angustifolium   Origin: South America
1907:   Matico
Uses: Aromatic astringent in inflammatory conditions of the urinary
        tract. Styptic.

Piper betle   Origin: India
1907:   Betel
Uses: Masticatory, stimulant and carminative.

Piper cubeba   Origin: Malay archipelago
1907:   Cubebae Fructus, Cubebs, Tailed Pepper
Uses: Similar action to copaiba. Antiseptic diuretic, uro-genital
        stimulant. Oil is a general stimulant, antiseptic of the mucous
        membranes.

Piper methysticum   Origin: Oceania
1907:   Kavae Rhizoma, Kava-Kava
Uses: Stimulant diuretic in gonorrhoea and cystitis; also used as an
        intoxicating drink.

Piper nigrum   Origin: Malay archipelago
1907:   Piper Nigrum, Black Pepper
Uses: Strong stimulant and carminative; condiment. Diuretic, also
         used for haemorrhoids.
Canon: Pepper, Black (Urdu: Kali mirch)
Parts used: Fruit.
Temperament: Hot and Dry in the Fourth Degree.

Piper officinarum   Origin: Malay archipelago
1907:   Piper Longum, Long Pepper
Uses: Stimulant and carminative.

Lizard Tail family – Saururaceae

Temperate and subtropical perennial herbs, 5 genera and 7 species
from East Asia and North America.
Amenopsis californica (Yerba Mansa) rootstock is made into ornamental beads; an infusion of the rootstock in water is used against
dysentery and malaria.

Pepper Elder family – Peperomiaceae

4 genera, about 1000 species, tropical and subtropical worldwide,
succulent herbs, many epiphytic or on rocky places.
Peperomia viridispica, young leaves and stems are eaten raw in
Central and South America.

ORDER ARISTOLOCHIALES

Asarum family – Aristolochiaceae

Some 625 species of herbs and shrubs and twisting lianas found in
tropical and warm temperate forest and scrubland throughout the
Near East and Australia.

Aristolochia indica   Origin: India
1907:   Aristolochia
Uses: Bitter – causes necrotic nephritis in rabbits.

Aristolochia serpentaria   Origin: North America
1907:   Serpentariae Rhizoma, Serpentary
Uses: Bitter, vehicle for tonics.

Pitcher Plant family – Nepenthaceae

Insectivorous plants, 1 genus of 7 species found in the rainforests of the Old World tropics including Madagascar and the Seychelles.

ORDER NYMPHAEALES

Hornwort family – Ceratophyllaceae

A cosmopolitan family of 1 genus of 2 (or perhaps more) species of rootless submerged water plants.

Water Lily family – Nymphaeaceae

9 genera, perhaps 90 or more species, cosmopolitan in temperate and tropical freshwater habitats. The seeds and rhyzomes of a number of Water Lilies are eaten and some when roasted yield arrowroot.

ORDER RANUNCULALES

May Apple family – Berberidaceae

Mainly found in the north temperate regions and the mountains of South America. Some 600 species in 13–16 genera, shrubs and perennial herbs.

Berberis vulgaris   Origin: Europe
1907: Berberidis Cortex, Barberry Bark
Uses: Source of berberine. Bitter tonic and stomachic (used in intermittent fevers).

Berberis aristata   Origin: India
1907: Berberis
Uses: Similar to Barberry Bark. Source of berberine. Bitter tonic and stomachic (used in intermittent fevers).
Canon: Berberin (Urdu: Rasaut)
Parts used: Extract.
Temperament: Hot, and Dry in the Second Degree.

Caulophyllum thalictroides   Origin: North America
1907: Caulophyllum, Blue Cohosh, Squaw Root
Uses: Diuretic, emmenagogue, anthelmintic.

Podophyllum hexandrum   Origin: India
1988:   Podophyllum Resin
Uses: Used in treatment of warts.
1979:   Podophyllum, Indian Podophyllum
Uses: Resin has a cytotoxic action; used as a treatment for venereal
        and other warts.
1907:   Podophylli Indici Rhizoma, Indian Podophyllum
Uses: Drastic purgative and cholagogue, twice as active as ordinary
        podophyllum.

Podophyllum peltatum   Origin: North America
1988:   Podophyllum Resin
Uses: Used in treatment of warts.
1979:   Podophyllum, American Mandrake
Uses: Resin has a cytotoxic action; used as a treatment for venereal
        and other warts.
1907:   Podophylli Rhizoma, May Apple, Mandrake
Uses: Drastic purgative, cholagogue.

Buttercup family – Ranunculaceae

World-wide distribution but having their main centre in the temperate
and cold parts of the northern hemisphere, some 50 genera with 1800
species.

Aconitum napellus   Origin: Europe
1907:   Aconite Leaf, Aconite Root
Uses: Diaphoretic, externally applied anodyne.
Canon: Aconite (Urdu: Mitha Taleya)
Parts used: Root.
Temperament: Hot and Dry in the Fourth Degree.
Comments: Referred to as *Aconitum ferox*.

Anemone pulsatilla   Origin: Europe
1907:   Pulsatilla, Pasque Flower
Uses: Powerful irritant similar to cantharides, has been given as a
        'sedative' for dysmenorrhoea, headache and neuralgia. No
        reliable evidence of value.

Cimicifuga racemosa   Origin: North America
1907:   Cimicifugae Rhizoma, Black Snakeroot
Uses: Bitter, mild expectorant

284

Delphinium staphisagria   Origin: western Asia
1907:   Staphisagriae Semina, Stavesacre Seed
Uses: Used as unguent to destroy pediculi.

Helleborus niger   Origin: Europe
1907:   Hellebori Nigri Rhizoma, Black Hellebore
Uses: Powerful hydragogue, cathartic and emmenagogue. Rarely used.

Hydrastis canadensis   Origin: North America
1907:   Hydrastis Rhizoma, Golden Seal Rhizome
Uses: Bitter, vasoconstrictor.

Nigella sativa
Canon: Cumin, Black (Fennel Seed) (Urdu: Kalwanji)
Parts used: Seeds.
Temperament: Hot and Dry in the Third Degree.
Comments: Fennel Flower, NOT Cumin.

Ranunculus ficaria   Origin: Europe
1907:   Ranunculus Ficaria, Pilewort
Uses: Old remedy for haemorrhoids.

Holboellia family – Lardizabalaceae

From Japan, the Himalayas, and Chile. 9 genera with 36 species of climbing shrubs, some erect. The fruit of some are eaten locally.

Curare family – Menispermaceae

Principally lianas, rarely trees, shrubs and herbs. Mainly in tropical rainforests, but some in warm temperate and subtropical areas across the New World and the Old.

Anamirta paniculata   Origin: Malaya
1907:   Cocculi Fructus, Levant Berries
Uses: Important as source of picrotoxin, a convulsive poison acting on the medulla. Powdered berries used in ointments for destroying pediculi. Fish poison. Once used to adulterate beer.

Chondrodendron tomentosum   Origin: South America
1907:   Pareirae Radix, Pareira
Uses: Simple bitter, and as an astringent for urinary tract disorders.

Cissampelos pareira   Origin: Caribbean
1907:   Cissampelos
Uses: Similar properties to Pareira Root (*Chondrodendron tomen-tosum*): simple bitter, and as an astringent for urinary tract disorders.

Coscinium fenestratum   Origin: India
1907:   Coscinium
Uses: Bitter, with similar properties to Calumba. (*Jateurhyza columba*): pure bitter, used in atonic dyspepsia and debility of digestive organs.

Jateurhyza columba   Origin: East Africa
1907:   Calumbae Radix, Calumba Root
Uses: Pure bitter, used in atonic dyspepsia and debility of digestive organs.

Tinospora cordifolia   Origin: India
1907:   Tinospora, Gulancha
Uses: Berberine-containing bitter.

ORDER PAPAVERALES

Poppy family – Papaveraceae

Temperate, mainly in the north, but also South Africa and eastern Australia. 26 genera and about 250 species of herbs, all of which produce coloured latex.

Papaver somniferum   Origin: Asia
1988:   Opium
Uses: Narcotic, analgesic.
1979:   Opium, Raw Opium
Uses: Similar effects to morphine, though slower and more con-stipating.
1907:   Opium, Papaveris Capsulae, Poppy Heads
Uses: Narcotic by depression of sensory nerve cells in the cerebrum; pain reducer, medullar depressant, antidiarrhoeic with a more prolonged action than morphine. Poppy heads are used as a mild sedative and analgesic.
Canon: Opium (Urdu: Ayfoon)
Parts used: Dried juice.

Temperament: Cool and Dry in the Fourth Degree.
Comments: Also as Poppy Seeds, Khashkhash, Cool and Dry in the
Second Degree.

Papaver rhoeas   Origin: Europe
1907:   Rhoedos Petala, Red Poppy Petals
Uses: Petals used for their colouring matter.

Sanguinaria canadensis   Origin: North America
1907:   Sanguinariae Rhizoma, Sanguinaria, Blood Root
Uses: Mild opiate; in small doses it is emetic, expectorant, and
mildly narcotic. Powdered, it is a violent irritant to the
respiratory passages.

Fumitory family – Fumariaceae

Mainly in north temperate region, with some in central and southern
Africa, a family of 16 genera with some 400 species of herbs.

Fumaria officinalis
Canon: Fumitory (Urdu: Shahtara)
Parts used: Plant.
Temperament: Cool and Dry in the First Degree.

Pitcher Plant family – Sarraceniaceae

3 genera with 17 species of Pitcher Plants found in coastal regions of
North America and northern South America.

Superorder Hamamelidae

ORDER TROCHODENDRALES

Trochodendron family – Trochodendraceae

1 genus with 1 species of forest trees found in Japan, Taiwan, and the
Ryu Kyu Islands.
Trochodendron aralioides, the aromatic bark of which is used for
making birdlime.

ORDER HAMAMELIDALES

Cercidiphyllum family – Cercidiphyllaceae

Coastal China and Japan, 1 genus with 1 species: *Cercidiphyllum japonicum*

Plane family – Platanaceae

Chiefly in North America with outliers in the Balkans, Himalayas and Indochina. The single genus presents the world with 10 species of handsome deciduous trees.
Plantanus orientalis, reputedly the tree under which the Hippocratic Oath was taken on the island of Kos.

Witch Hazel family – Hamamelidaceae

Spanning all continents except Australia, Greenland and Antarctica. 23 genera with 100 species of trees and shrubs show a discontinuous distribution across the subtropical and temperate zones.

Hamamelis virginiana   Origin: North America
1907:   Hamamelidis Cortex, Witch Hazel Bark, Leaves
Uses: Local astringent and haemostatic. Used for wounds, abrasions and piles.

Liquidambar orientalis   Origin: Turkey
1979:   Storax, Styrax
Uses: Ingredient in benzoin inhalations and tinctures.
1907:   Styrax Praeparatus, Styrax
Uses: An ointment is used as a parasiticide in scabies and other parasitic skin affections.

ORDER EUCOMMIALES

Chinese Rubber family – Eucommiaceae

Eucommia ulmoides is a small deciduous tree found in a small region of subtropical China, and is the single representative of this family. The bark is known as 'Tu-Chung' or 'Tze-Lien', and produces a tonic for arthritis. Its latex also provides a poor rubber.

Florida Corkwood family – Leitneriaceae

A single genus with a single species found in swamp forests in Florida.

ORDER MYRICALES

Sweet Gale family – Myricaceae

2 genera of aromatic shrubs and small trees with some 35 species found across the world except in Australia and the warm temperate parts of Africa and Eurasia. The fruits of a number of species are boiled to produce wax.
Myrica gale leaves and twigs are used in the brewing of Gale Beer in Scandinavia.

ORDER FAGALES

Birch family – Betulaceae

Trees and shrubs, 6 genera with some 170 species, widespread in the north temperate region pushing south into the mountains of South America. The family provides the world with hazelnuts, cobnuts and filberts.
Betula spp., the twigs of which are used for post-sauna flagellation.

Betula lenta   Origin: Europe
1907:   Oleum Betulae, Oil of Sweet Birch
Uses: Consists almost entirely of methyl salicylate. Given internally in acute rheumatism, though external use might give rise to eruptions – pure methyl salicylate is preferable. Flavouring agent.

Betula alba   Origin: Europe
1907:   Oleum Betulae Albae, Oil of White Birch, Birch Tar
Uses: Used in external applications for eczema, psoriasis, etc.

Corylus avellana
Canon: Hazel (Urdu: Fundaq)
Parts used: Nuts.
Temperament: Hot and Dry.

Beech family – Fagaceae

Hardwood trees of temperate and tropical forests. 8 genera with about 1000 species of cosmopolitan distribution. The family provides the world with sweet chestnuts and bottle corks.

Castanea sativa   Origin: Eurasia
Canon: Chestnut (Urdu: Baloot)
Parts used: Nuts.
Temperament: Cool and Dry in the Second Degree.

Quercus robur   Origin: Europe
1907:   Quercus Cortex, Oak Bark
Uses: Astringent, externally used in gonorrhoea, leucorrhoea and haemorrhoids, and as a gargle in sore throats.
Canon: Oak Galls (Urdu: Majoo)
Parts used: Galls.
Temperament: Cool in the First and Dry in the Second Degree.
Comments: Galla turcica Quercus infectoria.

Balanops family – Balanopsceae

1 genus with 12 species of trees confined to north Queensland, New Caledonia and Fiji.

ORDER CASUARINALES

She Oak family – Casuarinaceae

Trees and shrubs of dry places in Southeast Asia and the south-west Pacific, 1 genus with about 65 species.

Superorder Caryophyllidae

ORDER CARYOPHYLLALES

Cactus family – Cactaceae

A New World family of drought-resistant trees, shrubs and shrublets, mainly with spines and all except one with no leaves. 87 genera with over 2000 species making semi-deserts out of deserts.
Opuntia spp., fruits, the prickly pears, are eaten.

Mesembryanthemum family – Aizoaceae

Centred in South Africa, this family of succulent plants is of disjunct pantropical distribution, 143 genera with some 2300 species.

Carnation family – Caryophyllaceae

A large cosmopolitan family of about 80 genera with some 2000 species of herbaceous plants.

Bougainvillea family – Nyctaginaceae

30 genera and some 290 species of mainly tropical herbs, shrubs and trees, centred in America but of pantropical distribution.
Pisonia spp., the Cabbage and the Lettuce Trees, produce edible leaves. *Pisonia aculeata* leaves and *Pisonia capitata* fruits are used medicinally as decoctions.

Amaranth family – Amaranthaceae

Cosmopolitan, tropics to temperate zones, 65 genera with some 900 species of herbs and shrubs. Many are used as pot herbs; the seeds of the Grain Amaranth, which were once widely ground and used as flour in parts of the Americas, are now being researched as wheat substitutes for the many people who are allergic to cereals.

Amaranthus mangostanus
Canon: Amaranth (Urdu: Chaulai)
Parts used: Plant.
Temperament: Cool and Moist in the Second Degree.

Pokeweed family – Phytolaccaceae

Tropical and subtropical family, 2 genera with some 125 species of herbs, climbers, shrubs and trees.

Phytolacca decandra   Origin: North America
1907:   Phytolacca, Poke Root
Uses: Slow-acting emetic, purgative, narcotic.

Beet family – Chenopodiaceae

Some 100 genera with about 1500 species of mainly perennial herbs with a patchy distribution across the temperate and subtropical world, favouring saline habitats. The family provides the world with sugar beet, leaf beets, spinach beet and beetroot.

Beta vulgaris   Origin: Europe
1979:   Beet, Sugar
Uses: Sources for sucrose; sweetening agent, demulcent, syrup base
Canon: Beet (Urdu: Chuqandar)
Parts used: Seeds.
Temperament: Hot and Dry in the First Degree.

Chenopodium album
Canon: Goose Foot (Urdu: Bathwa)
Parts used: Leaves.
Temperament: Cool and Moist in the Second Degree.

Chenopodium ambrosoides   Origin: America
1907:   Chenopodium, American Wormseed
Uses: Vermifuge, anthelmintic.

Spinacea oleracea
Canon: Spinach (Urdu: Palak)
Parts used: Leaves.
Temperament: Cool and Moist in the First Degree.

Didiera family – Didiereaceae

4 genera with 11 species of tall cactus-like plants confined to the deserts of Madagascar.

Portulaca family – Portulacaceae

Succulent herbs and sub-shrubs; 19 genera with some 500 species, cosmopolitan.
Lewisia rediviva has starchy edible rootstocks; others are used as pot herbs.

Portulaca oleracea
Canon: Purselane (Urdu: Khurfa)
Parts used: Seeds.
Temperament: Cool and Moist in the Third Degree.

Madeira Vine family – Basellaceae

4 genera with 22 species of climbing vines, pantropical centring on America. Some are eaten as leaf vegetables and one produces small tubers which are eaten like potatoes.

ORDER BATALES

Saltwort family – Batidaceae

New World (including Hawaii) coastal salt marsh family of a single species. Saltwort leaves are eaten raw in salads.

ORDER POLYGONALES

Buckwheat family – Polygonaceae

Mainly in the north, but some in the south temperate regions, 30 genera with some 750 species, mainly herbs but a few shrubs and trees. They provide the world with Buckwheat and Rhubarb.

Rheum palmatum   Origin: China
1988:   Rhubarb
Uses: Laxative.
1979:   Rhubarb, Rheum
Uses: Mild anthraquinone purgative. The tannin present may exert an astringent action after purgation.
1907:   Rhei Radix, Rhubarb Root
Uses: Increases the flow of saliva when chewed, and acts as a stomachic. Large doses are purgative, used in diarrhoea.
Canon: Rhubarb (Urdu: Revand cheei)
Parts used: Root.
Temperament: Cool and Dry in the Second Degree.
Comments: Referred to as *Rheum emodi*.

Rumex acetosa
Canon: Sorrel (Urdu: Chooka)
Parts used: Leaves.
Temperament: Cool in the Second Degree and Dry.

ORDER PLUMBAGINALES

Sea Lavender family – Plumbaginaceae

> A cosmopolitan family of dry and saline habitats and thus expanding in distribution; 10 genera and about 560 species, herbs, shrubs and climbers. Sorrels have long been eaten as salads, also *Plumbago* spp. are used in dental treatment and in skin diseases, and *Limonium vulgare* (Sea Lavender) is used to treat bronchial haemorrhages.

Superorder Dilleniidae

ORDER DILLENIALES

Dillenia family – Dilleniaceae

> A pantropical family of 18 genera and some 530 species of shrubs, climbers and trees. The rough leaves of some trees are used as depilators.

Peony family – Paeoniaceae

> 1 genus, 33 species of perennial herbs and shrubs, chiefly in western temperate Eurasia and western North America.

> *Paeonia officinalis*   Origin: southern Europe
> *Canon*: Paeony (Urdu: Ood Saleeb)
> Parts used: Root.
> Temperament: Hot and Dry.

Crossosoma family – Crossosomataceae

> 1 genus with 4 species native of south-western North America, shrubs of dry habitats.

ORDER THEALES

Tea family – Theaceae

> Pantropical and subtropical; 29 genera with some 1100 species centred in Asia and America. The family provides us with tea.

Camellia sinensis   Origin: China
1979:   Caffeine
Uses: Source of caffeine, together with tea waste and coffee.
1907:   Caffeine (*Camellia thea*)
Uses: Source for caffeine. Central nervous system and cardiac
         stimulant, specific diuretic.

Camellia thea   Origin: China
1907:   Thea, Tea
Uses: Used as a source of caffeine, leaves are added to anti-
         asthmatic smoking compounds.

African Oak family – Ochnaceae

Pantropical family of some 40 genera with 600 species of trees, shrubs
and a few herbs, best represented in South America.

Shorea family – Dipterocarpaceae

An extremely important family of tropical hardwood trees found in
Southeast Asia, Asia, India and with an outlier in central Amazonas;
some 15 genera with some 580 species. One of the earth's most rapidly
disappearing resources.

Dammara orientalis   Origin: Malay Archipelago
1907:   Dammar, Amboyna Pine, Manilla Resin, occasionally Kauri
         Dammar
Uses: Dammar is a generic term for a series of East Asian resins,
         Dammara orientalis being the most important. Occasionally
         used for plaster masses.

Dryobalanops aromatica   Origin: Southeast Asia
1907:   Borneol
Uses: Source for borneol, with similar properties to camphor.

Mangosteen family – Guttiferae

A cosmopolitan family of trees and shrubs, some 40 genera with 1000
species spanning the world. Provides the Mangosteen and the
Mammey Apple.

Garcinia hanburyi   Origin: Southeast Asia
1907:   Cambogia, Gamboge
Uses: Powerful hydragogue cathartic, used in dropsy and cerebral
          congestion.

Garcinia morella   Origin: India
1907:   Cambogia Indica, Indian Gamboge
Uses: Powerful hydragogue cathartic, used in dropsy and cerebral
          congestion.

Garcinia mangostana
Canon: Mangosteen (Urdu: Joz jundam)
Parts used: Nuts.
Temperament: Cool and Dry.

Elatine family – Elatinaceae

Cosmopolitan; 2 genera and some 33 species in subtropical and
temperate regions. Herbs and shrubby herbs of aquatic to dry open
habitats.

Quiina family – Quiinaceae

4 genera with 52 species of trees and large shrubs, confined to the
moist tropical forests of South America and the West Indies. Little
appears to be known about them.

Marcgravia family – Marcgraviaceae

Of Central and South American tropical rainforests, the 5 genera with
some 125 species of climbers are perhaps related to the Theaceae.

ORDER MALVALES

Scytopetalum family – Scytopetalaceae

This is a small family of 5 genera with 20 species from tropical West
Africa.

Crinodendron family – Elaeocarpaceae

12 genera with about 350 species of the tropics and subtropics of East
Asia, Indomalaysia, Australasia and the Pacific with outliers in the

West Indies and in southern South America. The fruits and seeds of several species are eaten.
Elaeocarpus serratus gives Ceylon Olives; *Aristotelia chinensis* produces Macqui Berries which are used to produce a medicinal wine in China.

Lime family – Tiliaceae

Tropical and temperate trees and shrubs, some 41 genera with 400 species spread across the planet. It provides the world with some superb fibres including jute from *Corchorus* spp., while the leaves of *Corchorus olitorius* are used for food in the eastern Mediterranean.

Corchorus olitorius
Canon: Jute (Urdu: Bawphali)
Parts used: Pods.
Temperament: Cool in the First and Dry in the Second Degree.

Kola family – Sterculiaceae

Trees and shrubs with some climbers and herbs; some 60 genera with 700 species of pantropical distribution. Provides the world with Kola and Cocoa.

Cola vera   Origin: West Africa
1907:   Kolae Semina, Kola Seeds, Gooroo Nuts, Bissy Nuts
Uses: Same properties as caffeine, though slightly more astringent.

Sterculia urens   Origin: India
1988:   Sterculia
Uses: Gum, pharmaceutical aid.
1979:   Sterculia, Indian Tragacanth
Uses: Substitute for tragacanth. Also as surgical adhesive.

Theobroma cacao   Origin: Central America
1988:   Theobroma Oil (Cocoa Butter)
Uses: Suppository basis.
1979:   Theobroma Oil, Cocoa Butter
Uses: Basis for suppositories, pessaries and bougies.
1907:   Oleum Theobromatis, Cacao Butter; Theobromatis Semina, Cacao Seeds

Uses: Basis for suppositories, pessaries and bougies. Theobromine has properties similar to caffeine, though with a more marked effect on muscle fibres; it is also a diuretic.

Balsa family – Bombacaceae

Pantropical, a small family of 20 genera with some 180 species of trees, including some of the strangest in the world such as Balsa and the Baobab. Also provides Kapok, Jackfruit and Durian.

Cotton family – Malvaceae

A worldwide family of some 80 genera with more than 1000 species found in all but the coldest regions. Provides cotton, China jute and Okra fruits.

Althaea officinalis   Origin: Europe
1907:   Marshmallow Root, Althea
Uses: Demulcent, emollient.
Canon: Marsh Mallow (Urdu: Khatmi)
Parts used: Seeds.
Temperament: Cool and Moist in the First Degree.

Gossypium spp.   Origin: India
1988:   Absorbent Cotton
Uses: Dressings.
1907:   Gossypii Radicis Cortex, Cotton Root Bark, Cotton
Uses: Cotton bark has been used as an abortifacient and as an ergot substitute in labour, though the effect is fictitious. Cotton is used for dressings and absorbents. Oil used similarly to olive oil.

Rhopalocarpus family – Sphaerosepalaceae

Endemic to Madagascar; 2 genera with 14 species of trees and shrubs.

Sarcolaena family – Sarcolaenaceae

Endemic to eastern Madagascar; 8 genera with 39 species of trees of the now almost destroyed rainforests of the upper slopes of the high plateau.

ORDER URTICALES
Elm family – Ulmaceae

Tropical and temperate trees and shrubs, 16 genera with almost 2000 species spanning the world. Elms taught the world that trees too can suffer from disease. Huckleberries can be eaten and the mucilaginous inner bark of *Ulmus rubra* gives us slippery elm.

Ulmus campestris   Origin: Europe
1907:   Ulmi Cortex, Elm Bark
Uses: Bitter and astringent; given internally in intestinal catarrh and diarrhoea, and has been used in injections against leucorrhoea.

Ulmus fulva   Origin: Europe
1907:   Ulmi Fulvae, Slippery Elm
Uses: Mainly used as a demulcent mucilage.

Fig family – Moraceae

Tropical, subtropical and some temperate trees and shrubs. 75 genera with some 3000 species, cosmopolitan. An interesting family, providing us with Hops, Hemp, Mulberry bushes and Fig leaves.

Cannabis sativa   Origin: western Asia, India
1907:   Cannabis Indica, Indian Cannabis
Uses: Central nervous system stimulant, anodyne, hypnotic, sedative; smoked against asthma.
Canon: Hemp (Urdu: Bhang ke Beej)
Parts used: Seeds.
Temperament: Hot and Dry in the Third Degree.

Ficus carica   Origin: western Asia
1979:   Fig, Ficus
Uses: Demulcent, used in the confection of syrups.
1907:   Ficus, Figs
Uses: Dried figs are used as a mild laxative, sometimes in large quantities when a sharp object is swallowed. Interior can be applied to boils and abscesses.
Canon: Fig (Urdu: Anjir)
Parts used: Fruit.
Temperament: Hot and Moist.

Humulus lupulus   Origin: Europe
1907:   Lupulus, Hops
Uses: Aromatic bitter and stomachic. Mild sedative.

Morus alba
Canon: Mulberry (Urdu: Toot)
Parts used: Fruit.
Temperament: Hot and Moist.

Nettle family – Urticaceae

From tropical to temperate climes, 45 genera with more than 1000 species of herbs, shrubs, and some formidable stinging trees. *Boehmeria nivea* produces ramie fibre or China grass.

ORDER LECYTHIDALES

Brazil Nut family – Lecythidaceae

Tropical family centred in South America where the Brazil Nut is its most famous member; some 20 genera with 450 species of trees. *Lecythis zabucajo* provides the so-called Paradise nuts, claimed to be superior to Brazil nuts.

ORDER VIOLALES

Violet family – Violaceae

Cosmopolitan family but preferring the temperate climes. 22 genera and some 900 species of perennial or, rarely, annual plants, some shrubs. Violet petals are used in sweetmeats and for flavouring.

Viola odorata   Origin: Europe
1907:   Viola, Violet
Uses: Preparations of violet have been used, internally and externally, in the treatment of cancer.
Canon: Violets (Urdu: Banafsha)
Parts used: Flowers.
Temperament: Cool and Moist in the First Degree.

Chaulmoogra family – Flacourtiaceae

Pantropical and subtropical trees and shrubs, 89 genera with some 1250 species.

Hydnocarpus wightiana from India and *Taraktogenos kurzii* from Burma yield chaulmoogra oil, of use in the treatment of leprosy.

Taraktogenos kurzii   Origin: Burma
1907:   Oleo Gynocardiae, Gynocardia Oil, Chaulmoogra Oil
Uses: Employed externally in the treatment of rheumatism, psoriasis, eczema etc.; and both externally and internally in leprosy.

Lacistema family – Lacistemataceae

2 genera with 27 species in tropical America and the West Indies, all shrubs.

Passion Flower family – Passifloraceae

Pantropical vines, tree shrubs, and herbs; 20 genera with some 600 species, some 60 of which produce edible fruits, which are either eaten or used for flavouring drinks and sweets.

Turnera family – Turneraceae

Found in the tropical and subtropical regions of America and Africa, 8 genera with some 100 species of small trees and some herbs. The leaves of a number of species of *Turnera* spp. are used in medicine and in Mexico as a tea substitute.

Turnera diffusa   Origin: Mexico, USA
1907:   Damiana
Uses: Mild purgative, recommended for sexual debility. Contains damianin (bitter).

Malesherbia family – Malesherbiaceae

1 or 2 genera with 27 species of temperate herbs and undershrubs from western South America.

Ocotillo family – Fouquieriaceae

A small family of 2 genera and 8 species of semi-desert spiny trees and shrubs from the south-west of North America. Wax is extracted from the stem or bark of some species.

Papaw family – Caricaceae

Small trees with soft, latex-producing trunks; 4 genera with 30 species from tropical America and West Africa. Many fruits are eaten, the most famous being the Papaw, which is widely cultivated.

Annatto family – Bixaceae

1 genus, perhaps 4 species of shrubs and trees, from tropical America and West Indies.
Bixa orellana, an ornamental plant, but also grown on plantation scale, as the seeds provide a food colouring.

Rose Imperial family – Cochlospermaceae

Pantropical, preferring dry habitats, two genera with some 38 species of trees and shrubs.
Cochlospermum heteroneurum, from Queensland, provides a kapok; *Cochlospermum vitifolium* fibre for cordage; and *Cochlospermum religiosum* provides an amber-coloured medicinal gum, karaya gum.

Rockrose family – Cistaceae

Temperate, mainly in the northern hemisphere and favouring mediter-ranean climes, 8 genera with some 165 species of shrubs, subshrubs and herbs.
Cistus salviifolius has been used in Greece as tea, *Cistus ladaniferus* and *Cistus incanus* produce the aromatic ladanum gum.

Tamarisk family – Tamaricaceae

Heathy shrubs and small trees of the sandy subtropical and temperate Old World. 4 genera with some 120 species.
Tamarix mannifera: on insect attack, the twigs yield sweet manna gum, which could have been the manna of the Bible.

Tamarix gallica
Canon: Tamarisk (Urdu: Jhao)
Parts used: Leaves.
Temperament: Cool in the First and Dry in the Second Degree.

Tamarix mannifera
Canon: Manna (Urdu: Turanjbeen)

Parts used: Resin.
Temperament: Hot and Dry.
Comments: Given as *Alhagi manzorum*.

Ancistrocladus family – Ancistrocladaceae

A single genus with 20 species of tropical lianas from Africa, India, Burma and China.
Ancistrocladus extensus roots boiled are used against dysentery in Malaysia.

Frankenia family – Frankeniaceae

Small heath-like halophytes, of warm temperate and subtropical areas worldwide; 4 genera with some 90 species.
Frankenia ericifolia is used as a fish poison in Macronesia.

Acharia family – Achariaceae

Small shrubs, stemless or fine-stemmed climbing herbs, 3 mono-specific genera from South Africa.

Begonia family – Begoniaceae

Perennial herbs and shrubs, 5 genera with more than 900 species, widespread in the tropics and the subtropics.
Begonia spp. are used in the Moluccas as vegetables and as medicines.

Blazing Star family – Loasaceae

Rough herbs often with stinging hairs. 15 genera with 250 species, mainly in tropical and subtropical America, outliers in south-west Australia and Arabia.

Datisca family – Datiscaceae

3 genera with 4 species; a small family of tropical and subtropical trees and herbs, disjunct from east India to south-west America.
Datisca cannabina, roots and stem produce a yellow silk dye.

Gourd family – Cucurbitaceae

Tropics, subtropics to temperate, includes semi-desert plants; some 90 genera and 700 species of climbing and scrambling plants. Provides us with Gourds, Squashes, Melons, Pumpkins, Marrows, Cucumbers, Courgettes, Gherkins etc.

Bryonia dioica   Origin: Europe
1907:   Bryoniae Radix, Bryony Root
Uses: Similar to Jalap, large doses are cathartic and diuretic, small doses given against the pain and cough of pleurisy; also as a styptic.
Canon: Bryonia (Urdu: Fashara)
Parts used: Root.
Temperament: Hot and Dry in the Third Degree.

Carica papaya   Origin: South America
1907:   Papainum, Papain, Papayotin
Uses: Papain is employed to assist protein digestion in chronic dyspepsia, gastric fermentation and gastritis. Solutions are applied to diphteric membranes, and to digest dead tissue and promote healing of abscesses, ulcers and fissures of the tongue. Solutions have been recommended for injection into tumours.

Citrullus colocynthis   Origin: North Africa, Asia
1907:   Colocynthidis Pulpa, Bitter Apple
Uses: Strong purgative, irritant.

Cucumis sativus
Canon: Cucumber (Urdu: Kheera)
Parts used: Seeds.
Temperament: Cool and Moist in the Second Degree.

Cucumis melo
Canon: Melon (Urdu: Kharbooza)
Parts used: Fruit.
Temperament: Cool and Dry in the First Degree.

Cucurbita maxima   Origin: Mediterranean
1907:   Cucurbitae Semina, Melon Pumpkin Seeds
Uses: Anthelmintic.
Canon: Pumpkin (Urdu: Kadoo)
Parts used: Seeds.
Temperament: Cool and Moist in the Second Degree.

Ecballium elaterium   Origin: southern Europe
1907:   Elaterium
Uses: Main component is elaterin, a powerful hydragogue cathartic.

ORDER SALICALES

Willow family – Salicaceae

Worldwide 4 genera of trees and shrubs with some 350 species, favouring north temperate climes. The bark of some contains the chemical greenprint of aspirin, now finding value against heart attack.

Salix alba   Origin: Europe
1907:   Salicis Cortex, Willow Bark
Uses: Contains tannin and salicin; bitter and astringent.

Salix discolor   Origin: North America
1907:   Salicis Nigrae Cortex, Black Willow Bark, Pussy Willow Bark
Uses: Has been prescribed in gonorrhoea, and to relieve ovarian pain.

Salix aegyptica
Canon: Willow Bark (Urdu: Baid sada)
Parts used: Bark.
Temperament: Cool in the First Degree and Dry.
Comments: The leaves are also used.

ORDER CAPPARIDALES

Caper family – Capparidaceae

Pantropical and subtropical, some 45 genera with 700 species of herbs, shrubs, trees and lianas.
Capparis spp.; flower buds flavour the world with capers.

Capparis spinosa   Origin: Asia
Canon: Caper (Urdu: Kibr)
Parts used: Root.
Temperament: Hot and Dry in the Second Degree.

Tovaria family – Tovariaceae

1 genus with 2 species – a tropical shrub with an annual herb from America and the Caribbean.

Mustard family – Cruciferae

Wherever plants can grow, members of this family of some 380 genera with 3000 species are nearby. They provide the world with the ancestors of many cultivated vegetables.

Brassica oleracea is the ancestor of Cabbage, Kale, Sprouts, Kohlrabi, Cauliflower, Broccoli and such; *Brassica campestris* is the ancestor to Turnips, Chinese Cabbage and Oilseed Rape.

Brassica napus
1988:   Rape Seed Oil
Uses: Standard reagent.

Brassica nigra   Origin: Europe
1907:   Oleum Sinapis Expressum, Expressed Oil of Mustard
Uses: Rubefacient, lubricant. The volatile oil is an extremely powerful irritant and vesicant.
Canon: Mustard (Urdu: Rai)
Parts used: Seeds.
Temperament: Hot in the Second and Dry in the Fourth Degree.
Comments: Given as *Brassica juncea*.

Brassica sinapoides   Origin: Europe
1907:   Sinapis, Mustard
Uses: External counter-irritant, internally as a condiment and an emetic.

Brassica oleracea   Origin: Asia
Canon: Cabbage (Urdu: Band gobhi)
Parts used: Leaves.
Temperament: Hot in the First and Dry in the Second Degree.

Brassica campestris
Canon: Turnip (Urdu: Shaljam)
Parts used: Tuber.
Temperament: Hot in the Second and Moist in the First Degree.

Cheiranthus cheiri
Canon: Gilli Flower (Urdu: Phool, Khatmi)
Parts used: Flowers.
Temperament: Cool and Moist.

Cochlearia armoracia   Origin: eastern Europe
1907:   Horseradish Root
Uses: Stimulant, diuretic.

Eruca sativa
Canon: Herb Rocket (Urdu: Tarameera)
Parts used: Seeds.
Temperament: Hot in the Second and Dry in the First Degree.

Lepidium sativum
Canon: Watercress (Urdu: Haloon)
Parts used: Leaves.
Temperament: Hot and Dry in the Third Degree.

Raphanus sativus
Canon: Radish (Urdu: Mooli)
Parts used: Tuber.
Temperament: Hot in the Third and Moist in the Second Degree.

Mignonette family – Resedaceae

6 genera with some 5 species of herbs and shrubs favouring the mediterranean climates of the world.
Reseda odorata provides a perfumed oil.

Horseradish Tree family – Moringaceae

Small fast-growing trees, 1 genus with 12 species favouring mediterranean climates in south-east Africa, Europe, the Middle East, Madagascar and India.
Moringa oleifera produces ben oil, a watch lubricant oil also used as a salad oil, and its young swollen horseradish-like roots can be eaten.

ORDER ERICALES

Lily-of-the-valley Tree family – Clethraceae

Tropical and subtropical trees of America, East Asia and Madeira; 1 genus with some 120 species.

Grubbia family – Grubbiaceae

A South African family of 2 genera with 5 species of small heath-like shrubs.

Leatherwood family – Cyrillaceae

3 genera with 14 species of shrubs from tropical America.

Heath family – Ericaceae

Worldwide family of shrubs and small trees, some 100 genera with 3000 species. Provides the world with Cranberries, Blueberries and Bilberries.

Arcostaphylos uva-ursi   Origin: Europe
1907:   Uvae Ursi Folia, Bearberry Leaves
Uses: Diuretic and astringent, used in inflammatory diseases of the urinary tract.

Gaultheria procumbens   Origin: Pacific rim
1907:   Oleum Gaultherieae, Oil of Wintergreen
Uses: Consists almost entirely of methyl salicylate. Given internally in acute rheumatism, though external use might give rise to eruptions – pure methyl salicylate is preferable. Flavouring agent.

Epacris family – Epacridaceae

Heath-like shrubs and trees, 30 genera with some 400 species found in Australia, Indomalaysia and New Zealand, with an outlier in southern South America.
Styphelia malayana root and leaves are used as medicine.

Crowberry family – Empetraceae

Evergreen shrubs, circumboreal and cool temperate sub-arctic with disjunctions in southern South America and south-eastern USA; 3 genera with 4–6 species.

Wintergreen family – Pyrolaceae

Evergreen creeping perennials, 4 genera with 30 species of the temperate and arctic North. The leaves of some species are used to help the healing of wounds.

ORDER DIAPENSIALES

Shortia family – Diapensiaceae

Herbs and dwarf shrubs, 7 genera with 20 species from the cold North and the Himalayas.

ORDER EBENALES

Chicle family – Sapotaceae

Tropical trees, 35 to 75 genera with some 800 species which span the tropical belt in lowland and low montane forests. They provide the edible fruits Sapodilla Plum, Star Apple and Sapote.
Butyrospermum paradoxum, the Shea Butter Tree, provides an edible oil, *Ahcras zapota* the chicle and *Mimusops balata* the balata of original chewing gums.

Palaquium spp.   Origin: Malay Archipelago
1907:   Gutta Percha
Uses: Substitute for colloidon; covering for moist dressings; stopping for decayed teeth.

Persimmon family – Ebenaceae

Cosmopolitan tropical family with north temperate outliers; 2 genera with 400 to 500 species of trees including the Ebonies. They provide Persimmons and Date Plums; all fruits are very astringent before ripening.

Silverbell Tree family – Styracaceae

Shrubs and trees disjunct across the tropics with some in the mediterranean climate regions. 12 genera with 180 species.
Styrax officinale from the Mediterranean yields styrax resin, an antiseptic, inhalant and expectorant.

Styrax benzoin   Origin: Sumatra
1988:   Benzoin
1979:   Benzoin
Uses: Ingredient in inhalations against catarrh.

Styrax paralleloneurus   Origin: Sumatra
1988:   Benzoin
1979:   Sumatra Benzoin
Uses: Ingredient in inhalations against catarrh.

ORDER PRIMULALES

Primrose family – Primulaceae

Cosmopolitan in distribution but mainly north temperate and sub-tropical, although crossing the tropics.
Anagallis arvensis contains a saponin-like glycoside, *Lysimachia vulgaris* provides a yellow dye and a febrifuge.

Cyclamen europaeum
Canon: Maiden Weed (Urdu: Hathajori)
Parts used: Root.
Temperament: Hot in the Third and Dry in the Second Degree.

Myrsina family – Myrsinaceae

Trees and shrubs, 32 genera with some 1000 species, cosmopolitan in warm temperate to tropical regions.
Ardisia colorata (Malaysia) – the leaf infusion is a stomachic.
Ardisia fuliginosa (Java) – the sap is used against scurvy.
Ardisia squamulosa – the flowers and fruit are used to flavour fish.

Embelia robusta
Canon: Embelia Ribes (Urdu: Babarang)
Parts used: Seeds.
Temperament: Hot in the First and Dry in the Second Degree.

Superorder Rosidae

ORDER ROSALES

Weinmannia family – Cunoniaceae

Trees and shrubs; 26 genera and 250 species, centred on Australasia and Oceania with outliers in Africa and Central and South America.

Parchment-bark family – Pittosporaceae

Evergreen shrubs and trees from Australasia and the Old World tropics, 9 genera with more than 200 species.
Billardiera longiflora produces blue edible 'Apple Berries'.

Sundew family – Droseraceae

4 genera with 83 species of carnivorous plants, cosmopolitan, typically in semi-aquatic nitrogen-deficient habitats.

Brunellia family – Brunelliaceae

Tropical New World trees, 1 genus with some 45 species.

Eucryphia family – Eucryphiaceae

A single genus of 5 species of trees and shrubs, widely disjunct across the southern hemisphere, in Tasmania, south-east Australia, and Chile. The barks are a source of tannin.

Brunia family – Bruniaceae

12 genera with about 70 species of heath-like shrubs from the famous Cape flora of South Africa.

Rose family – Rosaceae

Cosmopolitan, 122 genera with 3370 species of woody and herbaceous plants. Provides the ancestral Apples, Pears, Plums and Cherries.

Brayeria anthelmintica   Origin: north-east Africa
1907:   Cusso, Kousso
Uses: Anthelmintic.

Crataegus azarola
Canon: Wild apple (?) (Urdu: Jangli seb)
Parts used: Berries.
Temperament: Cool and Moist.
Comments: In effect, it's a Hawthorn.

Potentilla nepalensis   Origin: Asia
Canon: Celtic juice (Urdu: Ratanjot)
Parts used: Juice.

Temperament: Hot and Dry in the Second Degree.
Comments: Referred to also as *Anchusa officinalis*

Prunus amygdalus var. *dulcis*   Origin: Mediterranean
1988: Almond Oil
1979: Almond Oil
Uses: Emollient, vehicle, to soften ear wax.
1907: Sweet Almonds
Uses: Demulcent, vehicle.
Canon: Almonds (Urdu: Badam)
Parts used: Nuts.
Temperament: Hot and Dry in the Second Degree.

Prunus amygdalus var. *amara*   Origin: Mediterranean
1907: Bitter Almonds
Uses: Cough mixtures, toiletry lotions.

Prunus serotina   Origin: North America
1979: Wild Cherry Bark, Virginian Prune
Uses: Flavouring agent, purported treatment of cough.
1907: Pruni Virginianae Cortex, Wild Cherry Bark
Uses: Mild sedative to relieve cough.

Prunus laurocerasus   Origin: western Asia
1907: Laurocerasi Folia, Cherry-Laurel Leaves
Uses: Used for preparation of Aqua Laurocerasi (0.1% hydrocyanic acid).

Prunus domestica   Origin: Europe
1907: Prunum, Prunes, French Plums
Uses: Mildly laxative, nutritious, and demulcent.
Canon: Plums (Urdu: Aloobuckara)
Parts used: Fruit.
Temperament: Cool and Moist in the Second Degree.
Comments: Referred to as *Prunus communis*.

Prunus armeniaca   Origin: Asia
Canon: Apricot (Urdu: Khobani)
Parts used: Fruit.
Temperament: Cool and Moist in the Second Degree.

Prunus persica   Origin: central Asia
Canon: Peach (Urdu: Aroo)
Parts used: Fruit.
Temperament: Cool and Moist in the Second Degree.

Pyrus cydonia   Origin: Europe
1907:   Cydoniae Semina, Quince Seeds
Uses: Soothing and demulcent mucilage.
Canon: Quince (Urdu: Bahi)
Parts used: Seeds.
Temperament: Cool in the First and Dry in the Second Degree.
Comments: Referred to as *Cydonia vulgaris*.

Pyrus malus   Origin: Eurasia
Canon: Apple (Urdu: Seb)
Parts used: Fruit.
Temperament: Hot and Moist in the First Degree.

Quillaja saponaria   Origin: South America
1988:   Quillaia
Uses: Emulsifying agent.
1979:   Quillaia, Panama Wood, Soap Bark
Uses: Saponin-rich emulsifying agent. As powder, sternutatory.
1907:   Quillaiae Cortex, Quillaja, Panama Bark
Uses: Reflex expectorant, emetic in large doses. Sternutatory.

Rosa damascena   Origin: western Asia
1907:   Oleum of Rosae, Otto of Rose
Uses: Perfuming agent.
Canon: Rose (Urdu: Ghulab)
Parts used: Flowers
Temperament: Cool in the First and Dry in the Second Degree.

Rosa canina   Origin: Europe, Asia
1907:   Rosae Caninae Fructus, Rose Hips
Uses: Used in the preparation of confections of hips.

Rosa gallica   Origin: Europe
1907:   Rosae Gallicae Petala, Red Rose Petals
Uses: Mildly astringent; colouring agent.

Rubus idaeus   Origin: Europe
1979:   Raspberry Juice
Uses: Flavouring agent in elixirs and mixtures.

Stonecrop family – Crassulaceae

Centred in South Africa, the weedy members of this family of succulent herbs and shrubs (some 35 genera with 1500 species) range across the world from hot dry to cold dry habitats; one is an aquatic.

Sempervivum arboreum
Canon: Houseleek (Urku: Sada bahar)
Parts used: Leaves.
Temperament: Cool and Dry in the Third Degree.

Flycatcher family – Cephalotaceae

1 genus with 1 species, a carnivorous plant from Western Australia.

Gooseberry family – Saxifragaceae

Patchy cosmopolitan family, avoiding large areas of the tropics; herbs and shrubs with a few annuals and trees, 80 genera with some 1250 species. Provides Gooseberries and Currants.

Ribes nigrum   Origin: Europe
1988:   Black Currant
Uses: Flavouring, vitamin C source.
1979:   Black Currant
Uses: Flavouring, vitamin C rich syrup.

Coco Plum family – Chrysobalanaceae

Cosmopolitan to the tropical and subtropical lowlands, 17 genera with some 400 species of trees and shrubs. Provides Coco Plums, Guinea Plum, Gingerbread Plum, Mobola Plum and Merecure Plum. *Licania rigida* (*oilica*), is grown in Brazil for its seed oil.

ORDER FABALES

Pea family – Leguminosae

Worldwide distribution but avoiding the colder areas; 700 genera with some 17,000 species of herbs, shrubs and trees. Thanks to nitrogen-fixing nodules in their roots, they help to keep the world supplied with usable nitrogen; they provide the Peas, Beans, Lentils, Chick Peas and other pulses, all important sources of amino acids. One of the most important families of medicinal plants.

Abrus precatorius   Origin: India
1907:   Abri Semina, Jequirity
Uses: Similar to ricin, but less toxic. Has been used for Lupus and
        ulcerations.

Acacia senegal   Origin: Africa
1979:   Gum Acacia, Gum Arabic
Uses: Suspending agent, binder.
1907:   Gum Acacia
Uses: Demulcent.

Acacia arabica   Origin: Arabia
1907:   Acacia Bark, Babul Bark
Uses: Tannic astringent
Canon: Acacia (Urdu: Babool ka Satt)
Parts used: Juice.
Temperament: Cool in the First and Dry in the Third Degree.

Acacia decurrens   Origin: Australia
1907:   Acacia Bark, Babul Bark
Uses: Tannic astringent

Acacia catechu   Origin: India
1907:   Catechu Nigrum, Cutch
Uses: Same uses as Gambier.

Aloe senegal   Origin: Africa
1988:   Acacia
Uses: Bulk-forming laxative.

Andira araroba   Origin: Brazil
1907:   Araroba, Goa Powder
Uses: Chrysarobin source. External use against psoriasis and skin
        parasites.

Arachis hypogaea   Origin: Brazil
1988:   Arachids Oil
1979:   Arachis Oil, Peanut Oil
Uses: Same properties and uses as olive oil.
1907:   Oleum Arachis, Arachis Oil, Peanut Oil, Groundnut Oil
Uses: Indian substitute for olive oil – oil is nutritious, demulcent
         and slightly laxative. Used to facilitate the removal of
         impacted faeces. Externally, lubricant and emollient.

Astragalus gummifer   Origin: western Asia
1988:   Tragacanth
1979:   Tragacanth
Uses: Lubricant and emulsifying medium, colloid medium.
1907:   Tragacantha, Tragacanth
Uses: Suspending agent, vehicle, colloid medium, exipient.
Canon: Tragacanth (Urdu: Gond kateera)
Parts used: Gum.
Temperament: Cool and Dry.

Astragalus sarcocolla
Canon: Anzaroot (Urdu: Anzaroot)
Parts used: Gum.
Temperament: Hot in the Second and Dry in the First Degree.

Butea frondosa
1907:   Butea Gum, Butea Seeds
Uses: Gum is strong astringent, seeds are aperient and anthelmintic.

Caesalpinia sappan   Origin: India
1907:   Sappan
Uses: Indian replacement for Logwood (*Haematoxylon campechi-*
         anum) as an astringent.

Cassia senna   Origin: Africa
1988:   Alexandrian Senna
Uses: Stimulant laxative.
1979:   Alexandrian Senna
Uses: Anthraquinone purgative.
1907:   Cassia Fistula, Cassia Pulp, Alexandrian Senna (*Cassia*
         acutifolia)
Uses: Simple laxative.

Cassia angustifolia   Origin: India
1988:   Tinnevelly Senna
Uses: Stimulant laxative.
1979:   Tinnevelly Senna
Uses: Anthraquinone purgative.
1907:   Cassia fistula. Cassia Pulp
Uses: Simple laxative.
Canon: Purging Cassia (Urdu: Amaltas)
Parts used: Pods.
Temperament: Hot and Moist.

Ceratonia siliqua
Canon: Carob Bean (Urdu: Kharnoob)
Parts used: Seeds.
Temperament: Cool and Dry.

Cicer arietinum
Canon: Chick Pea, Gram (Urdu: Chana)
Parts used: Seeds.
Temperament: Hot and Dry in the First Degree.

Copaifera lansdorfii   Origin: Brazil
1907:   Copaiba
Uses: Volatile oil; carminative, expectorant, urinary antiseptic.

Cytisus scoparius   Origin: Europe
1907:   Scoparii Cacumina, Broom Tops
Uses: Feeble diuretic. Source for sparteine – lowers blood pressure,
          in large doses paralyses sympathetic nerve cells.

Derris elliptica   Origin: Southeast Asia
1979:   Derris, Aker-Tuba, Tuba Root
Uses: External veterinary antiparasitary. Interchangeable with Lon-
          chocarpus.

Dipterix odorata   Origin: Southeast Asia
1907:   Tonco Semina, Tonka, Tonquin Bean
Uses: Origin: Main source for coumarin. Used in perfumery as a
          fixative.

Erythrophleum guineense   Origin: West Africa
1907:   Erythrophloei cortex, Sassy Bark, Mancona Bark, Casca Bark
Uses: Contains erythrophloeine, similar properties to digitaline.
         Cardiac tonic, local anaesthetic.

Glycine max
1988:   Soya Oil

Glycyrrhiza glabra   Origin: Europe, western Asia
1988:   Liquorice
Uses: Flavouring.
1979:   Liquorice, Liquorice Root
Uses: Demulcent, light expectorant. Flavouring agent.
1907:   Glycyrrhizae Radix, Liquorice Root
Uses: Demulcent, mild expectorant, flavouring agent.
Canon: Liquorice (Urdu: Mulathi)
Parts used: Root.
Temperament: Hot and Dry.

Haematoxylon campechianum   Origin: Central America
1907:   Haematoxyli Lignum, Logwood
Uses: Mild astringent in diarrhoea, dysentery, and to arrest intestinal
         haemorrhage.

Indigofera tinctoria   Origin: Asia
1907:   Indigo, Indigo Blue
Uses: Stain, laboratory reagent.

Lens culinaris
Canon: Lentil (Urdu: Masoor)
Parts used: Seeds.
Temperament: Hot, and Dry in the Second Degree.
Comments: Given as *Lens esculenta*

Lonchocarpus spp.   Origin: South America
1979:   Lonchocarpus, Barbasco, Cube Root, Timbo
Uses: Veterinary insecticide and larvicide, can be interchanged for
         Derris.

Lupinus termis
Canon: Lupin, bitter (Urdu: Turmas)

Parts used: Seeds.
Temperament: Hot in the First and Dry in the Second Degree.

Melilotus officinalis
Canon: Melilot (Urdu: Nakhoona)
Parts used: Pods.
Temperament: Hot and Dry in the First Degree.

Mucuna pruriens   Origin: Africa?
1907:   Mucuna, Cowhage, Cowitch
Uses: Hairs of the fruit formerly used as a mechanical vermifuge,
        also as an external irritant and rubefacient.

Myroxylon pereirae   Origin: South America
1907:   Balsam of Peru
Uses: Antiseptic, expectorant, external parasiticide.

Myroxylon toluifera   Origin: South America
1979:   Tolu Balsam
Uses: As Tolu Syrup, frequent component of cough mixtures.
1907:   Myroxylon toluifera, Balsam of Tolu
Uses: Antiseptic and expectorant.

Physostigma venenosum   Origin: West Africa
1979:   Calabar Bean
Uses: Source of physostigmine (eserine); inhibits cholinesterase
        activity and acetylcholine breakdown. Atropine antagonist.
        Miotic.
1907:   Phyostigmatis Semina, Calabar Bean, Ordeal Bean
Uses: Depresses central nervous system, slows pulse and increases
        blood pressure. Ophthalmic use: reduces intraocular pressure
        and pupil size. Used in tetanus, hemiplegia and paraplegia,
        strychnine poisoning.

Piscidia erythrina   Origin: South America
1907:   Piscidia, Jamaica Dogwood
Uses: Dilates the pupil, general sedative and antispasmodic. Fish
        poison.

Pterocarpus marsupium   Origin: southern India
1907:   Kino, Malabar Kino

Uses: Powerful astringent, both internal and external.
Canon: Indian Kino, Dragon's Blood (Urdu: Damul akhwain)
Parts used: Resin.
Temperament: Hot and Dry in the Second Degree.

Pterocarpus santalinus   Origin: India
1907:   Pterocarpi Lignum, Red Sanders Wood, Red Sandal Wood
Uses: Employed for its red colouring matter.

Tamarindus indica   Origin: Africa
1907:   Tamarindus, Tamarind
Uses: Mild laxative and febrifuge.
Canon: Tamarind (Urdu: Imli)
Parts used: Pulp.
Temperament: Cool and Dry in the Second Degree.

Trachilobium hornemannianum   Origin: Zanzibar
1907:   Copal
Uses: Occasional ingredient of plasters.

Trifolium pratense
Canon: Clover (Urdu: Barsim)
Parts used: Seeds.

Trigonella foenum-graecum   Origin: India
1907:   Foenum-Graeci Semina, Foenugreek Seeds
Uses: Source of mucilage. Seeds and leaves used in veterinary
            medicine and curries.

Trigonella corniculata   Origin: Asia
Canon: Blue Melitot (Urdu: Bhiskhapra)
Parts used: Root.
Temperament: Hot and Dry in the Second Degree.

ORDER PODOSTEMALES

Moss Plant family – Podostemaceae

Mainly tropical, found around the world in fast-flowing streams and waterfalls, the members of this family of 45 genera with some 130 species disguise themselves as mosses and hang on tightly to their substrate.

ORDER HALORAGALES

Theligonium family – Theligoniaceae

1 genus with 2 or 3 species, disjunct in the Mediterranean, China and Japan; all are annual or perennial herbs. The young shoots provide vegetables.

Gunnera family – Haloragaceae

Of temperate and subtropical distribution, centred in the southern hemisphere. 7 genera with some 180 species of aquatic and damp forest habitats. Delicate aquatics to giant herbs.
Gunnera chilensis (Chile) is used in tanning.

Mare's Tail family – Hippuridaceae

A single genus with a single species; *Hippuris vulgaris* is an emergent herbaceous water plant which spans the cool temperate western hemisphere.

ORDER MYRTALES

Sonneratia family – Sonneratiaceae

2 genera with 8 species of tropical trees in East Africa, India, Southeast Asia and Australia, either growing in littoral (mangrove swamp) or lowland forest. Some fruits are edible.

Water Chestnut family – Trapaceae

A single genus with 1 to maybe 30 species of floating aquatics found across the New World. The fruits contain much starch and fat and are eaten, but this is not the main Water Chestnut of commerce.

Henna family – Lythraceae

Mainly tropical with some temperate members worldwide in the three zones, 22 genera with some 450 species of herbs, shrubs and trees.

Lawsonia inermis   Origin: India
Canon: Henna (Urdu: Mendhi)
Parts used: Leaves.
Temperament: Cool in the First and Dry in the Second Degree.

Mangrove family – Rhizophoraceae

A circumtropical family of 16 genera with 120 species of shrubs, climbers and trees which include half of the world's Mangroves. The tannin from Mangrove bark is used in tanning and a number of species provide local medicines.

Penaea family – Penaeaceae

5 genera with 27 species of heathlike shrubs from South Africa. *Penaea mucronata* and *Saltera sarcocolla* yield medicinal gums (sarcocolla).

Daphne family – Thymelaeaceae

Widespread in the Old World, less so in the New, many genera in the Pacific Islands; mainly shrubs, 45 genera with some 500 species.

Daphne spp.   Origin: Europe
1907:   Mezerei Cortex, Mezereum, Mezereon
Uses: Formerly used internally in the treatment of syphilis. External use as an irritant and vesicant.
Canon: Mezereon (Urdu: Mazeryune)
Parts used: Resin.
Temperament: Hot and Dry in the Fourth Degree.

Eucalyptus family – Myrtaceae

Some 100 genera with 3000 species. Tropical and subtropical but mainly in the southern hemisphere, from small straggling shrubs to some of the tallest trees in the world.

Eucalyptus spp.   Origin: Australia
1988:   Eucalyptus Oil
1979:   Eucalyptus Oil, Oleum Eucalypti
Uses: External use as counter-irritant; inhalations relieve cough in chronic bronchitis; ingredient in cold remedies.

Eucalyptus globulus   Origin: Australia
1988:   Eucalyptus Oil
1907:   Eucalypti Folia, Eucalyptus. Eucalyptus Oil
Uses: Anti-asthmatic cigarettes, infusion prescribed against diabetes. Oil is antiseptic and germicidal in high concentration; it is an

external irritant and a rubefacient. Inhaled, it arrests profuse secretion and relieves bronchioles; salivatory, expectorant, diuretic and urinary stimulant. Weak irritant.

Eucalyptus rostrata   Origin: Australia
1907:   Eucalypti Gummi, Eucalyptus Gum, Red Gum
Uses: Astringent, both internal and external.

Eugenia caryophyllata   Origin: Moluccas
1907:   Cloves, Caryophyllum
Uses: Stimulating and carminative to the alimentary tract. Oil is antiseptic and antiputrescent; externally rubefacient, counter-irritant and slightly anaesthetic, given internally as antispasmodic and carminative.
Canon: Cloves (Urdu: Laung)
Parts used: Fruit.
Temperament: Hot and Dry in the Third Degree.
Comments: Given as *Caryophyllus aromaticus*.

Melaleuca cajaputi   Origin: Malay archipelago
1979:   Cajaput Oil
Uses: Mild counter-irritant.
1907:   Oeum Cajaputi, Oil of Cajaput
Uses: Stimulant and mild counter-irritant. Applied to inflamed and rheumatic joints. Internally, an antispasmodic, given for chronic rheumatism.

Melaleuca leucadendron   Origin: Moluccas
1979:   Cajaput Oil
Uses: Mild counter-irritant.

Myrtus communis
Canon: Myrtle (Urdu: Habul ass)
Parts used: Seeds.
Temperament: Cool in the First and Dry in the Second Degree.

Pimento officinalis   Origin: South America
1907:   Oleum Pimentae, Oil of Pimento, Oil of Allspice
Uses: Carminative to intestinal tract and an adjuvant to aperient medicines.

Syzygium aromaticum   Origin: Zanzibar
1988:   Clove, Clove Oil
Uses: Carminative, flavouring, local anaesthetic in dentistry.
1979:   Clove, Clove Oil
Uses: Carminative, flavouring agent.

Pomegranate family – Punicaceae

1 genus with 2 species of trees from Europe, the Himalayas and Socotra.
Punica granatum seeds have been eaten since antiquity.

Punica granatum   Origin: Europe
1907:   Granati Cortex, Pomegranate Bark; Granati Fructi Cortex,
        Pomegranate Rind
Uses: Bark is strong astringent, vermifuge – must be followed by a
        purgative. The fruit rind is a strong astringent used as an
        antidiarrhoeal.
Canon: Pomegrande (Urdu: Anar)
Parts used: Fruit.
Temperament: Cool and Dry in the Second Degree.

Clarkia family – Onagraceae

Cosmopolitan family of 18 genera with some 640 species; herbs, some shrubs, a few aquatics.
Oenothera spp. (Evening Primrose).

Olinia family – Oliniaceae

1 genus with 10 species of trees, native of eastern and southern Africa.

Dissotis family – Melastomataceae

Many shrubs and small trees, some vines, herbs, aquatics and epiphytes. Some 240 genera with 2000 species across the tropical and subtropical world, with some in the temperate zones.
Medinilla hasseltii leaves are eaten, as are the fruits of other species.

Terminalia family – Combretaceae

Circumtropical edging into the subtropics; 20 genera with some 475 species of trees, shrubs and lianas.
Terminalia catappa produces edible Indian Almonds.

Anogeissus latifolia   Origin: Inida
1907:   Gummi Indicum, Indian Gum, Ghatti Gum
Uses: Similar properties to Gum Arabic. Demulcent and emulsifying
         agent.

Terminalia chebula   Origin: India
1907:   Myrobalanum, Myrobalans
Uses: Indian replacement of galls as source of tannins.
Canon: Myrobalans (Urdu: Harr)
Parts used: Berries.
Temperament: Cool in the First and Dry in the Second Degree.

ORDER CORNALES

Tupelo family – Nyssaceae

3 genera with 8 species of small trees from India, China, Tibet and
north-east America.
Nyssa spp. (Tupelo) produces edible fruits.

Garrya family – Garryaceae

1 genus with 18 species of evergreen shrubs from Central America,
south-western North America and the West Indies.

Alangia family – Alangiaceae

A thin band across the tropics, 1 genus with 20 species in the Old
World and another with 3 species in north-west South America.

Dogwood family – Cornaceae

Widespread but mainly north temperate with some of the 13 genera
and their some 100 species of trees, shrubs and, rarely, herbs in the
tropics and subtropics.
Cornus mas fruits are used for jams and in France the tonic wine, Vin
de Cornouille, is produced from them.

ORDER PROTEALES

Sea Buckthorn family – Elaeagnaceae

A family of much-branched shrubs with silvery or golden scales; 3
genera with some 50 species, found on coasts and steppes of North

America, Europe, South Asia and eastern Australia. The fruits of a number of species are eaten as a good local source of vitamins.

Protea family – Proteaceae

An important family of the southern hemisphere; 62 genera with more than 1000 species in Central and South America, Asia, southern Africa, Australasia. Mainly of dry habitats, but derived from rainforest ancestors.
Macadamia integrifolia produces the Macadamia nut.

ORDER SANTALALES

Sandalwood family – Santalaceae

Widespread in the tropics and through the temperate regions, some 35 genera with around 400 species of herbs, shrubs and trees.

Santalum album   Origin: India
1907:   Oleum Santali, Oil of Santal, Oil of Sandalwood
Uses: Given in sub-acute stages of cystitis and gonorrhoea as urinary disinfectant; expectorant in chronic bronchitis.
Canon: Sandal Wood (Urdu: Sandal)
Parts used: Wood.
Temperament: Cool and Dry in the Second Degree.

Medusandra family – Medusandraceae

A single species of tree from the rainforest of the Cameroons and probably Nigeria.

African Walnut family – Olacaceae

Across the topics with some subtropical members; some 25 genera with 250 species. Several have wood and other parts smelling of garlic. *Ximenia* spp. provides a bitter bark containing prussic acid. *Olax gambecola* is used as a condiment in West Africa.

Mistletoe family – Loranthaceae

Semiparasitic plants appearing throughout the tropics and subtropics and extending into the temperate regions; more than 35 genera with some 1300 species.

Viscum album   Origin: Europe

1907:   Viscum Album, Mistletoe

Uses: Supposed to have properties similar to digitalis, and has been
         used in cardiac dropsy. Berries are purgative and emetic, and
         are said to have emmenagogue and ecbolic properties in large
         doses.

Misodendron family – Misodendraceae

A small family of semiparasitic shrubs; all grow on the Southern
Beeches of southern South America.

Cynomorium family – Cynomoriaceae

These obligate parasites are found from the Canaries through the
Mediterranean to central temperate Asia in very dry habitats.
Cynomorium coccineum roots are used as a condiment in Africa.

Balanophora family – Balanophoraceae

A pantropical family of obligate parasites, mainly in upland forests; 18
genera with some 120 species. In Java waxes are extracted from them
and used as fuel for torches. A number are thought to have aphrodisiac
properties.

ORDER RAFFLESIALES

Rafflesia family – Rafflesiaceae

500 species of totally parasitic plants, disjunct but widespread
throughout the tropics and subtropics. Only the flowering part and a
few scaly bracts appear outside the host tissues.
Rafflesia spp. produce the world's largest flower.

Hydnora family – Hydnoraceae

Root-feeding parasites found in Madagascar, tropical Africa and
South America; 2 genera with 18 species.

ORDER CELASTRALES

Geissoloma family – Geissolomataceae

1 genus with 1 species, a small scleromorphic shrub from South Africa.

Spindle Tree family – Celastraceae

Cosmopolitan, temperate to tropics, 55 genera with 850 species of trees and shrubs, many of which are climbing and twisting. *Catha edulis* leaves, cultivated, are used in Arabian tea and Ethiopian honey wine.

Euonymus atropurpureus   Origin: North America
1907:   Euonymus Bark
Uses: Digestive stimulant, increases the flow of bile.

Stackhousia family – Stackhousiaceae

3 genera with 27 species of herbs, many of which are xeromorphic; found mainly in Australasia.

Salvadora family – Salvadoraceae

Old World tropical and subtropical shrubs, 3 genera with 11 species.
Salvadora persica (Toothbrush Tree) shoots are used in salads, Kegr salt is obtained from its ash. *Doberia roxburghi* provides an essential oil in the Sudan.

Corynocarpus family – Corynocarpaceae

1 genus with 5 species of trees and shrubs from Australasia and Polynesia.
Corynocarpus levigatus fruits are eaten by the New Zealand Maoris.

Icacina family – Icacinaceae

Tropical rainforest trees, shrubs and lianas, found throughout the tropics with some of the 60 genera with about 600 species in the subtropics.
Citronella spp. leaves are used as a substitute for Yerba Mate tea.
Cassinopsis madagascariensis bark gives an antidysenteric.

Holly family – Aquifoliaceae

3 genera with some 400 species widespread in tropical through to temperate regions, trees and shrubs.

Ilex paraguensis   Origin: South America
1907:   Mate Folia, Mate
Uses: Infusion is a refreshing drink, containing caffeine and tannin.

Dichapetalum family – Dichapetalaceae

Family of 4 genera with some 200 species of shrubs, climbers and some trees. Found across the tropics and having one South African member. *Dichapetalum* spp. seeds produce a potent arrow poison, their active principle being fluoroacetic acid, a metabolic poison.

ORDER EUPHORBIALES

Box family – Buxaceae

6 genera with some 1000 species of evergreen shrubs, some trees; found across the tropical and subtropical to temperate world, absent from North Africa.

Panda family – Pandaceae

Tropical trees; 3 genera with some 28 species from West Africa, Asia and Indomalaysia.
Panda oleosa produces edible oily seeds.

Spurge family – Euphorbiaceae

A large cosmopolitan family, tropical, subtropical and temperate; some 300 genera with 5000 plus species. Provides us with Cassava, an increasingly important food crop, and with the novelty of Jumping Beans.

Acalypha indica   Origin: India
1907:   Acalypha
Uses: To remove mucus in the bronchitis of children. Emetic, laxative, expectorant, anthelmintic.

Croton eluteria   Origin: Bahamas
1907:   Cascarilla
Uses: Aromatic bitter, weak febrifuge.

Croton tiglium   Origin: India
1907:   Oleum Crotonis, Croton Oil, Oleum Tiglii

Uses: Extremely powerful cathartic, causes violent vomiting and purging in small doses. Externally, powerful counter-irritant and vesicant.

Euphorbia esula
Canon: Spurge-laurel (Urdu: Shibrum)
Parts used: Plant.
Temperament: Hot in the First and Dry in the Third Degree.

Euphorbia pilulifera   Origin: India
1907:   Euphorbia
Uses: Decoction or infusion used as an anti-asthmatic and against hay-fever.

Euphorbia resinifera   Origin: Morocco
1907:   Euphorbium
Uses: Resin is a violent emetic and a powerful cathartic. Externally it acts as a vesicant, used in veterinary practice. Powdered, it is a sternutic.
Canon: Orbium (Urdu: Farfayun)
Parts used: Resin.
Temperament: Hot and Dry in the Fourth Degree.

Hevea brasiliensis   Origin: Brazil
1907:   Caoutchouc, India Rubber
Uses: Basis of self-adhesive carrying plasters.

Mallotus philippensis   Origin: India
1907:   Kamala, Glandulae Rottlerae
Uses: Anthelmintic.

Manihot utilissima   Origin: South America
1988:   Tapioca Starch

Ricinus communis   Origin: Europe
1988:   Castor Oil
Uses: Stimulant laxative, emollient.
1979:   Castor Oil
Uses: Purgative, emollient.
1907:   Oleum Ricini, Castor Oil
Uses: Unirritating purgative; the most valuable laxative available in

medicine. Poisonous in large doses – two or three seeds have been known to be fatal.

ORDER RHAMNALES

Buckthorn family – Rhamnaceae

Cosmopolitan temperate-to-tropical herbs and shrubs; 58 genera with some 900 species. Provides Chinese Dates and perhaps the Lotus fruit of antiquity. Chemical analysis has shown that many members of the family contain quinine.

Ventilago oblongifolia bark extracts are used as a poultice to cure cholera.

Rhamnus purshiana   Origin: North America
1988:   Cascara
Uses: Stimulant laxative.
1979:   Cascara.
Uses: Anthraquinone purgative. Glycosides excreted in milk.
1907:   Cascara Sagrada, Sacred Bark
Uses: Mild laxative, suitable for elderly and delicate persons.

Rhamnus frangula   Origin: Europe
1988:   Frangula Bark
Uses: Stimulant laxative.
1907:   Frangulae Cortex, Frangula Bark, Alder Buckthorn Bark
Uses: Properties similar to Cascara Sagrada (*Rhamnus purshiana*); mild purgative.

Zizyphus sativa   Origin: Mediterranean
1907:   Zyzyphus, Jujuba
Uses: Berries are demulcent and nutritive, have been used as decoction for throat and bronchial irritation.
Canon: Medlar? (Urdu: Ber)
Parts used: Berries.
Temperament: Cool and Dry in the First Degree.

Grape Vine family – Vitaceae

A mainly tropical and subtropical family and cosmopolitan in these zones; 12 genera with some 700 species of climbers and some shrubs. The Grape Vine grows throughout the north temperate zone.

Cissus vitiginea
Canon: Hamama (Urdu: Hamama)
Parts used: Wood.
Temperament: Hot and Dry in the Second Degree.

Vitis vinifera   Origin: Europe
1907:   Uvae, Uvae Passae, Raisins
Uses: Raisins are demulcent, nutritive, and mildly laxative.
Canon: Grapes (Urdu: Angoor)
Parts used: Fruit.
Temperament: Ripe Hot and Moist in the First Degree, unripe Cool
      and Dry in the First Degree.

Bladder Nut family – Staphyleaceae

A mainly north temperate family but also present in Cuba, Hispaniola,
and the South American and Asian tropics; 5 genera with some 600
species of trees and shrubs.
Euscaphis japonica fruits are used in China and Japan as a drug.

Melianthus family – Melianthaceae

3 genera with 18 species of shrubs and trees from southern Africa.
Melianthus comosum root, bark and leaves are used against snake
venom in South Africa.

Zebra Wood family – Connaraceae

Pantropical trees and twining shrubs; 16 genera with some 350 species
yielding medicinals, tannins and fibres.
Cannarus africanus seeds give an anthelmintic, other species are emetic
and antidysenteric.

Litchi family – Sapindaceae

Tropical and subtropical cosmopolitans, some 150 genera with 2000
species. They provide the Litchi fruits and Rambutans; also the Akye
of Africa, the aril of which – though poisonous if eaten at the wrong
stage – tastes of scrambled egg, and which is grown as the national
fruit of Jamaica.

Paullinia cupana   Origin: Brazil
1907:   Guarana

332

Uses: Source of caffeine. Central nervous system and cardiac stimulant, specific diuretic. Guarana is the prepared seed, either as a drug or as a drink.

Sabia family – Sabiaceae

Tropical and subtropical, disjunct in East Asia and South America; 4 genera with some 80 species.

Juliana family – Julianaceae

From Mexico to Peru, 2 genera with 5 species of resinous trees and shrubs.
Amphipterygium adstringens (Cuachalala) bark is used as an astringent and as an antimalarial.

Horse Chestnut family – Hippocastanaceae

2 genera, 15 species of mainly north temperate trees in Europe and also into the subtropics in Asia and in the tropics of Central and South America.
Aesculus spp. fruits are used as medicine, in medicinal baths, and as a fish poison.

Maple family – Aceraceae

2 genera with between 100 and over 150 species of deciduous trees found throughout the temperate region. They produce maple sugar.

Frankincense family – Burseraceae

Circumtropical trees and shrubs, some 17 genera with 500 species, giving Frankincense and Myrrh.

Balsamodendron myrrha   Origin: north-eastern Africa, Arabia
1907:   Myrrha, Myrrh
Uses: Mild disinfectant and local stimulant in chronic skin diseases. Internally, carminative, mild expectorant, diaphoretic and diuretic.
Canon: Myrrh (Urdu: Mur Maki)
Parts used: Resin.
Temperament: Hot and Dry in the Second Degree.

Boswellia spp.   Origin: Arabia
1907:   Olibanum, Frankincense
Uses: Used in preparation of plasters, and is an ingredient of incense
         and fumigating powders.
Canon: Olibanum (Urdu: Kundar)
Parts used: Gum.
Temperament: Cool and Dry in the Third Degree.

Canarium commune   Origin: Philippines
1907:   Elemi, Manilla Elemi
Uses: Resin exudate, used externally as an ointment for ulcers and
         chronic skin diseases. Properties similar to turpentine.

Commiphora opobalsamum   Origin: western Asia
Canon: Balsam (Urdu: Bilsan)
Parts used: Oil.
Temperament: Hot and Dry in the Second Degree.

Cashew family – Anacardsiaceae

Mainly tropical and subtropical with a few temperate members; some
77 genera with 600 species of trees, shrubs and some lianas. Provides
Cashew, Pistachio and Dhobi nuts, Mangoes, Cashew Apples, Otahite
Apples, Hog Plums and Jamaica Plums.

Buchanania latifolia   Origin: Asia
Canon: Bugle Seed (Urdu: Chironji)
Parts used: Seed.
Temperament: Hot and Moist.

Pistacia lentiscus   Origin: Mediterranean
1979:   Mastic
Uses: Resin solution used as temporary tooth filling, compound
         paint used as protective covering for wounds.
1907:   Mastiche, Mastic
Uses: Masticatory. Temporary stopping for carious teeth.
Canon: Mastic (Urdu: Mastagi)
Parts used: Gum.
Temperament: Hot and Dry in the Second Degree.

Pistacia vera
Canon: Pistachio Gum (Urdu: Pista gond)
Parts used: Gum.
Temperament: Hot.

Pistacia terebinthus
Canon: Turpentine Resin (Urdu: Baroza)
Parts used: Gum.
Temperament: Hot in the Second and Dry in the Third Degree.

Rhus coriaria   Origin: southern Mediterranean
Canon: Sumach (Urdu: Somaq)
Parts used: Seeds.
Temperament: Cool in the First and Dry in the Second Degree.

Quassia family – Simaroubaceae

Circumtropical and subtropical family of some 20 genera with 120 species of trees and shrubs.

Picrasma excelsa   Origin: Central America
1979:   Quassia, Quassia Wood
Uses: Tannin-free bitter.

Picrasma excelsa   Origin: Jamaica
1907:   Quassiae Lignum, Quassia, Jamaica Quassia
Uses: Pure bitter, without astringency. Insect repellent.

Simaruba spp.   Origin: South America
1907:   Simarubae Cortex, Simaruba Bark
Uses: Bitter and astringent in chronic dysentery.

Coriaria family – Coriariaceae

Found in the warm temperate regions around the world; 1 genus with 8 species of shrubs.
Coriaria myrtifolia fruits crushed in water are used to poison flies in the Mediterranean area.

Mahogany family – Meliaceae

Circumtropical and subtropical trees and shrubs, some 50 genera with 550 species, producing Langsat and Santol fruits.

Guarea rusbyi   Origin: Caribbean
1988:   Cocillana
Uses: Expectorant.
1979:   Cocillana, Grape Bark, Guapi Bark
Uses: Expectorant and emetic; used in place of Ipecacuanha
(*Cephaelis ipecachuana*).

Melia azadirachta   Origin: India
1907:   Azadirachta Indica, Neem Bark, Margosa Bark
Uses: Simple bitter.
Canon: Persian Lilac (Urdu: Bakaine)
Parts used: Berries.
Temperament: Hot in the Third and Dry in the Second Degree.

Spurge Olive family – Cneoraceae

A single genus with 2 species of evergreen shrubs, found from the
Canaries to the western Mediterranean.
Cneorum tricoccum leaves and fruits provide a purgative and a
rubefacient.

Citrus family – Rutaceae

Circumtropical to warm temperate family; 150 genera with some 900
species of shrubs and trees. Provides citrus fruits such as Oranges,
Lemons and Limes and their cultivars.

Aegle marmelos   Origin: India
1907:   Bael Fructus
Uses: Mild astringent (mucilage and pectin in half-ripe fruit).

Barosma betulina   Origin: South Africa
1907:   Buchu Folia, Buchu Leaves
Uses: Diuretic, genito-urinary antiseptic.

Citrus limon   Origin: Europe
1988:   Lemon Oil
Uses: Flavouring.
1979:   Lemon Oil
Uses: Flavouring and perfumery agent.
1907:   Limonis Cortex, Lemon Peel

Uses: Bitter stomachic and tonic; flavouring substance. Oil is stimulant and carminative.
Canon: Lemon (Urdu: Bijora)
Parts used: Peel.
Temperament: Hot in the First and Dry in the Second Degree.

Citrus sinensis   Origin: Asia
1988: Orange Oil
Uses: Flavouring.
1979: Orange Oil, Sweet Orange Oil
Uses: Flavouring agent, perfume.
1907: Oleum Aurantii, Oil of Orange
Uses: Oil is used as flavouring and perfuming agent.

Citrus aurantium   Origin: Mediterranean
1988: Dried Bitter-Orange Peel
1979: Bitter Orange Peel
Uses: Flavouring agent.
1907: Bitter Orange (Peel); Oleum Neroli, Oil of Orange Flowers
Uses: Flavouring agent, bitter, stomachic, carminative. Oil is used as flavouring and perfuming agent. Oil of Neroli is largely employed in perfumery.

Citrus bergamia   Origin: Italy
1907: Oleum Bergamottae, Bergamot Oil
Uses: Oil is used as flavouring and perfuming agent.

Galipea officinalis   Origin: South America
1907: Cuspariae Cortex, Angostura Bark
Uses: Aromatic bitter.

Pilocarpus microphyllus   Origin: South America
1979: Pilocarpus
Uses: Pilocarpine source; similar action to physostigmine, but half as strong. Used to reduce intraocular pressure and constrict the pupil.
1907: Pilocarpus (jaborandi), Jaborandi
Uses: Pilocarpine source; stimulates nerves supplying unstriped muscle, heart and secretory glands. Powerful diaphoretic. In ophthalmic use, reduces intraocular pressure. Sialagogue, galactagogue, supposed to encourage hair growth.

Ruta graveolens   Origin: Europe
1907:   Oleum Rutae, Oil of Rue
Uses: Antispasmodic and emmenagogue in amenorrhoea.
Canon: Rue (Urdu: Sazab)
Parts used: Leaves.
Temperament: Hot and Dry in the Second Degree.

Lignum Vitae family – Zygophyllaceae

Largely tropical and subtropical family of trees and shrubs with a few temperate members; found around the world except for Central Africa.
Neoschroeteria tridentata, the Creosote Plant of Mexico, is used medicinally and its flower buds are eaten as capers.

Guaiacum offiçinale   Origin: Central America
1907:   Guaiaci Lignum, Guaiacum Wood; Guaiacum Resin
Uses: Mild purgative and diuretic. Used in acute tonsillitis for its supposed action on throat mucosae. Employed in chronic rheumatism and gout to relieve pain and inflammation.

ORDER JUGLANDALES

Walnut family – Juglandaceae

North temperate family, some tropical and subtropical members, found around the world except for Africa; 7 genera with some 50 species of deciduous trees. They provide Walnuts, Hickory nuts and Pecans.

Juglans regia   Origin: Asia
Canon: Walnut (Urdu: Akhrot)
Parts used: Nuts.
Temperament: Hot in the Third and Dry in the First Degree.

ORDER GERANIALES

Bastard Bullet Tree family – Houmiriaceae

Central and tropical South America, 8 genera with some 50 species, two of which occur in West Africa; trees and shrubs.
Sarcoglottis gabonensis fruits are fermented and drunk.

Flax family – Linaceae

Cosmopolitan except for the Far North, mainly temperate but some tropical members; 13 genera with some 300 species of herbs and a few shrubs.
Linum usitatissimum fibres give flax, its seeds give linseed oil. *Hugonia* spp. give edible fruits.

Linum usitatissimum   Origin: Europe
1988:   Linseed
Uses: Demulcent.
1979:   Linseed Oil, Flaxseed Oil
Uses: Veterinary laxative against cattle bloat.
1907:   Linum, Linseed, Flaxseed
Uses: Infusion is used as demulcent in coughs; crushed seeds are used in form of a poultice to apply heat locally. Oil is laxative, antihaemorrhoidal. Externally, the oil is used as a soothing ointment on burns.
Canon: Linseed (Urdu: Alsi)
Parts used: Seeds.
Temperament: Hot in the First Degree, and Moist.

Geranium family – Geraniaceae

11 genera with some 750 species of widespread herbs and a few shrubs, mainly temperate with some subtropicals.

Pelargonium spp.   Origin: Europe
1907:   Oleum Geranii, Oil of Pelargonium
Uses: Largely employed in perfumery; substitute for oil of rose.

Wood Sorrel family – Oxalidaceae

Widespread in the tropics, subtropics and temperate regions; 3 genera with some 900 species of herbs. The leaves of a number of species and the tubers of some are eaten as salads; most contain oxalic acid.

Coca family – Erythroxylaceae

Pantropical and subtropical trees and shrubs; four genera with some 260 species.
Erythroxylum coca gives Coca leaf and cocaine.

Erythroxylum coca   Origin: South America
1988:   Cocaine
Uses: Local anaesthetic.
1979:   Cocaine
Uses: Ophthalmic and ENT local anaesthetic.
1907:   Cocae folia, Coca Leaves
Uses: Stimulant, 'nervine' tonic.

Poached Egg Flower family – Limnanthaceae

2 genera with 11 species, annual herbs from North America, mainly California.

Balsam family – Balsaminaceae

Annual and perennial herbs; 4 genera with 500 to 600 species widespread in temperate and tropical regions except South Africa and Australia.

Nasturtium family – Tropaeolaceae

2 genera, some 90 species from South and Central America; climbing succulent herbs. Leaves, tubers, flowers and seeds of some species are eaten.

ORDER POLYGALALES

Malpighia family – Malpighiaceae

Pantropical but found especially in South America; 60 genera with some 800 species of climbers, shrubs and some trees. *Malpighia* spp. fruits are eaten; *Banisteria caapi* leaves and shoots provide a hallucinatory drug and *Hiptage benghalensis* is used to treat skin diseases.

Trigonia family – Trigoniaceae

A small tropical family with a disjunct distribution through America, Madagascar and Malaysia; 4 genera with some 35 species.

Tremandra family – Tremandraceae

An Australian family of 3 genera with 43 species of shrubs.

Vochysia family – Vochysiaceae

Trees, shrubs and climbers from Central and South America and West Africa, 6 genera with some 200 species.
Erisma calcaratum seeds give Jaboty Butter, used in soaps.

Milkwort family – Polygalaceae

Cosmopolitan except for large parts of the Far North; some 17 genera with 1000 species.

Polygala senega   Origin: North America
1988:   Senega Root
Uses: Expectorant.   .
1979:   Senega Root
Uses: Its saponins, though not absorbed, are irritants to the gastric mucosa and give rise to a reflex secretion of mucus in the bronchioles. Expectorant in chronic bronchitis.
1907:   Senegae Radix, Senega Root
Uses: Stimulating expectorant in chronic bronchitis.

Krameria family – Krameriaceae

A single genus with 25 species, of tropical America and the West Indies; shrubs and perennial herbs.

Krameria triandra   Origin: South America
1988:   Ratany Root
Uses: Astringent.
1907:   Krameriae Radix, Rhatany Root
Uses: Powerful astringent, both external and internal.

ORDER UMBELLALES

Ivy family – Araliaceae

Herbs, shrubs and trees, some 55 genera with 7000 species; worldwide except for India and North Africa.
Tetrapanax papyrifera pith yields 'rice paper'. *Panax* spp. give Ginseng.   .

Carrot family – Umbelliferae

A large, almost worldwide family of some 300 genera with 3000 species, herbs favouring temperate uplands. Provides Carrots, Celery, Lovage, Parsnips, Earthnuts, Pignuts, Angelica.

Anethum graveolens   Origin: Europe
1988:   Dill Oil
Uses: Carminative.
1979:   Dill Oil
Uses: Carminative, treatment for flatulence in children, flavouring.
1907:   Dill Fruit (*Peucedanum graveolens*)
Uses: Remedy for flatulence.
Canon: Dill (Urdu: Soya)
Parts used: Seeds.
Temperament: Hot in the Second and Dry in the First Degree.

Angelica archangelica   Origin: northern Europe
1907:   Angelica
Uses: Stimulating expectorant.

Apium graveolens   Origin: Eurasia
Canon: Apium, Wild Celery (Urdu: Ajmod)
Parts used: Seeds.
Temperament: Hot and Dry in the Third Degree.

Carum carvi   Origin: Europe
1988:   Caraway
Uses: Flavouring.
1979:   Caraway
Uses: Carminative, flavouring agent.
1907:   Carui Fructus; Oleum Carui, Caraway Oil
Uses: Aromatic, carminative, vehicle. The oil is an aromatic carminative to the gastro-intestinal tract.
Canon: Caraway (Urdu: Zeera-Siah)
Parts used: Seeds.
Temperament: Hot and Dry in the Second Degree.

Carum copticum   Origin: India
1907:   Oleum Ajowan, Ajowan, Ptychotis
Uses: Oil used as an antiseptic and carminative.
Canon: Ajowan (Urdu: Ajwain)

Parts used: Seeds.
Temperament: Hot and Dry in the Third Degree.
Comments: Other references – *Ptychotis coptica* and *Carum ajovan*.

Conium maculatum   Origin: Europe
1907:   Conii Folia, Conii Fructus, Hemlock
Uses: Sedative, antispasmodic; source of coniine: medullar depressant.
          Anal analgesic.
Canon: Hemlock (Urdu: Shookran)
Parts used: Seeds.
Temperament: Cool and Dry in the Third Degree.

Coriandrum sativum   Origin: southern Europe
1988:   Coriander
Uses: Flavouring.
1979:   Coriander
Uses: Carminative, flavouring agent.
1907:   Coriandri Fructus, Coriander
Uses: Aromatic, stimulant, carminative.
Canon: Coriander (Urdu: Dhania)
Parts used: Seeds.
Temperament: Hot in the First and Dry in the Second Degree.

Cuminum cyminum   Origin: North Africa
1907:   Cumini Fructus
Uses: Veterinary carminative.
Canon: Cumin (Urdu: Zeera)
Parts used: Seeds.
Temperament: Hot in the Second and Dry in the Third Degree.

Daucus carota
Canon: Carrot (Urdu: Gajar)
Parts used: Seeds.
Temperament: Hot in the Second and Moist in the First Degree.

Ferula foetida   Origin: central Asia
1907:   Asafetida
Uses: Expectorant, carminative. Used in hystrical conditions for its
          unpleasant smell and taste.
Canon: Asafoetida (Urdu: Heeng)
Parts used: Resin.

Temperament: Hot in the First and Dry in the Second Degree.
Comments: Referred to as *Ferula assafoetida*.

Ferula galbanifera   Origin: Persia
1907:   Galbanum
Uses: Resin used as stimulant and expectorant in chronic bronchitis.
Canon: Galbanum (Urdu: Ganda baroza)
Parts used: Resin.
Temperament: Hot in the Second and Dry in the Third Degree.

Ferula persica   Origin: Arabia, Persia
1907:   Sagapenum
Uses: Resin used as stimulant and expectorant in chronic bronchitis.

Ferula sumbul   Origin: Turkestan
1907:   Sumbul Radix, Sumbul
Uses: Employed as a stimulant and antispasmodic in hysterical conditions.

Foeniculum vulgare var. *vulgare*   Origin: Europe
1979:   Foeniculum, Fennel Fruit, Fennel
Uses: Carminative and flavouring agent.
1907:   Foeniculi Fructus, Fennel fruit; Oil of Fennel
Uses: Aromatic and carminative. Fennel water mixed with sodium bicarbonate and syrup constitutes 'gripe water'.
Canon: Fennel (Urdu: Sonf)
Parts used: Seeds.
Temperament: Hot in the Second and Dry in the First Degree.
Comments: Given as *Foeniculum officinale*.

Petroselinum spp.   Origin: Europe
1907:   Apiol, Parsley
Uses: Apiol is extracted from parsley; used in dysmenorrhoea and amenorrhoea (irritant), also as diuretic.
Canon: Parsley (Urdu: Karfas)
Parts used: Seeds.
Temperament: Hot and Dry in the First Degree.
Comments: Given as Celery (*Apium graveolens*) – probably refers to Mediterranean (smooth-leaved) Parsley.

Pimpinella anisum   Origin: Europe
1988:   Anise, Aniseed
Uses: Carminative, flavouring.
1979:   Anise
Uses: Carminative, expectorant.
1907:   Anise
Uses: Carminative, expectorant, cathartic. Oil is antiseptic, relieves
        flatulence.
Canon: Anise (Urdu: Anisoon)
Parts used: Seeds.
Temperament: Hot and Dry in the Second Degree.

Superorder Asteridae

ORDER GENTIANALES

Buddleia family – Loganiaceae

Widespread in the tropical, subtropical and temperate zones of the world; some 30 genera with 600 species of trees, shrubs and climbers, many highly poisonous.

Gelsemium nitidum   Origin: North America
1907:   Gelsemii Radix, Gelsemium Root, Yellow Jasmine Root
Uses: Effect like *Conium maculatum* in depressing heart functions
        and respiration, except that it paralyses the nerve centres first,
        and the motor nerve endings at higher doses. Used in migraine
        and neuralgia.

Spigelia marilandica   Origin: North America
1907:   Spigelia, Indian Pink, Pink Root
Uses: Action similar to Gelsemium, depressing heart functions and
        respiration. Anthelmintic and effective against roundworm.

Strychnos toxifera   Origin: South America
1907:   Curara, Curare
Uses: Parlayses motor nerve endings.

Strychnos nux-vomica   Origin: India, Southeast Asia
1979:   Nux Vomica
Uses: Similar effects to strychnine hydrochloride: stimulates the
        nervous system.

1907:   Nux Vomica
Uses: Used in atonic dyspepsia, and as a gastro-intestinal stimulant. Bitter; stimulates peristalsis. Used in surgical shock and cardiac failure.

Strychnos ignatii   Origin: Philippines
1907:   Ignatii Semina, St Ignatius Bean, Ignatia Amara
Uses: Similar effect to Nux Vomica seeds. Bitter stomachic tonic.

Gentian family – Gentianaceae

Cosmopolitan family of some 80 genera with 900 species of herbs and a few shrubs.

Erythraea centaurium
Canon: Centaury (Urdu: Quanturian)
Parts used: Flowers.
Temperament: Hot and Dry in the Third Degree.

Gentiana lutea   Origin: Europe
1988:   Gentian
Uses: Bitter.
1979:   Gentian, Gentianae Radix
Uses: Bitter and aperient.
1907:   Gentianae Radix, Gentian Root
Uses: Bitter and aperient.

Swertia chirata   Origin: North India
1907:   Chirata, Chiretta, Chirayta
Uses: Non-astringent bitter stomachic and tonic.

Periwinkle family – Apocynaceae

Mainly tropical and subtropical worldwide family of some 180 genera with 1500 species of trees, shrubs, lianas and a few temperate herbs.

Alstonia scholaris   Origin: India
1907:   Alstonia
Uses: Antimalarial (weaker than cinchona, but no side effects), bitter tonic, anthelmintic, antidiarrhoeal.

Apocynum cannabinum   Origin: America
1907:   Canadian Hemp
Uses: Cardiac tonic.

Aspidosperma quebracho-blanco   Origin: South America
1907:   Quebracho, White Quebracho
Uses: Bitter and tonic.

Catharanthus roseus   Origin: Madagascar
1979:   Vincristine, Vinca
Uses: Vincristine source; cytotoxic drug arresting mitosis in the metaphase. Used against leukaemia and other tumours.

Rauwolfia serpentina   Origin: India, Southeast Asia
1979:   Rauwolfia
Uses: Source of reserpine; central nervous system depressant, antihypertensive due to depletion of catecholamines. Also tranquillizer used in chronic psychoses, veterinary use in tranquillizing turkeys for transport.

Rauwolfia vomitoria   Origin: Africa
1979:   African Rauwolfia
Uses: Source of reserpine; central nervous system depressant, antihypertensive due to depletion of catecholamines. Also tranquillizer used in chronic psychoses, veterinary use in tranquillizing turkeys for transport.

Strophanthus kombe   Origin: East Africa
1907:   Strophanti Semina, Strophantus
Uses: Used instead of digitalis when cardiac stimulation alone is required, without increase of blood pressure.

Milkweed family – Asclepiadaceae

Worldwide, tropical and subtropical with temperate members, some 250 genera with 2000 species.

Calotropis procera   Origin: India
1907:   Calotropis
Uses: Resembles Ipecacuanha; small doses diaphoretic and expectorant, large doses cause vomiting and diarrhoea.

347

Gonolobus condurango   Origin: Ecuador
1907:   Condurango Cortex
Uses: Bitter substance used in dyspepsia.

Hemidesmus indicus   Origin: India
1907:   Hemidesmi Radix, Indian Sarsaparilla
Uses: Used as antisyphilitic in place of Sarsaparilla.

Tylophora asthmatica   Origin: India
1907:   Tylophorae Folia, Tylophora
Uses: Expectorant and emetic — Indian substitute for Ipecac (*Cephaelia acuminata*).

Olive family – Oleaceae

Trees and shrubs, 29 genera with some 600 species, almost cosmopolitan. Provides the world with olives and manna.

Fraxinus ornus   Origin: Mediterranean
1907:   Manna, Flake Manna
Uses: Gentle laxative for children and infants.

Olea europaea   Origin: Mediterranean
1988:   Olive Oil
1979:   Olive Oil
Uses: Nutritious, demulcent and slightly laxative. Used to facilitate the removal of impacted faeces. Vehicle.
1907:   Oleae Folia, Olive Leaves; Oleum Oliveae, Olive Oil
Uses: Tonic, febrifuge, antiperiodic. Leaves have been employed as a substitute for quinine in the treatment of obstinate fever. Oil is nutritious, demulcent and slightly laxative. Used to facilitate the removal of impacted faeces. Externally, lubricant and emollient.

ORDER POLEMONIALES

Nolona family – Nolonaceae

Found in Chile and Peru, 2 genera with 83 species of herbs and small shrubs, many of which are fleshy seashore plants.

Potato family – Solanaceae

Cosmopolitan except for the Far North, some 90 genera with between 2000 and 3000 species, many of which are herbs, a few shrubs and trees. The family provides Potato, Tomato, Capsicum, Aubergine, Husk Tomato, Tomatillo, Tree Tomato, Cape Gooseberry, Pepino, Cocona, Narafilla and Lulita.

Atropa belladonna   Origin: Europe

1988:   Belladonna
Uses: Antispasmodic.
1979:   Belladonna Leaf, Belladonna Root
Uses: Decreases secretion from Glands. Antispasmodic (hyoscyamine, atropine).
1907:   Belladonna Folia, Belladonna Fructus
Uses: Source for atropine and hyoscyamine; central nervous system stimulant, nerve-ending depressant.
Canon: Belladonna (Urdu: Yabrooj)
Parts used: Root.
Temperament: Cool and Dry in the Third Degree.

Capsicum annuum var. *minimum*   Origin: South America, Africa

1979:   Capsicum, Chillies
Uses: Carminative, rubefacient.
1907:   Capsicum Fructus
Uses: Stimulant and carminative, external irritant.
Canon: Pepper, Red (Urdu: Lal mirch)
Parts used: Pods.
Temperament: Hot and Dry in the Third Degree.

Datura stramonium   Origin: Europe

1988:   Stramonium Leaf
Uses: Antispasmodic.
1979:   Stramonium, Thornapple Leaf
Uses: Similar to Belladonna and Hyoscyamus. Used to control salivation, muscular rigidity and tremor in parkinsonism.
1907:   Source for daturine, mainly hyoscyamine with some atropine.
Uses: Mainly used as an ophthalmic preparation, drops or gelatin. Leaves used to relieve spasmodic contractions of bronchioles in asthma, either by tincture taken internally or by smoking.

Datura fastuosa   Origin: India
1907:   Datura leaf, seeds.
Uses: Also *Datura metel*. Used in India as a substitute for *Datura stramonium*.

Duboisia spp.
1979:   Atropine
Uses: Source for atropine.
1907:   Duboisia myoporoides
Uses: Source for hyoscyamine and hyoscine. Sedative, hypnotic, mydriatic. Some ophthalmic use.

Hyoscyamus niger   Origin: Europe
1988:   Hyoscyamus Leaf
Uses: Antispasmodic.
1979:   Hyoscyamus leaf, Henbane
Uses: Source for atropine; action similar to Belladonna, but less likely to cause cerebral excitement. Counteracts spasms and griping action of purgatives.
1907:   Hyosciami Folia, Henbane Leaf (and Seeds)
Uses: Cerebral and spinal sedative. Used in insomnia. Relieves the griping caused by purgatives, and pain from cystitis. Smoke from heated seeds used as a domestic remedy for toothache.
Canon: Hyusciamus (Urdu: Ajwain khurasani)
Parts used: Seeds.
Temperament: Cool and Dry in the Third Degree.

Mandragora officinarum   Origin: Europe, western Asia
Canon: Mandrake (Urdu: Astrang)
Parts used: Leaves.
Temperament: Cool in the Third Degree.

Nicotiana tabacum   Origin: America
1907:   Tabaci Folia, Tobacco
Uses: Smoked, as nervous relaxant. Liquid preparations as insecticide.

Solanum tuberosum   Origin: South America
1988:   Potato Starch
1907:   Amylum, Potato Starch
Uses: Dusting powder, mucilage.

Solanum dulcamara   Origin: Europe
1907:   Dulcamara, Bittersweet
Uses: Decoction was formerly a popular remedy for chronic
         rheumatism and for obstinate skin eruptions.

Solanum melongena   Origin: Asia
Canon: Aubergine, Brinjal (Urdu: Baingan)
Parts used: Fruit.
Temperament: Hot in the First and Dry in the Second Degree.

Solanum nigrum
Canon: Nightshade, Black (Urdu: Makoh)
Parts used: Plant.
Temperament: Cool in the First and Dry in the Second Degree.

Bindweed family – Convolvulaceae

Herbaceous and woody, mainly climbing plants, some 50 genera with
1800 cosmopolitan species except in the Far North. Provides the Sweet
Potato; the roots of many other species are also locally used.

Convolvulus scammonia   Origin: eastern Mediterranean
1907:   Scammoniae Resina, Scammony Resin
Uses: Drastic purgative, anthelminthic.
Canon: Scammony (Urdu: Saqmoonia)
Parts used: Resin.
Temperament: Hot and Dry in the Third Degree.

Cuscuta approximata
Canon: Dodder (Urdu: Akasbail)
Parts used: Seeds.
Temperament: Hot in the Third and Dry in the First Degree.

Ipomoea purga   Origin: Central America
1907:   Jalapa, Jalap
Uses: Powerful purgative, cathartic.

Ipomoea hederacea   Origin: India
1907:   Kaladana, Pharbitis Nil
Uses: Powerful purgative, cathartic. Indian equivalent of Jalap
         (*Ipomoea purga*).

Ipomoea turpethum   Origin: India
1907:   Turpethum, turpeth
Uses: Purgative – Indian substitute for Jalap (*Ipomoea purga*).
Canon: Turpeth (Urdu: Turbad)
Parts used: Root.
Temperament: Hot and Dry in the Second Degree.

Bogbean family – Menyanthaceae

5 genera with some 40 species of aquatic and wetland herbs, cosmopolitan. The leaves are eaten in the Far North. *Menyanthus* spp. contains the glycoside menyanthin used as a febrifuge.

Lennoa family – Lennoaceae

Fleshy parasitic herbs from south-west North America with an outlier in Colombia; 3 genera with 4 or 5 species, some formerly used as food.

Phlox family – Polemoniaceae

Trees and lianas to leafless annuals; 18 genera with some 300 species from much of the high latitudes throughout North America except eastern Canada, also throughout Asia except for the tropics and down the Andes to Tierra del Fuego.

Ehretia family – Ehretiaceae

13 genera, some 400 species of trees, shrubs and a few herbs; tropical and subtropical worldwide, especially in the southern hemisphere. The fruit of some species is edible, and a decoction of others is used against colds.
Ehretia philippensis leaves are used against dysentery.

Hydrophyllum family – Hydrophyllaceae

Widely distributed family of herbs and small shrubs, from the tropics to the subarctic, but absent from much of Canada, Eurasia and North Africa; some 18 genera with 250 species.

Forget-me-not family – Boraginaceae

Centred on the Mediterranean, some 100 genera with 2000 species of herbs, shrubs, a few trees and some lianas, worldwide in tropical through temperate zones. Provides Borage and Comfrey, long used as pot herbs.

Alkanna tinctoria   Origin: eastern Europe
1907:   Alkanna Root, Alkanet Root
Uses: Red colourings for lip salves and toiletry.

ORDER LAMIALES

Teak family – Verbenaceae

Tropical and subtropical with a few temperate members; some 75 genera with more than 3000 species of herbs, shrubs, trees (including Teak) and many lianas, distributed worldwide.
Lippia citriodora is the Lemon Verbena from South America, *Vitex agnus castus*, Monk's Pepper Tree, yields a valuable oil, while *Verbena officinalis*, the Vervain of Europe, is used in the treatment of skin diseases.

Mint family – Labiatae

Cosmopolitan, some 200 genera with 3000 species of herbs and undershrubs, mainly of open ground. Provide many culinary herbs which are also of medicinal value.

Collinsonia canadensis   Origin: North America
1907:   Collinsonia, Knob Root, Heal-All
Uses: Antispasmodic; diuretic and sedative for uro-genital disorders.

Hedeoma pulegioides   Origin: North America
1907:   Oleum Hedeomae, Oil of American Pennyroyal
Uses: Given as an emmenagogue. During excretion, it mildly irritates the kidneys and bladder, and reflexly excites uterine contractions.

Hyssopus officinalis
Canon: Hyssop (Urdu: Zoofa)
Parts used: Flowers.
Temperament: Hot in the Second and Moist in the First Degree when fresh, Hot and Dry in the Third Degree when dry.

Lavandula intermedia   Origin: Europe
1979:   Lavender Oil
Uses: Perfumery, as an odour corrective.
1907:   Oleum Lavandulae (*Lavandula vera*), Oil of Lavender
Uses: Aromatic and carminative. Used in perfumery and as flavouring agent.

Marrubium vulgare   Origin: Europe
1907:   Marrubium, Horehound
Uses: Expectorant, laxative in large doses.

Mentha arvensis var. *piperita*   Origin: Europe
1988:   Peppermint Leaf, Peppermint Oil
Uses: Carminative, flavouring.
1979:   Peppermint Oil
Uses: Menthol source; relieves symptoms of bronchitis. Oil is a carminative and antiseptic. Flavouring agent.
1907:   Oleum Menthae Piperiteae, Oil of Peppermint
Uses: Aromatic stimulant, carminative; it relieves gastric and intestinal flatulence and colic. Local anaesthetic, mild antiseptic, flavouring agent.
Canon: Mint, Wild (Urdu: Podina)
Parts used: Leaves.
Temperament: Hot and Dry in the Second Degree.

Mentha spicata   Origin: Europe
1988:   Spearmint Oil
Uses: Flavouring.
1979:   Spearmint Oil
Uses: Flavouring agent and carminative.
1907:   Oleum Menthae Viridis, Oil of Spearmint
Uses: Aromatic stimulant, carminative; it relieves gastric and intestinal flatulence and colic. Local anaesthetic, mild antiseptic, flavouring agent.

Mentha pulegium   Origin: Europe
1907:   Oleum Pulegii, Oil of Pennyroyal
Uses: Given as an emmenagogue. During excretion, it mildly irritates the kidneys and bladder, and reflexly excites uterine contractions.
Canon: Mint (Urdu: Podina)

Parts used: Leaves.
Temperament: Hot and Dry in the Second Degree.

Ocimum basilicum   Origin: Eurasia
*Canon:*Basil (Urdu: Tulsi)
Parts used: Seeds.
Temperament: Hot in the Second and Dry in the First Degree.

Ocimum canum   Origin: Eurasia
Canon: Wild Basil (Urdu: Jungli tulsi)
Parts used: Seeds.
Temperament: Hot in the First and Dry in the Second Degree.

Origanum hírtum   Origin: Europe
1907:   Carvacrol
Uses: Source of carvacrol (main component of Oil of Origanum).

Origanum majorana
Canon: Marjoram (Urdu: Marzanjosh)
Parts used: Leaves.
Temperament: Hot and Dry in the Third Degree.

Rosmarinus officinalis   Origin: southern Europe
1979:   Rosemary Oil
Uses: Perfumery agent, constituent of soap liniment.
1907:   Oleum Rosmarini, Oil of Rosemary, Oleum Anthos
Uses: Carminative, employed in hair lotions; perfuming agent.

Thymus vulgaris   Origin: Mediterranean
1907:   Oleum Thymi, Oil of Thyme
Uses: Rubefacient and counter-irritant in rheumatism etc. Internally
        it is an antiseptic, antispasmodic, and carminative. Thymol is
        a local analgesic, an antiseptic, and a vermifuge.
Canon: Wild Thyme (Urdu: Hasha)
Parts used: Leaves.
Temperament: Hot and Dry in the Third Degree.

Tetrachondra family – Tetrachondraceae

1 genus with 2 species, one each in New Zealand and in Patagonia, of
wet open habitats.

Water Starwort family – Callitrichaceae

A single genus with some 17 species of submerged aquatics, worldwide but favouring temperate climes. Indicators of a certain type of water pollution.

Phryma family – Phrymaceae

A single genus with perhaps 3 species of erect perennial herbs from eastern North America and north-east Asia.

ORDER PLANTAGINALES

Plantain family – Plantaginaceae

Annual and perennial herbs found throughout the world's temperate regions and in tropical mountains; 3 genera with some 253 species.

> *Plantago ovata*   Origin: Europe, Asia
> 1988:   Ispaghula Husk
> Uses: Antidiarrhoeal, bulk-forming laxative.
> 1979:   Ispaghula Husk
> Uses: Laxative.
> 1907:   Ispaghula
> Uses: Demulcent, antidiarrhoeal.
> *Canon*: Ispaghula (Urdu: Isbghole)
> Parts used: Seeds.
> Temperament: Cool and Moist in the Second Degree.
> Comments: Given as *Plantago psyllium*.
>
> *Plantago afra*   Origin: Mediterranean
> 1979:   Psyllium, Flea Seed
> Uses: Mucilaging and bulking agent.
>
> *Plantago indica*   Origin: India
> 1979:   Psyllium, Flea Seed
> Uses: Mucilaging and bulking agent.
>
> *Plantago major*   Origin: Europe, Asia
> *Canon*: Plantago (Urdu: Bartang)
> Parts used: Seeds.
> Temperament: Cool and Dry in the Second Degree.

ORDER SCROPHULARIALES

Columellia family – Columelliaceae

A single genus with 4 species of evergreen shrubs from the Andes of north-western South America.

Emu Bush family – Myoporaceae

Australian and South Pacific rim family, 4 genera with some 150 species of trees and shrubs.

Foxglove family – Scrophulariaceae

Mainly north temperate but cosmopolitan family; some 220 genera with 3000 species of herbs and some shrubs and lianas.

Digitalis purpurea   Origin: Europe
1988:   Digitalis Leaf
Uses: Cardiac glycoside.
1979:   Digitalis Leaf, Digitalis Folium
Uses: Increases excitability of cardiac muscle and strengthens contractions.
1907:   Digitalis Leaves, Foxglove Leaves, Digitalis Folia
Uses: Constituents are digitoxin, digitalin and possibly digitalein (all glycosides). Cardiac stimulant and vascoconstrictor.

Digitalis lanata   Origin: Europe
1979:   Digitalis Lanata Leaf, Austrian Foxglove
Uses: Source of digitoxin; cardiac glycoside.

Picrorhiza kurroa   Origin: Himalayas
1907:   Picrorhyzia
Uses: Bitter, tonic, antiperiodic.

Veronica virginica   Origin: North America
1907:   Leptandra, Culver's Root
Uses: Cholagogue, promoting the flow of bile without irritating the intestine.

Globularia family – Globulariaceae

2 genera with some 30 species of herbaceous or shrubby perennials, mainly Mediterranean but extending to Macronesia, Socotra, Somalia, the Alps and northern Europe.

African Violet family – Gesneriaceae

Tropical herbs and shrubs, worldwide, disjunct with some temperate species; some 125 genera with 2000 species. Many are used in rural medicine.

Broomrape family – Orobanchaceae

Mainly found in temperate Asia, but extending worldwide through the tropics though absent from the Far North, eastern South America and eastern Australia; some 14 genera with 180 species of total parasites.

Catalpa family – Bignoniaceae

Lianas, trees and shrubs; some 120 genera with 620 species, mainly pantropical.

Black-eyed Susan family – Acanthaceae

Tropical shrubs, with temperate outliers; some 250 genera with 2500 species, found worldwide.

Acanthus ebracteatus leaves, boiled, make a Malay cough medicine, *Acanthus mollis* roots are used to treat diarrhoea in Europe, and *Blechum pyramidatum*, leaves and flowers, are used as a diuretic and febrifuge in South America.

Adhatoda vasica   Origin: India
1907:   Adhatoda
Uses: Expectorant, antiasthmatic (cigarettes). Non-toxic to mammals, poisonous to insects and fish.

Andrographis paniculata   Origin: India
1907:   Andrographis
Uses: Bitter.

Hygrophila spinosa   Origin: India
1907:   Hygrophila
Uses: Demulcent and mild diuretic in catarrh of the urinary organs.

Sesame family – Pedaliaceae

Annual and perennial herbs and a few shrubs; 12 genera with some 50 species found in dry and sandy areas of Africa through Indomalaysia to Australia. The leaves of a number of species are used as vegetables in Africa. Sesame seeds are used in cooking and oil extraction.

Sesamum indicum   Origin: Asia
1988:   Sesame Oil
1979:   Sesame Oil
Uses: Vehicle for oily injections.
1907:   Oleum Sesami, Sesame Oil, Gingelly Oil, Teel Oil
Uses: Used in the preparation of additive compounds of iodine and bromine.
Canon: Sesame (Urdu: Til)
Parts used: Seeds.
Temperament: Hot and Moist in the First Degree.

Hydrostachis family – Hydrostachydaceae

A single genus with 22 species of aquatic herbs, centred in Madagascar but also found in southern Africa.

Unicorn Plant family – Martyniaceae

3 genera with some 13 species of herbs from the drier parts of tropical and subtropical South America and Mexico. The horned fruits of a number of species are eaten.

Bladderwort family – Lentibulariaceae

Carnivorous, aquatic or semiaquatic, sometimes epiphytic herbs; 4 genera with some 180 species, cosmopolitan except for the Far North.

ORDER CAMPANULALES

Bellflower family – Campanulaceae

Cosmpolitan except for Central Africa, some 35 genera with 300 species; mainly herbs, some shrubs and undershrubs, centred in the north temperate zone. Provides Rampion roots for salads.

Lobelia family – Lobeliaceae

Cosmopolitan family, but absent from the Far North and from large tracts of Eurasia; some 30 genera with 1200 species ranging from annuals through to weird trees in semi-desert areas. They provide the edible *Centropogon* and *Clermontia* berries.

Lobelia inflata   Origin: North America
1988:   Lobelia
Uses: Respiratory stimulant.
1907:   Lobelia, Indian Tobacco
Uses: Depresses vaso-motor centre and peripheral vagus, thus producing dilatation of the bronchioles. Used in spasmodic asthma and chronic bronchitis.

Trigger Plant family – Stylidiaceae

Subtropical and temperate annual or perennial herbs, some shrubs; 6 genera with some 150 species found in Australia, then disjunct in New Zealand, East Asia and the far south of South America.

Brunonia family – Brunoniaceae

1 genus with 1 species of a silky perennial herb from Australia.

Leschenaultia family – Goodeniaceae

14 genera of herbs and some shrubs with some 300 species centred in Australia and patchily distributed in coastal areas across the tropical and southern world.

ORDER RUBIALES

Gardenia family – Rubiaceae

One of the largest plant families, presenting some 500 genera with 7000 species; truly cosmopolitan, amongst them is the provider of coffee.

Cephaelis ipecacuanha   Origin: South America
1988:   Ipecacuanha
Uses: Expectorant, emetic.
1979:   Ipecacuanha, Ipecac
Uses: Contains emetine and cephaeline. In small doses, a reflex expectorant; in large doses, vomitory and emetic.

1907: Ipecachuanae Radix, Ipecac, Psychotria ipecachuana
Uses: Powerful expectorant. In large doses, vomitory, emetic and purgative. Powdered form is extremely irritant, and causes violent sneezing and coughing. Antiamoebic.

Cephaelis acuminata   Origin: India/Iran
1988: Ipecacuanha
Uses: Expectorant, emetic.
1979: Ipecacuanha, Ipecac
Uses: Contains emetine and cephaeline. In small doses, a reflex expectorant; in large doses, vomitory and emetic.

Cinchona spp.   Origin: South America
1907: Quinina, Quinine
Uses: General protoplasmic poison, in sufficient dosage paralyses all forms of living matter; especially lethal to undifferentiated protoplasm. Specific antimalarial, also used in headache, neuralgia, hay fever and catarrh as a metabolic retardant.

Cinchona pubescens   Origin: South America
1988: Cinchona Bark
Uses: Bitter.

Cinchona succirubra   Origin: South America
1907: Cinchonae Rubrae Cortex, Red Cinchona Bark
Uses: Bitter tonic and stomachic.

Coffea arabica   Origin: Arabia
1907: Caffeine
Uses: Source for caffeine. CNS and cardiac stimulant, specific diuretic.

Corynanthe yohimbi   Origin: South America
1907: Yohimbina, Yohimbehe
Uses: Sexual stimulant in impotence; ophthalmic local anaesthetic.

Uncaria gambier   Origin: Malay Archipelago
1988: Catechu
Uses: Intestinal astringent.
1979: Catechu

Uses: Astringent.
1907:   Catechu
Uses: Powerful internal and external astringent.

ORDER DIPSACALES

Adoxa family – Adoxales

A single monospecific genus, a perennial herb found from Europe across northern and central Asia to north-west North America.

Elder family – Caprifoliaceae

Cosmopolitan but missing from much of Africa, the Far North and the tip of South America; some 18 genera with 450 species of trees, shrubs and some climbers. Provides edible elderberries and elder flowers.

Sambucus nigra   Origin: Europe
1907:   Sambuci Flores, Elder Flowers; Sambuci Folia, Elder Leaves
Uses: Flowers used in the preparation of lotions and collyria. Leaves are used in a bruise ointment, as an emollient, and as wound treatment.

Viburnum prunifolium   Origin: North America
1907:   Viburnum, Black Haw
Uses: Depresses the medulla and spinal cord without affecting the higher cerebral centres; therefore it depresses respiration, and induces a large drop in blood pressure. Used for its supposed sedative effect in uterus to prevent threatened abortion. Used for asthma, dismenorrhoea and spasms.

Valerian family – Valerianaceae

Mainly herbs, but some shrubs and cushion plants; 13 genera with some 400 species, cosmopolitan except for the Far North, Central Africa and Australasia. Provides Lamb's Lettuce for salads, and the Spikenard of ancient trade.

Nardostachys jatamansi   Origin: Himalaya
Canon: Nard, Spikenard (Urdu: Nardeen)
Parts used: Oil.
Temperament: Hot in the First and Dry in the Second Degree.

Valeriana officinalis
1988:   Valerian
Uses: Sedative.
1907:   Valerianae Rhizoma, Valerian Root
Uses: Carminative and antispasmodic.

Valeriana wallichii   Origin: Himalayas
1907:   Valerianae Indicae Rhizoma, Indian Valerian Root
Uses: Carminative and antispasmodic.

Teasel family – Dipsacaceae

Herbs and subshrubs from the Old World subtropics with some temperate members; 11 genera with 350 species. The teasel is one of the only naturally occurring tools used in napping cloth.

Calycera family – Calyceraceae

6 genera with some 52 species of annual and perennial herbs, found in the southern Andes and the eastern South American Cono do Sul.

ORDER ASTERALES

Sunflower family – Compositae

One of the largest flower families, some 1100 genera with 25,000 species; mostly evergreen shrubs and subshrubs, but the whole range of plant forms including some trees and aquatic herbs is demonstrated by this truly cosmopolitan family. It provides Lettuce, Endive, Chicory, Scorzonera, Salsify, Globe Artichoke, Jerusalem Artichoke and Tarragon.

Anacyclus pyrethrum   Origin: Algeria
1907:   Pyrethri Radix, Pellitory Root
Uses: Masticatory; treatment of gums in toothache.

Anthemis nobilis   Origin: Europe
1988:   Chamomile Flowers, Roman Chamomile Flowers
1907:   Chamomile
Uses: Anti-inflammatory fomentation, aperient, tonic. Oil is an aromatic carminative.
Canon: Chamomile (Urdu: Baboona)

Parts used: Flowers.
Temperament: Hot in the First and Dry in the Second Degree.
Comments: Given as *Matricaria chamomilla.*

Arnica montana   Origin: Europe
1907:   Arnica
Uses: Dilute tincture sometimes used against sprains and bruises.

Artemisia absinthium   Origin: Europe
1907:   Wormwood, Absinthium
Uses: Stimulant of the cerebral cortex . . . could be used for
         neurasthenia.
Canon: Absinth (Urdu: Sheeh)
Parts used: Plant.
Temperament: Hot and Dry in the First Degree.

Artemisia maritima var. *stechmanniana*   Origin: Europe
1907:   Santonica
Uses: Source of santonin; vermifuge, remedy for roundworms and
         threadworms.

Artemisia dracunculus
Canon: Tarragon (Urdu: Tarkhoon)
Parts used: Root.
Temperament: Hot and Dry in the Third Degree.

Artemisia vulgaris
Canon: Wormwood (Urdu: Afsnteen)
Parts used: Plant.
Temperament: Hot in the First and Dry in the Second Degree.
Comments: Mugwort.

Calendula officinalis   Origin: eastern Mediterranean
1907:   Calendula
Uses: Believed once to aid in the absorption of blood effusions.
         Lotion for sprains and bruises.

Carthamus tinctorius
Canon: Safflower (Urdu: Kasumbah)
Parts used: Seeds.
Temperament: Hot and Dry in the Second Degree.

Cichorium intybus
Canon: Chicory (Urdu: Kasni)
Parts used: Plant.
Temperament: Cool and Dry in the First Degree.

Chrysanthemum cinerariaefolium   Origin: Balkans
1979:   Pyrethrum Flower, Insect Flowers, Dalmatian Insect Flowers
Uses: Contact insecticide.
1907:   Pyrethri Flores, Insect Flowers
Uses: Contact insecticide.
Canon: Pyrethrum (Urdu: Aquarqara)
Parts used: Root.
Temperament: Hot and Dry in the Third Degree.

Chrysanthemum parthenium   Origin: Europe
1907:   Feverfew
Uses: Anti-inflammatory fomentation, aperient, tonic. The oil is an
        aromatic carminative.

Dahlia variabilis   Origin: Central America
1988:   Inulin
Uses: The ground tuber is used for measurement of glomerular
        filtration rate.

Erigeron canadensis   Origin: North America
1907:   Oleum Erigerontis, Oil of Canadian Fleabane
Uses: Antiseptic, germicidal in high concentration. External irritant
        and rubefacient. Inhaled, arrests profuse secretion and relieves
        bronchioles; salivatory, expectorant, diuretic and urinary
        stimulant. Less irritating than oil of turpentine.

Grindelia camporum   Origin: North America
1907:   Grindelia
Uses: Action resembles atropine, probably dependent on depression
        of vagal endings. Used in spasmodic asthma, whooping
        cough, bronchitis and hay fever. Also recommended for
        cystitis.

Helianthus tuberosus   Origin: North America
1988:   Inulin

Uses: The ground tuber is used for measurement of glomerular filtration rate.

Helianthus annuus
1988:   Sunflower Oil
Uses: Standard reagent.

Inula helenium   Origin: Europe
1907:   Inula, Elecampane
Uses: Decoction has been recommended in chronic bronchitis and tuberculosis. Helenin, its bitter active principle, is a powerful antiseptic.
Canon: Roman Ginger (Urdu: Zanjbil-e-roomi)
Parts used: Root.
Temperament: Hot and Dry in the Second Degree.

Lactuca virosa   Origin: Europe
1907:   Lactuca, Lettuce
Uses: Mild sedative and hypnotic, used chiefly in irritable cough.
Canon: Lettuce (Urdu: Kahu)
Parts used: Roots.
Temperament: Cool in the Second Degree and Moist.
Comments: Given as *Lactuca scariola*.

Matricaria chamomilla   Origin: Europe
1907:   German Chamomile
Uses: Anti-inflammatory fomentation, aperient, tonic. Oil is an aromatic carminative.

Taraxacum officinale   Origin: Europe
1907:   Taraxaci Radix, Dandelion Root
Uses: Bitter in atonic dyspepsia and as a mild laxative.

Tussilago farfara   Origin: Europe
1907:   Tussilaginis Flores, Foliae; Coltsfoot, Farfara
Uses: Demulcent to relieve chronic and irritable cough.

SUB-CLASS MONOCOTYLEDONAE

Superorder Alismatidae

ORDER ALISMATALES

Flowering Rush family – Butomaceae

Found in Europe and temperate Asia, 1 genus with a single perennial herbaceous aquatic species. The rhizome is eaten in Russia.

Water Poppy family – Limnocharitaceae

Present in aquatic habitats throughout the tropics and subtropics, 3 genera with some 12 species.
Limnocharis flava leaves are eaten as 'spinach' or 'endive' in India.

Water Plantain family – Alismataceae

11 genera with some 100 species of aquatic and amphibious plants, found worldwide except for the Far North and the southern tip of South America. Provides edible roots and corms; some species are cultivated in China and Japan.

ORDER HYDROCHARITALES

Canadian Pondweed family – Hydrocharitaceae

Cosmopolitan except for the Far North and the southern tip of South America; 15 genera with some 106 species of marine and freshwater aquatics.

ORDER NAJADALES

Water Hawthorn family – Aponogetonaceae

A single genus with some 45 species from the tropics and the warmer regions of the Old World; freshwater aquatics providing edible tubers.

Arrowgrass family – Scheuchzeriaceae

A single genus with 2 species, found from a circumboreal fringe into the cold temperate regions and the Alps.

Triglochin family – Juncaginaceae

From temperate and cold regions, in marshy habitats in both northern and southern hemispheres, annual and perennial herbs. The leaves of the Sea Arrowgrass are edible and the roots of *Triglochin procerum* are eaten in Australia.

Lilaea family – Lilaeaceae

A single genus with 1 species, a herb of aquatic and marshy places along most of the Pacific seabord of the New World.

Najas family – Najadaceae

Appears worldwide in temperate and warm regions of the world, spanning the tropics; 1 genus with 50 species of small submerged aquatics. They provide a good green fertilizer.

Pondweed family – Potamogetonaceae

Freshwater aquatic herbs, 2 genera with some 100 species found throughout the world except for the furthest North. Provides edible turions (overwintering buds).

Horned Pondweed family – Zannichelliaceae

Submerged, freshwater and brackish aquatics, 4 genera with some 7 species found worldwide in the correct habitat except in the Far North.

Ditch Grass family – Ruppiaceae

Monogeneric family with 7 species found in brackish coastal waters worldwide, with some freshwater members in South America.

Eel Grass family – Zosteraceae

Marine grass-like herbs, 3 genera with 18 species found mainly in temperate seas but also in the tropics; worldwide except for South America. The seeds provide an edible flour.

Posidonia family – Posidoniaceae

Single genus with 3 species of marine herbs found around the Mediterranean Sea and along the southern Australian coasts. Provides Posidonia fibre (Cellonia) in Australia, and is used for insulating panels in the Mediterranean.

Cymodocea family – Cymodoceaceae

The tropical and subtropical 'sea grasses', marine herbs whose 5 genera with 16 species are found worldwide in those climates, with a few outliers in the temperate zone.

ORDER TRIURIDALES

Triuris family – Triuridaceae

Tropical herbs; 7 genera with 80 species growing on dead and decaying wood throughout tropical America, Africa and Asia.

Superorder Commelinidae

ORDER COMMELINALES

Yellow-eyed Grass family – Xiridaceae

Herbaceous marsh herbs, 2 genera with some 240 species, pantropical and subtropical.
Xiris ambigua and *Xiris caroliniana* leaves and roots are used against skin diseases and colds.

Rapatea family – Rapateaceae

Perennial herbs native to tropical eastern South America with an outlier in Liberia; 16 genera with some 80 species.

Mayaca family – Mayacaceae

Aquatic, amphibious mat-growing herbs; 1 genus with some 10 species found from the south-western USA to Paraguay, with an outlier in Angola.

Spiderwort family – Commelinaceae

Cosmopolitan in tropical, subtropical and warm temperate zones; 38 genera with some 600 species, providing edible leaves and roots.
Aneilema beninense is a laxative, and *Floscopa scandens* gives a leaf sap used to treat eye irritations.

ORDER ERIOCAULALES

Pipewort family – Eriocaulaceae

Perennial herbs with a few annuals, centred in the New World, though pantropical and subtropical with temperate outliers; 13 genera with some 1200 species.

ORDER RESTIONALES

Flagellaria family – Flagellariaceae

Found throughout the Old World tropics and subtropics; one to 3 genera with 3–7 species of herbs, often climbers. Some of the stems are used for basket-making.

Centrolepis family – Centrolepidaceae

Spread through New Zealand to Southeast Asia and the tip of South America, 5 genera with some 30 species; small, even moss-like annual or perennial herbs.

Thatching Weeds family – Restionaceae

Disjunct through the southern hemisphere: New Zealand, Australia, Madagascar, southern Africa, Chile, and one species in northern Vietnam; some 30 genera with 320 species which provide stems for thatching and matting.

ORDER POALES

Grass family – Gramineae

Truly cosmopolitan, of some 650 genera with 9000 species, the world's most dominant plant family and of extreme economic importance. The family provides the all-important cereals, Rice, Corn, Wheat, Barley, Rye, Oats, Millet, Pearl Millet, Sorghum, Finger Millet, Fundi, Tef, as well as Sugar Cane and others.

Agropyron repens
1907:   Couch Grass
Uses: Demulcent diuretic, treatment of catarrhal diseases of the genito-urinary tract.

Andropogon schoenanthus   Origin: India
1907:   Oleum Graminis Citrati, Oil of Lemon Grass
Uses: Formerly used internally as a carminative; mainly used in
        perfumery and as a source for citral.
Canon: Bogrush, Lemon Grass (Urdu: Azkhar)
Parts used: Root.
Temperament: Hot and Dry in the Second Degree.

Cymbopogon nardus   Origin: Sri Lanka
1979:   Citronella Oil
Uses: Main source of Citronella Oil.

Hordeum spp.   Origin: Europe
1979:   Malt Extract
Uses: Vehicle for Cod Liver Oil, flavouring agent.
1907:   Hordeum Decorticatum, Pearl Barley
Uses: Decoction (barley water) is demulcent and is used for diluting
        cow's milk for young infants (flocculates the casein).
Canon: Barley (Urdu: Jao)
Parts used: Seeds.
Temperament: Cool and Dry in the Second Degree.

Lolium spp.
Canon:Darnel (Urdu: Sheelam)
Parts used: Seeds.
Temperament: Hot in the First and Dry in the Third Degree.

Oryza sativa   Origin: Asia
1988:   Rice Starch
1907:   Amylum, Rice Starch
Uses: Dusting powder, mucilage.

Panicum miliaceum
Canon: Millet (Urdu: Bajra)
Parts used: Seeds.
Temperament: Cool and Dry in the Third Degree.

Saccharum officinarum   Origin: Asia
1979:   Sugar, Sucrose
Uses: Source of sucrose; sweetening agent, demulcent, syrup base.

Triticum aestivum   Origin: western Asia
1988:   Wheat Starch
1907:   Amylum, Wheat Starch
Uses: Dusting powder, mucilage.

Triticum sativum   Origin: western Asia
1907:   Farina Tritici, Wheaten Flour
Uses: Dusting powder, not as good as Wheat Starch.

Zea mays   Origin: America
1988:   Maize Starch
Uses: Lubricant for surgeon's gloves
1979:   Maize Starch
Uses: Tablet binding agent, lubricant for surgeon's gloves.
1907:   Amylum, Maize Starch; Maidis Stigmata, Maize Stigmas
Uses: Dusting powder, mucilage. Maize stigmas are diuretic and slightly anodyne. Used to alleviate urinary tract disorders.
Canon: Maize (Urdu: Jawar)
Parts used: Seeds.
Temperament: Cool.
Comments: Given as *Triticum romanum*.

ORDER JUNCALES

Rush family – Juncaceae

Found in damp habitats, mainly in cold temperate and mountainous regions worldwide; 9 genera with some 400 species. Provides material for rushwork matting.

Thurnia family – Thurniaceae

Endemic to Guyana and the adjacent parts of the Amazon, 1 genus with 3 species of perennial sedge-like herbs.

ORDER CYPERALES

Sedge family – Cyperaceae

Worldwide except for the furthest North, especially in damp temperate and subarctic climes; some 90 genera with 4000 species. They provide the papyrus on which early prescriptions were written, and the storage organs are eaten as Tiger nuts and Chinese Water Chestnut.

Scirpus grossus and *Scirpus articulatus* roots are used as a purgative and against diarrhoea in India, *Mariscus sieberianus* rhizomes are used as a vermifuge in Sumatra.

ORDER TYPHALES

Cattail family – Typhaceae

1 genus with some 15 species of emergent perennial aquatic herbs, found worldwide in open aquatic habitats except in tropical America, Asia and Australasia.

Bur-reed family – Sparganiaceae

A single genus with some 15 species of perennial aquatic amphibious plants, mainly north temperate and arctic, also found in Southeast Asia, south-east Australia and New Zealand.

ORDER BROMELIALES

Pineapple family – Bromeliaceae

A distinctive tropical to warm temperate family of some 50 genera with 2000 species, endemic to the New World with an outlier in West Africa; many are epiphytes.
Ananas comosus provides, apart from the edible fruit, pineapple stems and fronds which are a source of the proteolytic enzyme bromelain.

ORDER ZINGIBERALES

Banana family – Musaceae

2 genera with some 40 species of evergreen perennial herbs of lowland wet tropical forests from Africa through to the Pacific and northern Australia. Provides Bananas and Plantains.

Bird of Paradise plant family – Strelitziaceae

4 genera with some 55 species of banana-like herbs and trees, disjunct from tropical America to South Africa and Madagascar.

Ginger family – Zingiberaceae

Perennial, aromatic forest plants, 49 genera with some 1300 species, circumtropical but centred in Indomalaysia. Provides Ginger, Cardamom, Turmeric and Arrowroot.

Aframomum melegueta   Origin: West Africa
1907:   Paradisi Grana, Grains of Paradise, Guinea Grains, *Amomum melegueta*.
Uses: Used in veterinary practice as a substitute for cardamoms.

Alpinia officinarum   Origin: southern China
1907:   Galangae Rhizoma, Galangal Root, Lesser Galangal
Uses: Aromatic and carminative, used for flatulence and dyspepsia.
Canon: Galingale (Urdu: Nagar motha)
Parts used: Root.
Temperament: Hot and Dry in the Third Degree.
Comments: Given as *Cyperus rotundus*.

Costus spp.
Canon: Costus Root (sweet) (Urdu: Qust)
Parts used: Root.
Temperament: Hot in the Third and Dry in the Second Degree.
Comments: Given as *Aucklandia costos*.

Curcuma longa   Origin: India
1907:   Curcuma, Turmeric
Uses: Aromatic, colouring agent.

Elettaria cardamomum var. *minuscola*   Origin: southern India
1988:   Cardamom
Uses: Carminative, flavouring.
1979:   Cardamom
Uses: Carminative, flavouring agent.
1907:   Cardamomi Semina, Cardamom
Uses: Carminative, flavouring agent.
Canon: Cardamom (Urdu: Bari Ilachi)
Parts used: Seeds.
Temperament: Hot and Dry in the Third Degree.

Zingiber officinale   Origin: Asia
1988:   Ginger
Uses: Flavouring.
1979:   Ginger

Uses: Carminative and flavouring agent.
1907:   Zingiber, Ginger
Uses: Carminative and aromatic stimulant to the gastro-intestinal tract.
Canon: Ginger (Urdu: Adrak)
Parts used: Root.
Temperament: Hot in the Third and Dry in the Second Degree.

Queensland Arrowroot family – Cannaceae

From tropical America and the West Indies; a single genus with 30 to 35 species of large herbs with very showy flowers. Provides Queensland Arrowroot, an easily digestible starch finding wide dietary use.

Arrowroot family – Marantaceae

Pantropical and subtropical, centred in America; 30 genera with some 350 species of herbaceous perennials. Provides Maranta starch and sweet corn root in the West Indies, while in Mexico some flowers are cooked and eaten. Maranta starch is now being cultivated for invalid dietary use.

Maranta arundinacea   Origin: Central America
1979:   Arrowroot, Maranta
Uses: Starchy medium, treatment of diarrhoea (gruel).
1907:   Amylum, Arrowroot Starch
Uses: Mucilage.

Superorder Arecidae

ORDER ARECALES

Palm family – Palmae

Pantropical, subtropical and with a few warm temperate members; some 212 genera with 2780 species, usually found in moist areas. Palms are palms, not trees, and they provide Coconut, Dates, Sago and Palm oil.

Areca catechu   Origin: India, eastern Asia
1907:   Areca Nuts, Betel Nut
Uses: Veterinary vermifuge for tapeworm. Astringent, used in toothpaste.

Calamus draco   Origin: Sumatra
1907:   Sanguis Draconis
Uses: Sometimes used for colouring plasters, but it is much more
          widely used for colouring lacquers and varnishes.

Cocos nucifera   Origin: Indian Ocean
1988:   Coconut Oil
1979:   Coconut Oil
Uses: Ointment basis, vehicle.
1907:   Oleum Cocos, Coconut Oil, Coprah Oil
Uses: Massage lubricant, ointment. Given as substitute for cod liver
          oil.

Copernicia cerifera
1988:   Carnauba Wax

Elaeis guineensis   Origin: Africa
1988:   Fractionated Palm Kernel Oil
Uses: Suppository basis.
1979:   Fractionated Palm Kernel Oil
Uses: Suppository basis.

ORDER CYCLANTHALES

Panama Hat Plant family – Cyclanthaceae

11 genera with 180 species confined to tropical America and the West
Indies, mainly perennial herbs and stemless climbers. Provide at least a
million Panama hats a year, ideal protection against holes in the ozone
layer.

ORDER PANDANALES

Screw Pine family – Pandanaceae

Originating in the Old World tropics and subtropics; 3 genera with
some 700 species of trees, shrubs and climbers. The family provides
edible starchy fruits highly regarded in Micronesia.
Pandanus odoratissimus flowers produce Kewda Attar, and the leaves
of *Pandanus odorosus*, which never flowers, are used in potpourris.
Pandanus leram is the edible Nicobar Breadfruit.

ORDER ARALES

Duckweed family – Lemnaceae

Cosmopolitan in freshwater habitats except for the Far North and much of north Asia; 6 genera with some 43 species of flowering or submerged aquatic herbs.

Aroid family – Araceae

Cosmopolitan except for the Far North; some 110 genera with 2000 species, mainly herbaceous plants of great variety. They provide edible Yams, Taro, Cocoyam, Eddo, Dasheen, Tanier etc.; these are mainly swollen tuberous corms. The leaves of some species are also eaten. The starch grains of *Colocasia esculenta* are small and readily digested, and used for invalid food.

Acorus calamus   Origin: eastern Europe
1907:   Calamus, Sweet Flag
Uses: Aromatic bitter, digestive, carminative.

Superorder Liliidae

ORDER LILIALES

Water Hyacinth family – Pontederiaceae

9 genera with 34 species of pantropical freshwater aquatics. They provide a green vegetable in China.

Philydra family – Philydraceae

Perennial herbs from Southeast Asia, New Guinea and Australia.

Iris family – Iridaceae

Found worldwide except for the Far North and much of North Asia, some 70 genera with 1800 species of perennial herbs, Saffron amongst them.

Crocus sativus   Origin: Europe
1907:   Crocus, Saffron
Uses: Colourant, flavouring.
Canon: Saffron (Urdu: Zaffran)

Parts used: Flowers.
Temperament: Hot in the Second and Dry in the First Degree.

Iris ensata
Canon: Iris (Urdu: Eersa)
Parts used: Root.
Temperament: Hot and Dry in the Second Degree.

Iris germanica   Origin: Europe
1907:   Iridis Rhizoma, Orris
Uses: Mild cathartic and diuretic. Perfumery component.
Canon: Orris, Lily (Urdu: Sosan)
Parts used: Root.
Temperament: Hot and Dry in the Second Degree.

Iris versicolor   Origin: North America
1907:   Iris, Blue Flag
Uses: Cathartic and diuretic, common ingredient of antisyphilitic
         nostrums.

Drimia indica   Origin: India
1988:   Indian Squill
Uses: Expectorant.
1979:   Indian Squill, Urginea
Uses: Cardiac stimulant, action on heart similar to digitalis (increases
         excitability and causes a more forceful contraction). In small
         doses, expectorant; in large doses, emetic.

Drimia maritima   Origin: Mediterranean
1988:   Squill
Uses: Expectorant.
1979:   Squill, Scilla
Uses: Cardiac stimulant, action on heart similar to digitalis (increases
         excitability and causes a more forceful contraction). In small
         doses, expectorant; in large doses, emetic.
1907:   Scilla, Squill (*Urginea scilla*)
Uses: Heart stimulant and vasoconstrictor similar to digitalis, but
         stronger; expectorant.

Schoenocaulon officinale   Origin: Central America
1907:   Cevadilla, Sabadilla

378

Uses: Parasiticide; source for the alkaloid mixture veratrine. Similar properties to atropine, used as external analgesic.

Veratrum album   Origin: Europe
1907:   Veratri Albi Rhizoma, White Hellebore
Uses: Formerly used internally in dropsy and other disorders, and externally as a parasiticide in scabies etc. Also used as insecticide for furs and woollens.
Canon: Hellebore (Urdu: Kutki)
Parts used: Wood.
Temperament: Hot and Dry in the Third Degree.

Lily family – Liliaceae

One of the largest families, cosmopolitan except for the Far North and much of North Asia; some 70 genera with 1800 species of perennial herbs. Provides Onions, Garlic, Chives and Asparagus.

Allium cepa
Canon: Onion (Urdu: Pyaz)
Parts used: Bulb.
Temperament: Hot in the Second and Dry in the Third Degree.

Allium porrum
Canon: Leek (Urdu: Gandana)
Parts used: Seeds.
Temperament: Hot in the Third and Dry in the Second Degree.

Allium sativum
Canon: Garlic (Urdu: Lashan)
Parts used: Tuber (bulb).
Temperament: Hot and Dry in the Second Degree.

Aloe barbadensis   Origin: Caribbean
1988:   Aloes, Barbados Aloes, Curacao Aloes
Uses: Laxative.
1979:   Aloes, Barbados Aloes
Uses: Purgative. Colours urine red.
1907:   Aloes
Uses: Purgative, emmenagogue.

Aloe ferox   Origin: South Africa
1988:   Aloes, Cape Aloes
Uses: Laxative.
1979:   Aloes, Cape Aloes
Uses: Purgative. Colours urine red.
Canon: Aloes (Urdu: Elwa)
Parts used: Juice.
Temperament: Hot and Dry.
Comments: Refers to *Aloe vera*.

Colchicum autumnale   Origin: Europe
1988:   Colchicine
Uses: Used in the treatment of gout.
1979:   Colchicum Corm, Meadow Saffron
Uses: Relieves pain and inflammation of gout – used with care.
1907:   Colchici Flores, Colchici Semina
Uses: Slow poison, excites kariokinesis. Specific for treatment of gout.

Convallaria majalis   Origin: Europe
1907:   Convallaria Flores, Lily-of-the-valley
Uses: Digitalis-like action. Cardiac tonic and diuretic.

Daffodil family – Amaryllidaceae

Large warm temperate, subtropical and tropical family with occasional temperate outliers, some 75 genera with about 1100 species of herbs, found throughout the world.

Sisal Hemp family – Agavaceae

Pantropical and subtropical, found mainly in arid regions; 20 genera with some 700 species of woody plants, some climbing. Provides the national drink of Mexico, pulque, which is then distilled into mescal; the family is also important as a source of fibres.

Grass Tree family – Xanthorrhoeaceae

8 genera with some 66 species of woody perennials found in Australia, New Caledonia and New Zealand. Many produce gums.

Vellozia family – Velloziaceae

4 genera with some 300 species of tropical and subtropical fibrous shrubs, found in arid regions in South America, Central Africa and Madagascar.

Kangaroo Paw family – Haemodoraceae

Tropical to warm temperate herbs found in Australia (not in New Zealand), Central Africa, Madagascar, and eastern Central and South America; 17 genera with some 100 species.

Aletris farinosa   Origin: North America
1907:   Starwort, Aletris, Colic Root
Uses: Uterine tonic; also recommended as of service in chronic rheumatism and in dropsical conditions.

Hawaiian Arrowroot family – Taccaceae

2 genera with 31 species of pantropical, perennial herbs, some in subtropical China. The family produces Hawaiian and East Indian arrowroot.
Tacca fatsifolia and *Tacca palmata* leaves have a stomachic, urinary and dermal use.

Stemona family – Stemonaceae

Perennial erect or climbing herbs found in eastern Asia, Indomalaysia, northern Australia, disjunct in eastern North America.
Stemona tuberosa has insecticidal roots.

Tecophilaea family – Cyanastraceae

6 genera with some 22 species of perennial herbs, disjunct in Chile, South Africa, Central Africa and California.

Smilax family – Smilacaceae

Pantropical and subtropical family with a few temperate members; 4 genera with some 375 species, most of which are climbing herbs.
Smilax spp. are the source of sarsaparilla, which is used as a tonic and for treating rheumatism; *Smilax china* (China Root) dried rhizomes

are used as a stimulant, and *Rhipogonum scandens* is used as a sarsaparilla substitute in New Zealand.

Smilax ornata   Origin: Central America
1907:   Sarsae Radix, Sarsaparilla
Uses: Used as a vehicle for mercurials in syphilis treatment.

Yam family – Dioscoreaceae

Pantropical family, some members subtropical; 6 genera with some 630 species, mainly shrubby climbers with a few dwarf shrubs. They provide the edible Yams, of which some 60 species are cultivated across the world.
Dioscorea spp. yield a steroidal saponin, diosgenin, which is the starting chemical for the production of oral contraceptives.

ORDER ORCHIDALES

Burmannia family – Burmanniaceae

5 or 6 genera with some 125 species of pantropical and subtropical forest herbs, many of which are colourless saprophytes.

Orchid family – Orchidaceae

Cosmopolitan except for the Far North, some 750 genera with 18,000 species of perennial herbs.

Vanilla planifolia   Origin: Mexico
1988:   Vanillin
Uses: Flavouring.
1979:   Vanillin
Uses: Flavouring and perfuming agent.
1907:   Vanilla
Uses: Flavouring and perfuming agent.

TABLE 2
SUMMARY OF THE SIMPLES
MENTIONED IN VARIOUS SOURCES
OF MATERIA MEDICA

The relative frequencies of medicinal plants occurring in families has been noted. In the Division Anthophyta, all Families have been listed; in the other groups only those Orders and Families in which cited genera appear. The sources are the 1988 edition of the *British Pharmacopoeia* (BP88),[1] the 1979 (BPC79) and 1907 (BPC07) editions of the *(British) Pharmaceutical Codex*,[2] and a 1966 edition of the first Book of Avicenna's *Canon* as used in Unani Medicine (CAN).[3] In addition, the last two columns show the number of species within the family which are mentioned in two major catalogues of materia medica referring to the two other principal medical systems, Chinese Traditional Medicine as represented by the medical flora of Hong Kong (HK),[4] and Ayurveda, based on the medicinal flora of Sri Lanka.[5]

Notes

1 The British Pharmacopoeia Commission, *The British Pharmacopoeia* (London: HMSO, 1988).
2 The Pharmaceutical Society, *The Pharmaceutical Codex*, 11th edn (London: The Pharmaceutical Society, 1979, repr. 1988); and The Pharmaceutical Society, *The British Pharmaceutical Codex* (London: The Pharmaceutical Society, 1907).

3 Mazar H. Shah (ed.), Avicenna, *The General Principles of Avicenna's Canon of Medicine* (Karachi: Naveed Clinic, 1966).

4 Cheung Siu-Cheong and Li Ning-hon (eds), *Chinese Medical Herbs of Hong Kong*, vols 1–5 (Hong Kong, 1978).

5 D. M. A. Jayaweera, *Medicinal Plants (Indigenous and Exotic) Used in Ceylon*, 5 vols (Colombo: The National Science Council of Sri Lanka, 1981).

	BP88	BPC79	BPC07	CAN	HK	SK
	1	2	3	4	5	6

KINGDOM: PROTISTA

PHYLUM PHAEOPHYTA

	BP88	BPC79	BPC07	CAN	HK	SK
Fucaceae			1 (0.3%)			

PHYLUM RHODOPHYTA

	BP88	BPC79	BPC07	CAN	HK	SK
Gelidiaceae	1 (1.3%)		1 (0.3%)			
Gigartinaceae			1 (0.3%)			

KINGDOM: FUNGI

DIVISION EUMYCOPHYTA

Class Ascomycetes

SUB-CLASS EUASCOMYCETIDEAE

Series Hymenoascomycetes

SUB-SERIES PYRENOMYCETES

ORDER CLAVICIPITALES

	BP88	BPC79	BPC07	CAN	HK	SK
Clavicipetaceae			1 (0.3%)			

	BP88 1	BPC79 2	BPC07 3	CAN 4	HK 5	SK 6
Class Basidiomycetes						
SUB-CLASS HETEROBASIDIOMYCETIDEAE						
ORDER TREMELLALES						
Tremellaceae					1(0.2%)	1(0.2%)
Auriculariaceae					1(0.2%)	1(0.2%)
SUB-CLASS HOMOBASIDIOMYCETIDEAE						
Series Hymenomycetes						
ORDER APHYLLOPHORALES (POLYPORALES)						
Poliporaceae					1(0.2%)	1(0.2%)
ORDER AGARICALES						
Agaricaceae				1(0.7%)		
DIVISION LICHENES			2(0.7%)			

KINGDOM: PLANTAE			
DIVISION LYCOPHYTA			
ORDER LYCOPODIALES			
Lycopodiaceae	1 (0.3%)	2 (0.4%)	3 (0.5%)
ORDER SELAGINELLALES			
Selaginellaceae		3 (0.6%)	1 (0.2%)
DIVISION SPHENOPHYTA			
ORDER EQUISETALES			
Equisetaceae		1 (0.2%)	
DIVISION PTEROPHYTA			
CLASS EUSPORANGIATE			
ORDER OPHIOGLOSSALES		1 (0.2%)	
Ophioglossaceae			2 (0.3%)
Class Osmundideae			
ORDER OSMUNDALES			
Osmondaceae		1 (0.2%)	

	BP88 1	BPC79 2	BPC07 3	CAN 4	HK 5	SK 6
Class Leptosporangiata						
ORDER FILICALES						
Gleichenaceae		1(1.1%)			1(0.2%)	
Dennstaedtiaceae			1(0.3%)		6(1.2%)	
Adiantaceae				1(0.7%)	1(0.2%)	2(0.3%)
Polypodiaceae				1(0.7%)	7(1.4%)	1(0.2%)
DIVISION CONIFEROPHYTA						
ORDER CONIFERALES						
Pinaceae	1(1.3%)		6(2.0%)	1(0.7%)	1(0.2%)	2(0.3%)
Cupressaceae			5(1.7%)	2(1.3%)	1(0.2%)	
DIVISION CYCADOPHYTA						
ORDER CYCADALES						
Cicadaceae					1(0.2%)	1(0.2%)
DIVISION GNETOPHYTA						
ORDER GNETALES						
Gnetaceae					1(0.2%)	

DIVISION ANTHOPHYTA

Class Angiospermae

SUB-CLASS DICOTYLEDONEAE

Superorder Magnoliidae

ORDER MAGNOLIALES

Magnoliaceae				3(0.6%)	2(0.3%)
Winteraceae					
Himantandraceae					
Canellaceae		1(1.1%)			
Annonaceae					
Myristicaceae	1(1.3%)	1(1.1%)	1(0.3%)		
Degeneriaceae				2(0.4%)	1(0.2%) 4(0.6%)

ORDER ILLICIALES

Illiciaceae	1(1.3%)	1(1.1%)	1(0.3%)
Schisandraceae			1(0.3%)

ORDER LAURALES

Austrobaileyaceae	
Eupomatiaceae	
Gormotegaceae	
Monimiaceae	1(0.3%)
Calycanthaceae	

	BP88 1	BPC79 2	BPC07 3	CAN 4	HK 5	SK 6
Chloranthaceae						
Lauraceae	2(2.7%)	1(1.1%)	8(2.7%)	3(1.9%)	2(0.4%)	5(0.8%)
Hernandiaceae					6(1.2%)	
ORDER PIPERALES						
Piperaceae			4(1.3%)	1(0.7%)	2(0.4%)	5(0.8%)
Saururaceae					2(0.4%)	
Peperomiaceae						
ORDER ARISTOLOCHIALES						
Aristolochiaceae			2(0.7%)		1(0.2%)	2(0.3%)
Nepenthaceae					1(0.2%)	
ORDER NYMPHAEALES						
Ceratophyllaceae						
Nymphaeaceae					1(0.2%)	3(0.5%)
ORDER RANUNCULALES						
Berberidaceae	2(2.7%)	2(2.2%)	5(1.7%)	1(0.7%)	2(0.4%)	1(0.2%)

Ranunculaceae			7(2.3%)	2(1.3%)	2(0.4%)	
Lardizabalaceae					1(0.2%)	
Menispermaceae			6(2.0%)		4(0.8%)	5(0.8%)

ORDER PAPAVERALES

Papaveraceae	1(1.3%)	1(1.1%)	3(1.0%)	1(0.7%)		3(0.5%)
Fumariaceae				1(0.7%)		
Sarraceniaceae						

SUPERORDER HAMAMELIDAE

ORDER TROCHODENDRALES

Trochodendraceae

ORDER HAMAMELIDALES

Cercidiphyllaceae			
Platanaceae			
Hamamelidaceae	1(1.1%)	2(0.7%)	2(0.4%)

ORDER EUCOMMIALES

Eucommiaceae
Leitneriaceae

	BP88	BPC79	BPC07	CAN	HK	SK
	1	2	3	4	5	6
ORDER MYRICALES						
Myricaceae					1(0.2%)	
ORDER FAGALES						
Betulaceae			2(0.7%)	1(0.7%)		1(0.2%)
Fagaceae			1(0.3%)	2(1.3%)		1(0.2%)
Balanopsceae						
ORDER CASUARINALES						
Casuarinaceae						
Superorder Caryophyllidae						
ORDER CARYOPHYLLALES						
Cactaceae					3(0.6%)	1(0.2%)
Aizoaceae						6(0.9%)
Caryophyllaceae					2(0.4%)	
Nyctaginaceae					1(0.2%)	3(0.5%)
Amaranthaceae				1(0.7%)	6(1.2%)	8(1.3%)
Phytolaccaceae			1(0.3%)		1(0.2%)	
Chenopodiaceae		1(1.1%)	1(0.3%)	2(1.3%)	1(0.2%)	

Didiereaceae						
Portulacaceae				1(0.7%)	3(0.6%)	2(0.3%)
Basellaceae						1(0.2%)
ORDER BATALES						
Batidaceae						
ORDER POLYGONALES						
Polygonaceae	1(1.3%)	1(1.1%)	1(0.3%)	2(1.3%)	6(1.2%)	3(0.5%)
ORDER PLUMBAGINALES						
Plumbaginaceae					2(0.4%)	2(0.3%)
Superorder Dilleniidae						
ORDER DILLENIALES						
Dilleniaceae					1(0.2%)	2(0.3%)
Paeoniaceae						
Crossosomataceae				1(0.7%)		
ORDER THEALES						
Theaceae		1(1.1%)	2(0.7%)		3(0.6%)	2(0.3%)
Ochnaceae						2(0.3%)

	BP88 1	BPC79 2	BPC07 3	CAN 4	HK 5	SK 6
Dipterocarpaceae			2(0.7%)		4(0.8%)	3(0.5%)
Guttiferae			2(0.7%)	1(0.7%)		7(1.1%)
Elatinaceae						
Quiinaceae						
Marcgraviaceae						

ORDER MALVALES

	BP88 1	BPC79 2	BPC07 3	CAN 4	HK 5	SK 6
Scytopetalaceae						
Elaeocarpaceae						
Tiliaceae	1(1.3%)			1(0.7%)	3(0.6%)	4(0.6%)
Sterculiaceae		2(2.2%)	3(1.0%)		3(0.6%)	5(0.8%)
Bombacaceae					1(0.2%)	3(0.5%)
Malvaceae	1(1.3%)		2(0.7%)	1(0.7%)	8(1.6%)	
Sphaerosepalaceae						
Sarcolaenaceae						

ORDER URTICALES

	BP88 1	BPC79 2	BPC07 3	CAN 4	HK 5	SK 6
Ulmaceae			2(0.7%)			3(0.5%)
Moraceae		1(1.1%)	3(3.2%)	3(1.9%)	9(1.8%)	8(1.3%)
Urticaceae					3(0.6%)	1(0.2%)

ORDER LECYTHIDALES

Lecythidaceae				4(0.6%)

ORDER VIOLALES

Violaceae	1(0.3%)	1(0.7%)		
Flacourtiaceae	1(0.3%)		2(0.4%)	6(0.9%)
Lacistemataceae				
Passifloraceae				
Turneraceae	1(0.3%)	2(0.4%)		
Malesherbiaceae				
Fouquieriaceae				
Caricaceae	1(0.3%)			1(0.2%)
Bixaceae				
Cochlospermaceae				
Cistaceae				
Tamaricaceae		2(1.3%)	1(0.2%)	
Ancistrocladaceae				
Frankeniaceae				
Achariaceae				
Begoniaceae			2(0.4%)	
Loasaceae				
Datiscaceae				
Cucurbitaceae	4(1.3%)	4(2.6%)	7(1.4%)	21(3.3%)

395

	BP88 1	BPC79 2	BPC07 3	CAN 4	HK 5	SK 6
ORDER SALICALES						
Salicaceae			2(0.7%)	1(0.7%)		
ORDER CAPPARIDALES						
Capparidaceae				1(0.7%)	1(0.2%)	6(0.9%)
Tovariaceae						
Cruciferae	1(1.3%)		3(1.0%)	7(4.5%)	3(0.6%)	3(0.5%)
Resedaceae						
Moringaceae						1(0.2%)
ORDER ERICALES						
Clethraceae						
Grubbiaceae						
Cyrillaceae						
Ericaceae			2(0.7%)		1(0.2%)	2(0.3%)
Epacridaceae						
Empetraceae						
Pyrolaceae						

	Col 1	Col 2	Col 3	Col 4	Col 5	Col 6
ORDER DIAPENSIALES						
Diapensiaceae						
ORDER EBENALES						
Sapotaceae	2(2.7%)		1(0.3%)			5(0.8%)
Ebenaceae						1(0.2%)
Styracaceae		2(2.2%)				
ORDER PRIMULALES						
Primulaceae				1(0.7%)		1(0.2%)
Myrsinaceae				1(0.7%)	4(0.8%)	1(0.2%)
Superorder Rosidae						
ORDER ROSALES						
Cunoniaceae						
Pittosporaceae					1(0.2%)	
Droseraceae						
Brunelliaceae						
Eucryphiaceae						
Bruniaceae						
Rosaceae	2(2.7%)	4(4.4%)	11(3.7%)	9(5.8%)	9(1.8%)	1(0.2%)
Crassulaceae				1(0.7%)	2(0.4%)	1(0.2%)
Cephalotaceae						

	BP88 1	BPC79 2	BPCo7 3	CAN 4	HK 5	SK 6
Saxifragaceae						
Chrysobalanaceae	1(1.3%)	1(1.1%)			2(0.4%)	
ORDER FABALES						
Leguminosae	7(9.5%)	9(9.9%)	27(9.0%)	14(9.0%)	30(6.0%)	61(9.7%)
ORDER PODOSTEMALES						
Podostemaceae						
ORDER HALORAGALES						
Theligoniaceae						
Haloragaceae						
Hippuridaceae						
ORDER MYRTALES						
Sonneratiaceae						
Trapaceae						
Lythraceae				1(0.7%)	1(0.2%)	3(0.5%)
Rhizophoraceae						

Penaeaceae						3(4.0%)
Thymelaeaceae	3(0.5%)	2(0.4%)	1(0.7%)	1(0.3%)		
Myrtaceae	7(1.1%)	6(1.2%)	2(1.3%)	5(1.7%)	4(4.4%)	
Punicaceae	1(0.2%)		1(0.7%)	1(0.3%)		
Onagraceae	1(0.2%)	1(0.2%)				
Oliniaceae						
Melastomataceae	3(0.5%)	4(0.8%)				
Combretaceae	6(0.9%)	1(0.2%)	1(0.7%)	2(0.7%)		

ORDER CORNALES

Nyssaceae		1(0.2%)				
Garryaceae						
Alangiaceae	1(0.2%)	1(0.2%)				
Cornaceae						

ORDER PROTEALES

Elaeagnaceae		1(0.2%)				
Proteaceae						

ORDER SANTALALES

Santalaceae	1(0.2%)	1(0.2%)	1(0.7%)	1(0.3%)		
Medusandraceae						
Olacaceae	1(0.2%)	2(0.4%)				
Loranthaceae		1(0.2%)		1(0.3%)		

	BP88 1	BPC79 2	BPC07 3	CAN 4	HK 5	SK 6
Misodendraceae						
Cynomoriaceae						
Balanophoraceae						
ORDER RAFFLESIALES						
Rafflesiaceae						
Hydnoraceae						
ORDER CELASTRALES						
Geissolomataceae						
Celastraceae			1(0.3%)			3(0.5%)
Stackhousiaceae						
Salvadoraceae						1(0.2%)
Corynocarpaceae						
Icacinaceae						
Aquifoliaceae			1(0.3%)		4(0.8%)	
Dichapetalaceae						

ORDER EUPHORBIALES

Family						
Buxaceae						
Pandaceae						
Euphorbiaceae	1(1.3%)	1(1.1%)	8(2.7%)	2(1.3%)	24(4.8%)	27(4.3%)

ORDER RHAMNALES

Rhamnaceae	2(2.7%)	1(1.1%)	3(1.0%)	1(0.7%)	3(0.6%)	8(1.3%)
Vitaceae			1(0.3%)	2(1.3%)	2(0.4%)	5(0.8%)
Staphyleaceae						
Melianthaceae						
Connaraceae						
Sapindaceae			1(0.3%)		3(0.6%)	7(1.1%)
Sabiaceae						
Julianaceae						
Hippocastanaceae						
Aceraceae						
Burseraceae			3(1.0%)	3(1.9%)	1(0.2%)	3(0.5%)
Anacardiaceae		1(1.1%)	1(0.3%)	4(2.6%)	2(0.4%)	13(2.1%)
Simaroubaceae		1(1.1%)	2(0.7%)		1(0.2%)	4(0.6%)
Coriariaceae						
Meliaceae	1(1.3%)	1(1.1%)	1(0.3%)	1(0.7%)	1(0.2%)	8(1.3%)
Cneoraceae						
Rutaceae	3(4.0%)	4(4.4%)	9(9.5%)	2(1.3%)	12(2.4%)	19(3.0%)
Zygophyllaceae			1(0.3%)			1(0.2%)

	BP88 1	BPC79 2	BPCo7 3	CAN 4	HK 5	SK 6
ORDER JUGLANDALES						
Juglandaceae				1(0.7%)		
ORDER GERANIALES						
Houmiriaceae						
Linaceae	1(1.3%)	1(1.1%)	1(0.3%)	1(0.7%)	1(0.2%)	
Geraniaceae			1(0.3%)			
Oxalidaceae					2(0.4%)	4(0.6%)
Erythroxylaceae	1(1.3%)	1(1.1%)	1(0.3%)			2(0.3%)
Limnanthaceae						
Balsaminaceae					2(0.4%)	1(0.2%)
Tropaeolaceae						
ORDER POLYGALALES						
Malpighiaceae						
Trigoniaceae						
Tremandraceae						
Vochysiaceae						
Polygalaceae	1(1.3%)	1(1.1%)	1(0.3%)		2(0.4%)	
Krameriaceae	1(1.3%)		1(0.3%)			

ORDER UMBELLALES

Araliaceae	4(5.4%)				4(0.8%)	
Umbelliferae		5(5.5%)	15(5.0%)	13(8.3%)	6(1.2%)	12(1.9%)

Superorder Asteridae

ORDER GENTIANALES

Loganiaceae	1(1.3%)	1(1.1%)	5(1.7%)		2(0.4%)	2(0.3%)
Gentianaceae		1(1.1%)	2(0.7%)		2(0.4%)	3(0.5%)
Apocynaceae		3(3.3%)	4(1.3%)	1(0.7%)	8(1.6%)	13(2.1%)
Asclepiadaceae			4(1.3%)		6(1.2%)	13(2.1%)
Oleaceae	1(1.3%)	1(1.1%)	2(0.7%)			4(0.6%)

ORDER POLEMONIALES

Nolonaceae	4(5.4%)					
Solanaceae		5(5.5%)	9(3.0%)	6(3.8%)	6(1.2%)	11(1.7%)
Convolvulaceae			4(1.3%)	3(1.9%)	6(1.2%)	15(2.4%)
Menyanthaceae						
Lennoaceae						
Polemoniaceae						
Ehretiaceae						
Hydrophyllaceae					1(0.2%)	
Boraginaceae						3(0.5%)

	BP88 1	BPC79 2	BPC07 3	CAN 4	HK 5	SK 6
ORDER LAMIALES						
Verbenaceae					18(3.6%)	16(2.5%)
Labiatae	2(2.7%)	5(5.5%)	11(3.7%)	7(4.5%)	22(4.4%)	16(2.5%)
Tetrachondraceae						
Callitrichaceae						
Phrymaceae						
ORDER PLANTAGINALES						
Plantaginaceae	1(1.3%)	3(3.3%)	1(0.3%)	2(1.3%)	1(0.2%)	1(0.2%)
ORDER SCROPHULARIALES						
Columelliaceae						
Myoporaceae						
Scrophulariaceae	1(1.3%)	2(2.2%)	3(1.0%)		9(1.8%)	7(1.1%)
Globulariaceae						
Gesneriaceae					1(0.2%)	
Orobanchaceae					3(0.6%)	
Bignoniaceae			3(1.0%)		10(2.0%)	2(0.3%)
Acanthaceae						11(1.7%)
Pedaliaceae	1(1.3%)	1(1.1%)	1(0.3%)	1(0.7%)		2(0.3%)

	A	B	C	D	E	F
Hydrostachydaceae						
Martyniaceae						
Lentibulariaceae						

ORDER CAMPANULALES

	A	B	C	D	E	F
Campanulaceae	1(1.3%)				5(1.0%)	
Lobeliaceae		1(1.1%)				
Stylidiaceae						
Brunoniaceae						
Goodeniaceae						1(0.2%)

ORDER RUBIALES

	A	B	C	D	E	F
Rubiaceae			4(1.3%)		19(3.8%)	26(4.1%)

ORDER DIPSACALES

	A	B	C	D	E	F
Adoxales						
Caprifoliaceae			2(0.7%)			
Valerianaceae			2(0.7%)	1(0.7%)	2(0.4%)	
Dipsacaceae						
Calyceraceae	1(1.3%)					2(0.3%)

ORDER ASTERALES

	A	B	C	D	E	F
Compompositae	4(5.4%)	1(1.1%)	15(5.0%)	8(5.1%)	39(7.8%)	19(3.0%)

	BP88	BPC79	BPC07	CAN	HK	SK
	1	2	3	4	5	6
SUBCLASS MONOCOTYLEDONAE						
Superorder Alismatidae						
ORDER ALISMATALES						
Butomaceae						
Limnocharitaceae						
Alismataceae						
ORDER HYDROCHARITALES						
Hydrocharitaceae						
ORDER NAJADALES						
Aponogetonaceae						1 (0.2%)
Scheuchzeriaceae						
Juncaginaceae						
Lilaeaceae						
Najadaceae						
Potamogetonaceae						
Zannichelliaceae						
Ruppiaceae						

Zosteraceae
Posidoniaceae
Cymodoceaceae

ORDER TRIURIDALES

Triuridaceae

Superorder Commelinidae

ORDER COMMELINALES

Xiridaceae		
Rapateaceae		
Mayacaceae	2(0.4%)	
Commelinaceae		1(0.2%)

ORDER ERIOCAULALES

Eriocaulaceae   1(0.2%)

ORDER RESTIONALES

Flagellariaceae
Centrolepidaceae
Restionaceae   2(0.3%)

| | BP88 | BPC79 | BPC07 | CAN | HK | SK |
	1	2	3	4	5	6
ORDER POALES						
Gramineae	3(4.0%)	4(4.4%)	7(2.3%)	5(3.2%)	7(1.4%)	21(3.3%)
ORDER JUNCALES						
Juncaceae						
Thurniaceae						
ORDER CYPERALES						
Cyperaceae					2(0.4%)	1(0.2%)
ORDER TYPHALES						
Typhaceae						
Sparganiaceae						
ORDER BROMELIALES						
Bromeliaceae						1(0.2%)
ORDER ZINGIBERALES						
Musaceae						

Strelitziaceae						
Zingiberaceae	2(2.7%)	2(2.2%)	5(1.7%)	4(2.6%)	8(1.6%)	14(2.2%)
Cannaceae						1(0.2%)
Marantaceae		1(1.1%)	1(0.3%)		1(0.2%)	
Superorder Arecidae						
ORDER ARECALES						
Palmae	3(4.0%)	2(2.1%)	3(1.0%)		1(0.2%)	8(1.3%)
ORDER CYCLANTHALES						
Cyclanthaceae						
ORDER PANDANALES						
Pandanaceae						
ORDER ARALES						
Lemnaceae					1(0.2%)	2(0.3%)
Araceae			1(0.3%)		8(1.6%)	13(2.1%)
Superorder Liliidae						
ORDER LILIALES						
Pontederiaceae						

	BP88 1	BPC79 2	BPC07 3	CAN 4	HK 5	SK 6
Philydraceae						
Iridaceae	2(2.7%)	2(2.2%)	6(2.0%)	4(2.6%)	2(0.4%)	1(0.2%)
Liliaceae	3(4.0%)	3(3.3%)	3(1.0%)	4(2.6%)	15(3.0%)	6(0.9%)
Amaryllidaceae					3(0.6%)	5(0.8%)
Agavaceae						
Xanthorrhoeaceae						
Velloziaceae						
Haemodoraceae			1(0.3%)			
Taccaceae					1(0.2%)	
Stemonaceae					1(0.2%)	
Cyanastraceae						
Smilacaceae						
Dioscoreaceae					2(0.4%)	
ORDER ORCHIDALES						
Burmanniaceae						
Orchidaceae	1(1.3%)	1(1.1%)	1(0.3%)		5(1.0%)	4(0.6%)
Total (100%)	74	91	298	156	500	630
Maximum number of species per family	7	9	27	14	39	61

GLOSSARY
OF PHARMACEUTICAL / APOTHECARY
TERMS

Anthelmintic	Of use against intestinal worms.
Carminative	Having the quality of expelling wind.
Cathartic	Cleansing the bowels, purgative.
Cholagogue	A medicine that carries off bile.
Cicatrizant	Healing by means of producing a cicatrice, or scar-like tissue.
Demulcent	Soothing.
Emmenagogue	An agent which promotes the menstrual discharge.
Febrifuge	A medicine used against fever.
Galactagogue	A medicine inducing a flow of milk.
Hydragogue	A medicine removing water from the body.
Rubefacient	A medicine which produces slight inflammation, a counter-irritant.
Sialagogue	A medicine which produces a flow of saliva.
Sternutatory	Causing or tending to cause sneezing.
Vermifuge	Causing the expulsion of worms and other parasites from the intestines.
Vesicant	Causing blisters on the skin.

BIBLIOGRAPHY

Abithel, John Williams, *The Physicians of Myddvai* (London, 1891)

Appleby, John H., 'Ginseng and the Royal Society', *Notes and Records of the Royal Society of London*, 37, no.2 (1983)

Aristotle, *The Works of Aristotle*, 2 vols (Chicago: Encyclopedia Britannica Inc., 1952 edn)

Avicenna, ed. Mazar H. Shah, *The General Principles of Avicenna's Canon of Medicine* (Karachi: Naveed Clinic, 1966)

Avicenne, trans. Henry Jahier and Abdelkader Noureddine, *Poème de la medicine (Urguza Fi 'T-Tibb – Cantica Avicennae)* (Paris: Les Belles Lettres, 1956)

Bellamy, David J., *Bellamy's New World* (London: British Broadcasting Corporation, 1983)

Boulinois, L., *La Route de la soie* (Paris: Arthaud, 1963)

British Pharmaceutical Codex, The (London: The Pharmaceutical Society, 1907)

Budge, Sir E. A. Wallis, *The Divine Origin of the Craft of the Herbalist* (London: Culpeper House – The Society of Herbalists, 7 Baker St, 1928)

Chapman, Stanley, *Jesse Boot of Boots the Chemist* (London, 1974), in Griggs, *Green Pharmacy*, p. 243

Charlesworth, M. A., *Trade Routes and Commerce of the Roman Empire* (1926)

Cheung Siu-cheong and Li Ning-hon (eds), *Chinese Medical Herbs of Hong Kong*, vols 1–5 (Hong Kong: , 1978)

Corcellet, Paul and Bernard *et al.*, *La via delle spezie* (Milan: RCS Rizzoli Libri S.p.A., and Singapore: Times Editions, 1987, 1988)

Culpeper, Nicholas, *Pharmacopoeia Londinensis or, the London Dispensatory* (London, 1675)

Cuppy, Will, *The Decline and Fall of Practically Everybody* (New York: Holt) in Leake, *The Old Egyptian Medical Papyri*, p. 3

Davis, Wade, 'Hallucinogenic plants and their use in traditional societies – An Overview', *Cultural Survival Quarterly*, 9.4 (1985), pp. 2–5

Diehl, C., *La République de Venise* (Paris: Flammarion, 1985)

Disanayaka, J. B., *Mihintale – Cradle of Sinhala Buddhist Civilization* (Colombo: Lake House Investments, 1987)

Driver, Harold E., *Indians of North America* (Chicago: University of Chicago Press, 1969, 2nd edn)

Drury, Nevill, *The Elements of Shamanism* (Longmead, Shaftesbury: Element Books, 1986)

Encyclopedia Britannica, 15th edn (Chicago: Encyclopedia Britannica Inc., 1985)

Farnsworth, 'The Plant Kingdom – suppliers of steroids', *Tile & Till*, 53 no. 55 (Sept. 1967)

Fischer, H., *Mittelalterliche Pflanzenkunde* (Munich: Verlag der Münchener Drucke, 1929)

Fratkin, Jake, *Chinese Herbal Patent Formulas* (Institute of Traditional Medicine and Preventive Health Care, 2442 SE Sherman St, Portland, OR 97214, USA, 1986)

Gillon, Edmund V., *The Middle Ages* (New York, Dover Publications, 1971)

Goldin, Hyman E., *The Jew and his Duties – The Essence of the Kitzur Shulhan Arukh* (1953; New York: Hebrew Publishing Co, 1984)

Gordon, M. B., Medicine in Colonial New Jersey and Adjacent Areas (*Bulletin of Health and Medicine*, 17, 1945)

Grew, Nehemiah, *Experiments in Consort of the Luctation arising from the affusion of several Menstruums upon all sorts of Bodies*, Exhibited to the Royal Society of London, April 13th and June 1st, 1676 (1676)

Griggs, Barbara, *Green Pharmacy – A History of Herbal Medicine* (London: Robert Hale, 1981, 1987)

Grossinger, Richard, *Planet Medicine: From Stone Age Shamanism to Post-industrial Healing* (Boulder, CO, and London: Shambhala, 1982)

Gulbenkian Museum of Oriental Art and Archaeology, Durham University, Co. Durham, *Oman and the Sindbad Project*, expedition pamphlet (1980)

Gunaratna, Rohan, *Sino-Lankan Connection: 2000 Years of Cultural Relations* (Colombo: Department of Information, Ministry of State, 1987)

Hatton, Richard G., *The Craftsman's Plant-Book: or Figures of Plants* [from sixteenth- and seventeenth-century herbals] (1909), repr. as

Handbook of Plant and Floral Ornament (New York: Dover Publications, 1960)

Hawker, Lilian E., *Fungi, an Introduction* (London: Hutchinson University Library, 1966)

Herodotus, trans. George Rawlinson, *The History of Herodotus* (Chicago: Encyclopedia Britannica Inc., 1952)

Heywood, V. H. (ed.), *Flowering Plants of the World* (Oxford: Oxford University Press, 1978)

Hillary, Sir Edmund (ed.), *Ecology 2000 – The Changing Face of Earth* (New York: Beaufort Books, 1984)

Hippocrates, *Hippocratic Writings* (Chicago: Encyclopedia Britannica Inc., 1952 edn)

Holmyard, E. J., *Alchemy* (1957; New York, Dover Publications, 1990)

Homer, *The Iliad*, trans. S. Butler (Chicago: Encyclopedia Britannica Inc., 1952)

Hou, Joseph P., 'The development of Chinese herbal medicine and the Pen-ts'ao', *Comparative Medicine East and West*, 5.2 (1977), pp. 117–22

Hsu, Hong-Yen and William G. Peacher, *Chinese Herb Medicine and Therapy* (Hawaiian Garden, CA: Oriental Healing Arts Institute of the USA, 1976)

Hui-Lin Li *Nan-fang ts'ao-mu chuang – A Fourth Century Flora of Southeast Asia* (Hong Kong: The Chinese University Press, 1979)

Jacobovits, Immanuel, *Jewish Medical Ethics* (New York: Bloch Publishing Co., 1975)

Jayaweera, D. M. A. *Medicinal Plants (Indigenous and Exotic) Used in Ceylon*, 5 vols (Colombo: The National Science Council of Sri Lanka, 1981)

Ji Zhongpu, 'Review and prospect of integration of Traditional Chinese and Western Medicine in past 30 years', *Chinese Journal of Integrated Medicine*, 8 (1988), pp. 88–9 (Special Issue 2)

Jiang Tinglian, 'Research on Chinese materia medica with Traditional Chinese and Western Medicine', *Chinese Journal of Integrated Medicine*, 8 (1988), pp. 193–6 (Special Issue 2)

Kao, Frederick K., 'China, Chinese Medicine, and the Chinese medical system', *American Journal of Chinese Medicine*, 1.1 (1973), pp. 1–59

Keys, John D., *Chinese Herbs* (Rutland, VT and Tokyo: Charles E. Tuttle Co., 1976)

Kreig, Margaret, *Green Medicine* (London, 1965)

Kudlien, Fridolf, *Der Beginn des Medizinischen Denkens bei den Griechen von Homer bis Hippokrates* (Zürich: Artemis Verlag, 1967)

414

Lambo, T. A., in *Proceedings of the Joint Istituto Italo–Africano/World Health Organization Meeting on Research and Training in Traditional Systems of Medicine in Developing Countries, Rome, 2–6 April 1979*, ed. G. B. Marini–Bettolo

Lawn, Brian, *The Salernitan Questions* (Oxford: Clarendon Press, 1963)

Le Strange, Richard, *A History of Herbal Plants* (New York: Arco Publishing Co., 1977)

Leake, Chauncey D., *The Old Egyptian Medical Papyri*, Logan Clendening Lectures on the History and Philosophy of Medicine, Second Series (Lawrence, KAN: University of Kansas Press, 1952)

Leigh, Denis, *Medicine, the City and China*, The Monckton Copeman Lecture, given at the Apothecaries' Hall on 31 January 1973, *Medical History*, 18 (1974), pp. 51–67

Leroi-Gourhan, Arlette, 'The flowers found with Shanidar IV, a Neanderthal burial in Iraq', *Science*, 190 (7 Nov. 1975), p. 562

Leung, Albert Y., *Chinese Herbal Remedies* (London: Wildwood House, 1985)

Linnel, 'Further examples of the misuse of common remedies', *The Practitioner* (1936), p. 212

Liu Chang-Xiao, 'Development of Chinese Medicine based on pharmacology and therapeutics', *Journal of Ethnopharmacology*, 19 (1987), pp. 119–23

Liu, Frank and Liu Yan Mau, *Chinese Medical Terminology* (Hong Kong: The Commercial Press, 1980)

McGraw, Eric, *Population: The Human Race* (London: Bishopsgate Press, 1990)

Mendis, Vernon L. B., *Foreign Relations of Sri Lanka From Earliest Times to 1965*, Ceylon Historical Journal Monograph Series, vol.2 *Dehiwela* (Sri Lanka: Tisara Prakasakayo, 1983)

Moldenke, Harold N. and Alma L. Moldenke, *Plants of the Bible* (Waltham, MA: Chronica Botanica Co., 1952)

Mortimer, W. Golden, *History of Coca – The 'Divine Plant' of the Incas* (1901; San Francisco: Fritz Hugh Ludlaw Memorial Library Edition, 1974)

Munting, A., *Nauwerkeurige Beschryving der Aard-Gevassen* (Leyden, 1696; ed. T. Menten, New York, Dover Publications, 1975)

Obeyesekere, Gananath, 'The theory and practice of psychological medicine in the Ayurvedic tradition', *Culture, Medicine and Psychiatry*, 1 (1977), pp. 155–81

Ornstein, R. and David Sobel, *The Healing Brain* (Macmillan, London, 1988)

Paracelsus, *The Archidoxes of Magic* (1656; London, Askin Publishers, 1975)

Pharmaceutical Codex, The (11th edn, London: The Pharmaceutical Society, 1979; repr. 1988)

Pharmacopoeia, The British (London: HMSO, 1988)

Rainey, Froelich, 'Quinine hunters of Equador', *National Geographic Magazine*, 89.3 (1946), pp. 341–63

Raven, Peter H. and George B. Johnson, *Biology* (St Louis, MO: Times Mirror/Mosby College Publishing, 1986)

Reid, Daniel P., *Chinese Medicine* (Wellingborough, Northants: CWF Publications/Thorsons, 1987)

Richardson, Sir Benjamin Ward, Asclepiad, vols V–VI, p. 174, 183, in C. J. S. Thompson, *The Mystic Mandrake*, pp. 225–6

Rosner, Fred, *Medicine in the Bible and the Talmud* (New York: Ktav Publishing House Inc., Yeshiva University Press, 1977)

Sacks, Oliver, *Migraine: Understanding a Common Disorder* (Berkeley, CA: University of California Press, 1985)

Savnur, H. V., *Ayurvedic Materia Medica* (1950; Dehli: Sri Satuguru Publications, 1988)

Schiffler, John W., 'An essay on some of the fundamental philosophical tenets found in Traditional Chinese Medicine', *American Journal of Chinese Medicine*, 7.3 (1979), pp. 285–94

Schultes, Richard Evans and Albert Hofmann, *Plants of the Gods* (New York: Alfred van der Marck Editions, 1987)

Shi Jizong and Chu Feng Zhu, trans. Shi Jiaxin, *The ABC of Traditional Chinese Medicine* (Hong Kong: Hai Feng Publishing Co., 1985)

Shiu Ying Hu, 'The genus *Panax* (Ginseng) in Chinese medicine', *Economic Botany*, 30 (January–March 1976), pp. 11–28

Singer, Charles, *From Magic to Science* (London: Ernest Benn, 1928)

Singh, Dharamit, 'The traditional medicine in India', *Impact of Science on Society*, 26.4 (1976)

Smith, A. J. E., *The Moss Flora of Britain and Ireland* (Cambridge: Cambridge University Press, 1978)

Solecki, Ralph S., 'Shanidar IV, a Neanderthal flower burial in northern Iraq', *Science*, 190 (28 Nov. 1975), p. 880

Sporne, K. R., *The Morphology of Pteridophytes* (London: Hutchinson University Library, 1962, 4th edn)

Sporne, K. R., *The Morphology of Gymnosperms* (1965; London: Hutchinson University Library, 1974, 2nd edn)

Svrcek, Mirko, *The Hamlyn Book of Mushrooms and Fungi* (London: Hamlyn, 1983)

Teeguarden, Ron and Caroline Davies, *Chinese Tonic Herbs* (Tokyo: Japan Publications Inc., 1984)

The Holy Bible, King James' Authorized Version (London: Oxford University Press)

Thompson, C. J. S., *The Mystic Mandrake* (London: Ryder & Co., 1934)

Thompson, Campbell, *Assyrian Medical Texts* (Oxford, 1923), and *Assyrian Herbal* (London, 1924), in Leake, *The Old Egyptian Medical Papyri*, p. 3

Ullman, Manfred, *Islamic Medicine* (Edinburgh: Edinburgh University Press, 1978), Islamic Surveys II

Unschuld, Paul U., 'The development of medical-pharmaceutical thought in China', *Comparative Medicine East and West*, 5.2 (1977), pp. 109–15 (Part I); 5.3–4, pp. 211–321 (Part II)

Unschuld, Paul U., *Medicine in China – A History of Ideas* (Berkeley, CA: University of California Press, 1985)

Uragoda, C. G., *A History of Medicine in Sri Lanka* (Colombo: Sri Lanka Medical Association, 1987)

Vernant, Jean-Pierre, *Les Origines de la pensée grecque* (Paris: Presses Universitaires de France, 1962)

Walahfrid Strabo *Hortulus* (872; Munich: Verlag Münchner Drucke, 1926)

Wallace, A. R., *Vaccination – A Delusion; Its Penal Enforcement – A Crime*, in Harry Clements, *Alfred Russel Wallace* (London: Hutchinson, 1983)

Wanninayaka, P. B., *Ayurveda in Sri Lanka* (Sri Lanka: Ministry of Health, 1982)

Wesley, John, *Primitive Physic, or an Easy and Natural Method of Curing Most Diseases* (London, 1781), in Griggs, *Green Pharmacy*

Wohl, Anthony S., *Endangered Lives – Public Health in Victorian Britain* (London: Dent, 1983)

Woodward, Marcus, *Gerard's Herball – The Essences Thereof Distilled* [from 1636 edn] (1927; London: Spring Books, 1964)

Worldwide Fund for Nature (*advertisement*), International Herald Tribune, 13 June 1990

Wren, R. C., *Potter's Cyclopedia of Botanical Drugs and Preparations* (London: Potter & Clarke, 1941)

Xinru Liu, *Ancient India and Ancient China – Trade and Religious Exchanges AD 1–600* (Delhi, Oxford University Press, 1988)

INDEX

INDEX

435